ACLS Review made Incredibly Easy!

Fourth Edition

Laura M. Willis, DNP, APRN-CNP
Family Nurse Practitioner
Mercy Health
Springfield, Ohio

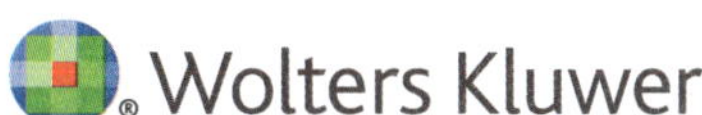

Wolters Kluwer

Philadelphia • Baltimore • New York • London
Buenos Aires • Hong Kong • Sydney • Tokyo

Acquisitions Editor: Joyce Berendes
Product Development Editor: Devika Kishore
Editorial Coordinator: Priyanka Alagar
Production Project Manager: Matthew West
Design Coordinator: Stephen Druding
Manufacturing Coordinator: Bernard Tomboc
Marketing Manager: Amy Whitaker
Prepress Vendor: Straive

Fourth Edition

9 8 7 6 5 4 3 2 1

Printed in United States of America

Cataloging-in-Publication Data available on request from the Publisher

ISBN: 978-1-9752-1840-9

---

shop.lww.com

MPP0923

Dedication

Andrew, Thank you for always letting me do more.

And, For all those who provide emergency and critical care to those in need-You are seen and valued. This is for you.

Contributors

Cheryl Brown, DNP, MEd, ENP, FNP-BC
Family Nurse Practitioner
Urgent Care and Village Medicine
Anchorage, Alaska

Jacob "Tyler" Callahan, BSN
Registered Nurse
Denver, Colorado

Jane Von Dohre, MSN, Ed
Registered Nurse Clinical Faculty
Kettering College
Kettering, Ohio

Joseph Gucwa, EMT-P, BSN, CCRN, CFRN
Flight Nurse
Trauma One Flight Services
Jacksonville, Florida

Kelly Schlotterbeck, AAS, BS Respiratory Education
RRT, RCP
Dayton, Ohio

Jeffrey W. Schultz, MS, APRN, ACNP-BC, CCNS, CV-BC, CCRN-CSC, CEN, NE-BC, NR-P, Senior APRN
CVICU
HCA Florida North Florida Hospital
Florida Heart & Lung Institute
Flight Nurse
University of Florida Health Shands Hospital
ShandsCair Critical Care Transport Program
Gainesville, Florida

Previous Edition Contributors

Marguerite Ambrose, PhD, RN, ACNS-BC

Louise Colwill, RN, MSN

Kathleen M. Hill, RN, MSN, CCNS-CSC

Jared Kutzin, RN, DNP, MPH

Margaret McAtee, RN, MN, ACNP-BC, CCRN

Deborah Murphy, RN, MSN, CRNP, CNRN, SCRN

Antoinette Pretto-Sparkle, RN, MSN

Kerry Rinato, PharmD

Foreword

Emergency situations can cause anxiety in even the most experienced health care workers. It can be overwhelming to think that someone's life is in your hands. The American Heart Association (AHA) has provided evidence-based interventions for many critical situations to optimally improve patient outcomes. *ACLS Review Made Incredibly Easy*, fourth edition, provides information that follows AHA guidelines to assist with preparing for Advanced Cardiovascular Life Support (ACLS) certification. This book provides current treatment algorithms as well as information regarding oxygen delivery, critical medications, and how to care for patients in other life-threatening situations, such as anaphylaxis and submersion. Don't stress too much while preparing for your certification—you will get through it with diligent studying and guidance from ACLS instructors, who truly want you to succeed. Once certified, your knowledge in a critical situation may be the difference between life and death for the person you are caring for.

Laura M. Willis, DNP, APRN-CNP
Family Nurse Practitioner
Mercy Health
Springfield, Ohio

Contents

Chapter 1

ACLS essentials

Just the facts

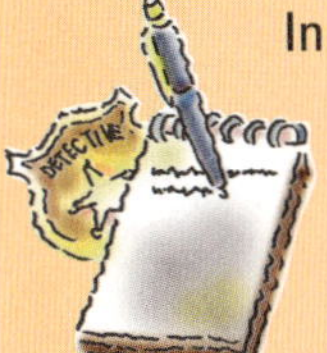

In this chapter, you'll learn:

- core concepts of advanced cardiovascular life support (ACLS)
- basic components of the ACLS course
- study strategies to help you prepare for the ACLS examination

What is ACLS?

Advanced cardiovascular life support (ACLS) is a systematic approach to advanced resuscitation efforts. ACLS training gives rescuers a coordinated way to approach critically ill patients, regardless of response team size. (See *ACLS core concepts*.)

Health care workers seeking ACLS training include physicians, registered nurses (RNs), emergency medical services (EMS) personnel, and dental and surgical care professionals.

ACLS training

The foundation of ACLS is high-quality basic life support (BLS) measures. A current BLS card is required of ACLS certification participants.

ACLS certification is obtained after an individual successfully completes a certification course, either online or in person. ACLS education involves information on ACLS concepts, algorithms, and medications, followed by hands-on practice and testing using simulated ACLS case studies and scenarios. Certification cards are issued only to active health care providers who demonstrate the appropriate skills and knowledge of ACLS.

Keep in mind that the certification card, which verifies that you've successfully completed the ACLS course, isn't a license to perform techniques discussed or reviewed in the course (such as endotracheal intubation or intravenous catheter insertion). Instead, each person's scope of practice and state license determine the specific

ACLS core concepts

Here are the core concepts and skills you'll need for ACLS certification.

General skills

For cardiopulmonary resuscitation (CPR):

- identification of need for CPR
- demonstration of CPR

For devices and procedures, you need to know:

- indications
- precautions
- proper use

Airway management

You need to know ventilation techniques, such as how to use a bag valve mask device, how to perform and assist with endotracheal intubation, and use of supraglottic devices.

Early management

You need to know how to manage the first 30 minutes of emergencies that result from such causes as:

- acute coronary syndrome
- cardiac arrest associated with trauma
- cardiac arrest involving a pregnant patient
- cardiac tamponade
- drowning and near-drowning
- electrocution and lightning strike
- hypothermia
- pneumothorax
- possible drug overdose
- stroke
- thrombosis

Electrical therapy

You need to know how to safely use electrical devices, such as an automated external defibrillator, conventional defibrillator, and pacemakers.

Emergency conditions

You need to know cardiac rhythms that may require ACLS treatment, such as bradycardia, asystole, pulseless electrical activity, tachycardias, ventricular tachycardia, and ventricular fibrillation.

Intravenous (IV) and invasive techniques

You need to be familiar with IV and invasive therapeutic techniques, such as peripheral and central IV line insertion and intraosseous cannulation.

Pharmacology

You need to know the action, indication, dosages, and precautions for the major drugs used during ACLS, such as epinephrine, atropine, adenosine, amiodarone, and dopamine.

individual's ability to perform these techniques. ACLS certification renewal is required every 2 years.

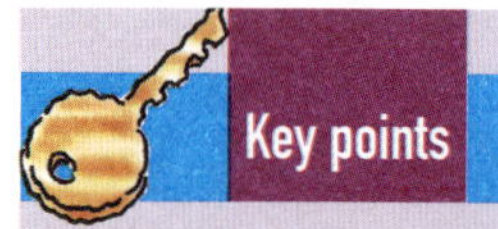

Taking the examination

- The examination consists of written and practical sections.
- The passing grade is 84%.
- Participation in established case scenarios is required.
- A team approach is used for the Megacode.

Born to teach

After successfully completing an ACLS course, participants who display exemplary understanding of the core concepts and are interested in teaching ACLS can obtain additional education to become an ACLS instructor.

ACLS testing

The ACLS examination is required in both live and online courses. The test, issued by the American Heart Association (AHA), contains 30 to 50 multiple choice questions and generally takes about 1 hour.

To pass the test, you must answer 84% of the questions correctly.

"Mega" practice

The skills section must be completed with an authorized instructor at a training center and consists of performing adult CPR accurately and completing a Megacode scenario successfully. A Megacode is a simulation of an emergency situation in which a team approach is used to provide appropriate treatment. Each team member will have the opportunity to provide the correct actions associated with a described scenario and assigned role, following the appropriate algorithm.

Study strategies

Preparation is needed to pass ACLS testing successfully. Testing assesses both knowledge of ACLS concepts and the ability to apply those concepts during emergency situations. As a trained health care professional, you should view the ACLS certification as another step in your professional development. Preparing effectively creates confidence about being tested.

Several strategies may be utilized to study. Not all strategies are appropriate for every student. A combination of strategies may help you learn ACLS concepts and be enthusiastic about the material.

Determining your strengths and weaknesses

ACLS training focuses on a broad range of skills, from airway management to pharmacology to leadership during emergency situations. Chances are, some areas are more familiar than others.

Make a list and check it twice

One good way to begin your studying is to look at the list of ACLS core concepts provided in this chapter. On a sheet of paper, create two columns. Title one column "know well." Title the other "need review." Now go through the list of ACLS core concepts and place each one in either the "know well" or "need review" column. Don't worry if one column is longer than the other. This will provide an initial guide to how much time may be needed for each topic.

Remember, although time will be spent studying the topics listed in the "know well" column, more will be needed for the topics in the "need review" column.

Setting your schedule

Most people can identify a period in the day when they feel most alert. Topics that need more review should be studied at the "high-energy" time of day. Topics that need less review can be studied at the "low-energy" time of day, if needed. Plan your schedule accordingly.

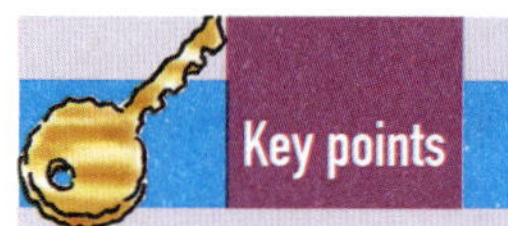

Study tips

- Use a combination of study strategies to help learn effectively.
- Create a guide of "know well" and "needs review."
- Devise a study schedule.
- Use additional materials to maintain motivation.

Eight days a week

Set up a basic study schedule. Using a calendar or organizer, determine how many days there are before ACLS testing. Fill in those dates with specific times and topics to study.

Keep in mind that studying all day or for extended periods of time may not be helpful. Set aside time for regular activities. Personal study capabilities should be considered to set realistic goals. (See *Creating an effective study space.*)

Get creative

Even the most determined student needs an occasional change of pace to stay motivated. Consider studying with a group or using audiovisual or other devices to make study time more effective.

Study buddies

Studying with a partner or group can be an excellent way to increase energy and motivation. Working with a partner provides the opportunity to test one another and encourage and motivate each other. When choosing a partner, select someone with similar goals, motivation, and knowledge; otherwise, valuable time may be wasted chatting or needlessly reviewing basic material.

Creating an effective study space

When preparing for the ACLS examination, it's important to use your time and space effectively. Time is wasted when studying in places where it's hard to concentrate. Look for a study space that:

- is quiet, convenient, and away from traffic
- has soft lighting to prevent eye strain
- has a temperature between 65°F and 70°F (18.3°C and 21.1°C)
- contains a solid chair that facilitates good posture
- contains flowers, green plants, familiar photos, paintings, or other elements that provide a sense of comfort

Virtual studying

Many websites offer study materials to help with preparing for the ACLS examination. For example, several sites offer ACLS simulators that facilitate practice of ACLS skills on virtual patients and offer immediate feedback as well as a fun approach to studying. Remember, ACLS information and recommendations may change, so check to see when a site was last updated before relying on it too heavily.

In addition, many professional sites (such as the American Medical Association, the AHA, and various other nursing and medical sites) offer materials that provide specific concepts and up-to-date information on the changing field of health care.

Always beware of online ACLS courses that may not be approved by the AHA. Your health care facility may not find them to be acceptable courses, and you may waste time and money on unreliable sources.

Visualize success

Audiovisual tools can also enhance a study routine. Flash cards, flowcharts, drawings, and diagrams all provide images that may improve retention of studied material. Even the process of creating these materials may help learning. (See *Virtual studying.*)

Do you hear what I hear?

If understanding and retaining information occurs more effectively by listening rather than seeing, consider using a handheld recording device (such as a tape recorder or cell phone) to record key ideas. Like flash cards, a recording is portable and perfect for short study periods during the day.

Quick quiz

1. What's the meaning of "advanced cardiovascular life support?"
   A. A systematic approach to life support
   B. Life support with the use of a ventilator
   C. A 2-day course with 6 to 8 hours of lecture
   D. A written and practical examination

Answer: A. ACLS is a systematic approach to resuscitation that provides rescuers with memory aids for the treatment of critically ill patients.

2. To prepare for ACLS testing, you should:
   A. study all day the day prior to the examination.
   B. determine a study strategy that works for you.
   C. not study at all.
   D. study for several weeks prior to the examination.

Answer: B. Not all study strategies are appropriate for every student. Determine a study strategy or combination of strategies that works for you to adequately prepare for ACLS testing.

3. ACLS certification is a professional advancement for which groups of health care professionals?
   A. RNs, physicians, and advanced EMS personnel
   B. Physicians, licensed practical nurses (LPNs), and nursing students
   C. Certified nursing assistants, nursing students, and RNs
   D. LPNs, physician assistants, and surgical care professionals

Answer: A. Health care professionals seeking ACLS training may include physicians, RNs, EMS personnel, and dental and surgical care professionals.

Scoring

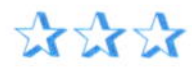 If you answered all three questions correctly, way to go! You really know your essentials.

 If you answered two questions correctly, keep up the good work! You're "essentially" on the right track.

 If you answered fewer than two questions correctly, nice try! Next time, you're sure to get an "A" on ACLS.

Suggested references

American Heart Association. (2020). *2020 handbook of emergency cardiovascular care for healthcare providers*. Dallas, TX: American Heart Association.

American Heart Association (2020). *Advanced cardiovascular life support provider manual*, E-book edition.

American Heart Association. (2020). *Highlights of the 2020 American Heart Association guidelines update for CPR and ECC*. Dallas, TX: American Heart Association.

Chapter 2

ACLS in practice

Just the facts

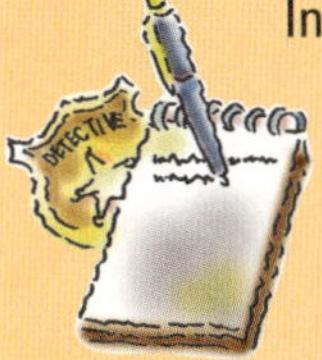

In this chapter, you'll learn:

- American Heart Association's "chains of survival"
- BLS and ACLS surveys that form the basis of advanced cardiac life support actions
- phased-response approach to emergency response team management
- purpose of treatment algorithms

The chain of survival

The chain of survival describes a chain of events—each interdependent—that plays a crucial role in helping a patient survive cardiac arrest. Just like a real "chain," each link must be strong for the process to work. If one link is weak or missing, poor survival rates will result even if the rest of the emergency cardiac care system is excellent. The American Heart Association (AHA) instituted two separate chains of survival to reflect the two separate processes for in-hospital cardiac arrest (IHCA) and out-of-hospital cardiac arrest (OHCA).

The links in each adult chain of survival are similar. The in-hospital chain includes a link regarding surveillance and prevention of cardiac arrest (such as utilizing a rapid response system). The out-of-hospital chain includes a link regarding utilizing basic and advanced emergency medical services. (*See IHCA and OHCA chains of survival*).

Both chains include the following:

- recognition of cardiac arrest and activation of an emergency response system
- immediate cardiopulmonary resuscitation (CPR) with high-quality chest compressions
- rapid defibrillation
- effective advanced cardiovascular life support (ACLS) interventions
- integrated post–cardiac arrest care
- recovery

IHCA and OHCA Chains of Survival

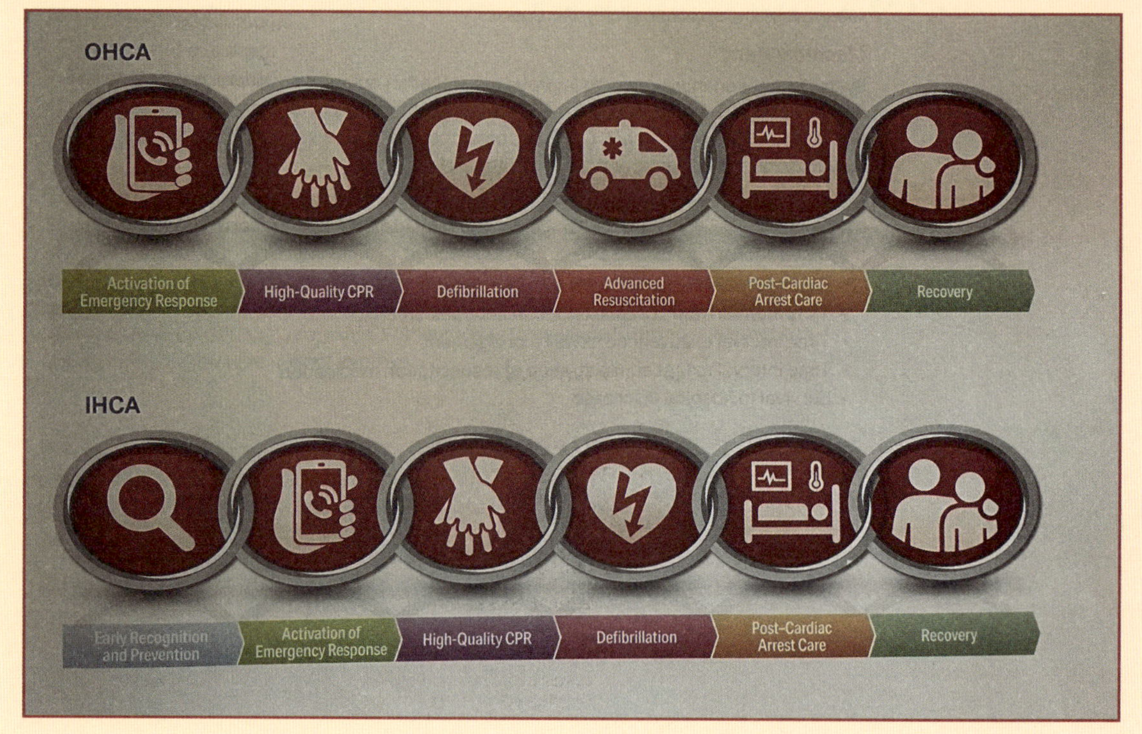

Recognition and activation

Recognition of cardiac arrest begins with identifying the patient's collapse, establishing unresponsiveness, absence of effective breathing, and pulselessness. Activation of the emergency response system, whether in hospital or out of hospital, and the arrival of ACLS trained response personnel improve the patient's chance for survival.

Immediate CPR

Immediate, high-quality CPR bridges the gap between the patient's collapse and the arrival of ACLS trained personnel with emergency equipment. Even with an effective emergency response system, a delay between the out-of-hospital patient's collapse and the arrival of EMS personnel may be unavoidable.

Many studies show that CPR is most effective when started immediately after a person collapses. Whether in hospital or in the community, non–health care personnel can easily be trained in the techniques of CPR to be able to provide this lifesaving technique to victims of cardiac arrest. Some communities have even begun to incorporate social media to notify people trained in CPR who are in close proximity to the victim of cardiac arrest.

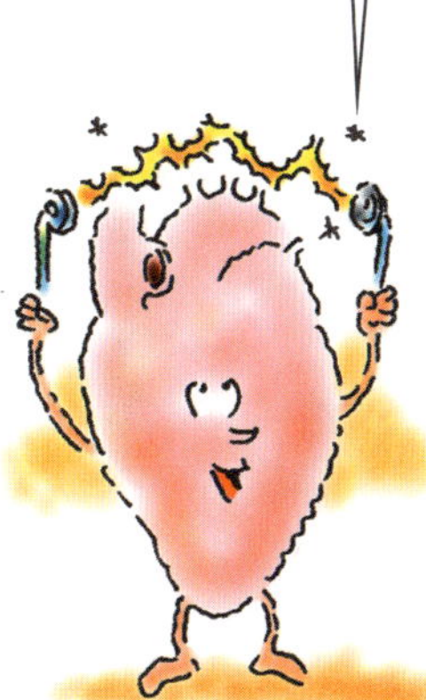

Rapid defibrillation

When performed correctly, rapid defibrillation is the most effective way to improve the patient's chance for survival. Because early defibrillation is so important, any action that safely shortens the time between collapse and defibrillation can have a significant impact. Public access automated external defibrillator (AED) programs exist in many communities and are available in areas where there is a relatively high risk of witnessed cardiac arrest such as airports, gyms, sports stadiums, and public buildings, such as hotels and malls. Typically, EMS personnel equipped with either an AED or a manual defibrillator perform defibrillation as soon as possible after they arrive on the scene.

Effective ACLS interventions

After defibrillation, effective ACLS interventions performed by trained personnel, including advanced airway management and the administration of rhythm-appropriate IV medications, is the next step in patient care.

For out-of-hospital emergencies, EMS systems should provide a minimum of two responders trained in ACLS for all emergencies. Studies show that an ideal response team consists of two members trained in ACLS supported by two members trained in basic life support (BLS). For in-hospital emergencies, cardiac arrest teams are typically made up of many different health care providers, including physicians, nurses, pharmacists, electrocardiogram (ECG) technicians, and lab personnel, with many members being ACLS providers.

Integrated post–cardiac arrest care

Following return of spontaneous circulation (ROSC), integrated post–cardiac arrest care emphasizes the importance of comprehensive, multidisciplinary care, including interventions to optimize oxygenation and ventilation, and hemodynamic, neurologic, and metabolic function. Consideration must also be given to initiation of therapeutic hypothermia, if appropriate. (See *Post–cardiac arrest care.*)

BLS vs. ACLS

A thorough understanding of BLS principles will prepare you to learn more advanced ACLS skills. BLS includes such skills as high-quality compressions, airway management, and the abdominal thrust. Any trained person who recognizes a cardiac emergency can initiate BLS interventions before ACLS-trained personnel arrive. These interventions form an important bridge between the patient's collapse and the initiation of ACLS interventions.

ACLS is an advanced version of BLS that adds more complex interventions, such as advanced airway management, initiating IV access, giving medications, and attempting to identify the cause of the emergency to provide further interventions.

Initial rescue steps

Understanding the systematic approach of ACLS will help you use ACLS skills effectively in a cardiac emergency.

ACLS uses a two-pronged approach: Initial BLS survey followed by progressive ACLS survey. You should use this approach with all potential cardiac arrest patients and at all major decision points during a difficult resuscitation effort.

Initial BLS survey focuses on basic CPR and defibrillation. Remember these four steps:

1. Check for responsiveness and adequate breathing.
2. Activate the emergency response system.
3. Check for a pulse for 5 to 10 seconds. If no pulse—perform chest compressions and administer breaths at a ratio of 30:2. If a pulse is present but the patient is not breathing—give rescue breaths—one every 5 to 6 seconds.
4. Defibrillate as soon as possible with either an AED or a manual defibrillator. Resume CPR immediately after administering a shock.

Carrying out the steps

Assess the patient and determine unresponsiveness by tapping and shouting, "Are you OK?" Look at the patient's chest to detect breathing. This scanning of the chest should only take 5 to 10 seconds. If the patient is not breathing, or is not breathing normally (gasping), call for help; then place the patient in the supine position on a hard, flat surface.

Pulse detection is unreliable, even when performed by trained rescuers, so only attempt a pulse check over 5 to 10 seconds, and then proceed to performing chest compressions if you are unable to detect a pulse or are uncertain of a pulse.

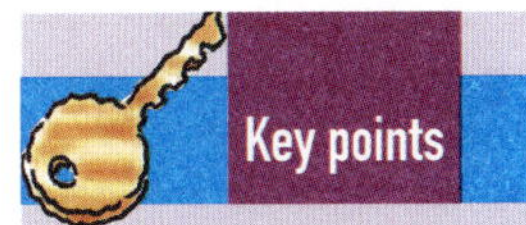

Initial BLS survey
- Assess the patient for responsiveness and adequate breathing.
- Call for help.
- Check for a pulse. If none found, begin chest compressions and provide 2 breaths after every 30 compressions.
- Deliver shocks as soon as possible after an AED or conventional defibrillator arrives on the scene.

BLS to the rescue

If the patient is unresponsive and not breathing normally and a pulse is not detected, perform high-quality compressions using BLS techniques:

- Stand or kneel next to the patient with your knees apart for a wide base of support.
- Place the heel of one hand over the lower half of the patient's sternum (center of the chest) at the nipple line, and then place your other hand on top of the first with your hands overlapped.
- Lock your elbows and keep your shoulders directly over the patient. Your body will now act as a fulcrum as you apply chest compressions.
- Give chest compressions hard and fast. Compress at least 2.0 to 2.4″ (5 to 6 cm) for an adult at a rate of 100 to 120/minute. Remember to allow the chest to completely recoil after each compression and avoid leaning on the chest. Minimize interruptions in compressions to no more than 10 seconds, and rotate the task of compressions every 2 minutes (five cycles of CPR).
- Give 30 compressions and 2 breaths for both one- and two-person CPR until an advanced airway is in place. Give each breath over 1 second each, ensuring that each breath makes the patient's chest rise.
  - For two-person CPR, one team member performs compressions while the other provides breaths. Deliver ventilations at 8 to 10 breaths/minute. The rescuer providing breaths can also monitor the quality of CPR by checking for a pulse during compressions.
- After an advanced airway is in place, deliver compressions at a rate of at least 100 to 120/minute continuously without interruptions for ventilations. The team member providing ventilations gives 1 breath every 6 seconds (10 breaths/minute).

Airway

To open the patient's airway, open the patient's mouth using the basic CPR head-tilt, chin-lift maneuver. As a health care provider, if you suspect neck injury, use the jaw-thrust maneuver. If the jaw-thrust maneuver doesn't effectively open the airway, use the head-tilt, chin-lift maneuver.

Breathing

Once you have opened the patient's airway, begin ventilations with a barrier device or bag valve mask device. Deliver each breath over 1 second and allow 2 seconds for exhalation. If the patient's chest doesn't rise with provided breaths, reposition the airway and reattempt ventilation. If you're still unsuccessful, follow the AHA's steps for obstructed airway.

Defibrillation

Defibrillation must occur as soon as possible. For example, a person in ventricular fibrillation (VF) has almost no chance of survival if defibrillation doesn't occur within 10 minutes of cardiac arrest. You must move swiftly and efficiently through the steps of the BLS survey in order to proceed quickly to defibrillation.

The AED advantage

Current ACLS training emphasizes the use of AEDs for defibrillation both in the community and hospital settings. AEDs are computerized, low-maintenance defibrillators that analyze the patient's heart rhythm to determine if a shockable rhythm is present. If an AED detects a shockable rhythm (VF or ventricular tachycardia [VT]), it recommends a shock or automatically charges and shocks, based on the model of AED used.

All AEDs operate using four steps:

1. Power—Turn the AED on.
2. Attachment—Attach the pads to the patient.
3. Analyze—Place the AED into analyze mode (if it does not do it automatically) to detect a shockable rhythm.
4. Shock—Press the shock button when indicated, or stand back if the AED voice announces that it will do so.

After a shock is delivered, immediately resume CPR beginning with compressions. Perform for 2 minutes until the AED begins another rhythm analysis. If an AED isn't available, continue the steps of CPR. If an AED determines that no shock is advised and the patient remains pulseless, continue CPR.

Conventional (or manual) defibrillators are present in many EMS vehicles and most hospital settings. Conventional defibrillators operate in a similar manner to AEDs. Staff must turn on the machine and attach pads to the patient. Trained staff then analyzes the patient's rhythm and determines if a shock is needed. If so, the machine is charged and the shock administered by pushing the "Shock" button. (See *Conventional defibrillators.*)

The BLS survey adds defibrillation to the CAB approach to emergency care. Thanks, I needed that!

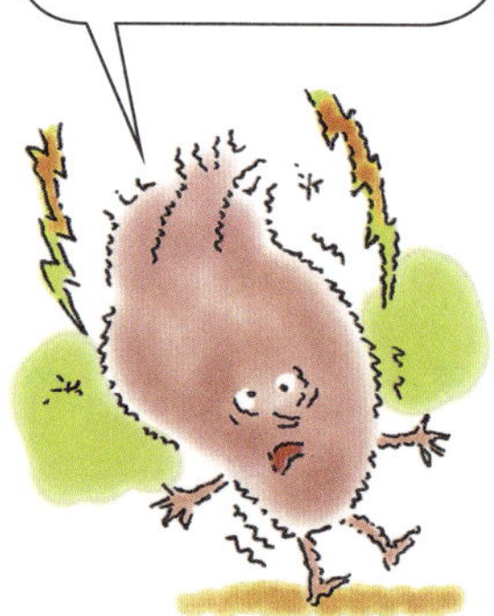

ACLS survey

The ACLS survey may be conducted for both conscious and unconscious patients. For the conscious patient, the BLS survey is bypassed. For the unconscious patient, the BLS survey is completed prior to ACLS actions being initiated. Think of the ACLS survey as "ABCD."

Steps in the ACLS survey include the following:

- Airway—Assess for a patent airway. If needed, insert an advanced airway and ensure proper placement and securement.
- Breathing—Assess bilateral chest movement and adequacy of ventilation. Administer oxygen and breaths as needed.
- Circulation—Gain IV or intraosseus (I/O) access, determine the heart rhythm, and give medications appropriate to that rhythm. Assess for high-quality CPR if being performed.
- Differential diagnosis—Search for, find, and treat reversible causes of the arrest.

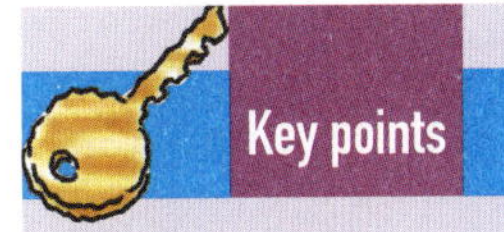

ACLS survey

- **A**—Reassess the airway; intubate as soon as possible if bag valve mask ventilations are ineffective.
- **B**—Check for breath sounds; confirm tube placement.
- **C**—Perform interventions to deliver medications, identify heart rhythm, and monitor blood pressure.
- **D**—Determine what caused the event.

Airway

Assess the airway to make sure that it's open. If needed, use a bag valve mask device for providing adequate airway management. You may defer insertion of an endotracheal (ET) tube until after return of spontaneous circulation, or after CPR and defibrillation have been provided, as long as the airway is patent.

Breathing

When using a bag valve mask device, assess chest movement with each breath. The chest should rise as a breath as given. After insertion of an ET tube, confirm placement by using an end-tidal carbon dioxide detector or exhaled esophageal detector device, and auscultating for bilateral breath sounds using a five-point technique (over the stomach, left and right anterior chest, left and right midaxillary points, and over the stomach). Also assess for equal chest movement during ventilation. Monitor oxygenation and ventilation with an oxygen saturation monitor and waveform capnography, if available. Make any necessary adjustments to ensure that the patient is breathing adequately, including removing the tube, if necessary, and starting over.

When you're confident that the ET tube is in place, secure it to prevent dislodgment. A chest X-ray and arterial blood gas levels help to accurately evaluate tube placement and adequate ventilation.

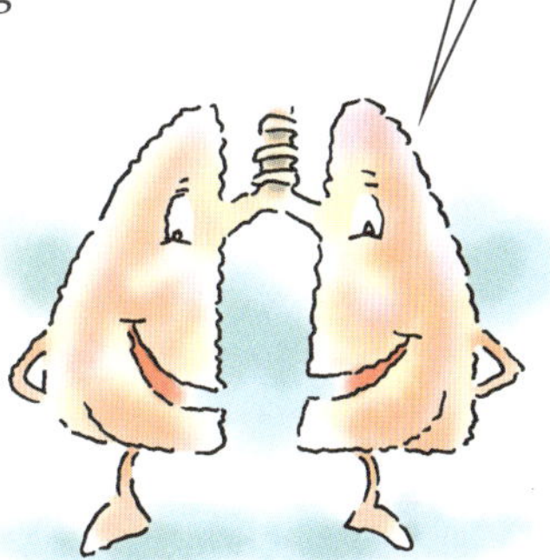

Circulation

The circulation component of the ACLS survey involves several interventions ultimately designed to identify arrhythmias and determine and deliver appropriate medication to the patient. As one person obtains IV access, another attaches cardiac monitor leads, identifies the heart rhythm, and measures blood pressure.

Knowing the patient's vital signs will help you determine if they are stable or unstable. Proper identification of their heart rhythm will help you decide which medication or treatment (such as cardioversion or defibrillation) to administer to help restore a normal heart rate and rhythm.

Differential diagnosis

Consider potentially reversible causes of the cardiopulmonary emergency, such as hypovolemia, hypoxia, hydrogen ion excess (acidosis), hyperkalemia, hypokalemia, hypothermia, toxins (drug overdose), cardiac tamponade, tension pneumothorax, coronary thrombosis, or pulmonary thrombosis. These are often referred to as the H's and T's. Even if you succeed in establishing a perfusing rhythm, cardiac arrest can recur if the underlying cause isn't identified and appropriately treated.

Using a team approach

The BLS and ACLS surveys provide an overall structure for patient care before, during, and after a cardiopulmonary emergency. Similarly, using an effective team approach allows for clear communication and guidance as the team functions through all phases of an emergency.

Components of an team approach include the following:

- showing respect
- communicating clearly
- knowing roles and responsibilities
- sharing knowledge
- summarizing actions
- debriefing

Showing respect

Emergency situations can be quite stressful. Aggressive or uncontrolled behavior tends to create more stress. Team members should speak in a controlled tone of voice and provide support to each other in a professional manner. Being respectful of the situation and each other promotes team cohesiveness.

Communicating clearly

Emergency situations can be quite chaotic. Miscommunication with one another may occur, causing more chaos. Team leaders should use closed-loop communication when communicating with team members. This means that when they give a message, order, or assignment to another team member, that team member confirms receiving that message and also communicates when the order or assignment has been completed. Communication should occur with a calm, controlled voice and distinctive speech. Poor communication techniques can impair team interaction.

Knowing roles and responsibilities

Each team member's role is important for effective resuscitation. Tasks should be delegated to the team members who are qualified to complete them. Team members should communicate if they are unable to handle the task, so it can be reassigned to another team member capable of completing the task. Crucial roles during resuscitation may include team leader, compressor, airway manager, recorder, and administrator of drugs and fluids.

Knowledge sharing

Information is a critical component of the resuscitation event. Team members need to share information about the patient (such as history, symptoms, or events), interventions, diagnostics and outcomes, in order to direct decisions about care. If an intervention is recognized by a team member as inappropriate, they need to intervene with constructive criticism. Confrontation should be avoided as it can impede resuscitation efforts.

Summarization

An effective team leader will ask for a reevaluation and summarization of interventions and patient response before deciding to terminate resuscitation efforts. The code recorder is an essential part of this process as they can concisely summarize actions and time frames.

Debriefing

Every emergency situation should finish with a debriefing of the event. This debriefing exercise should occur away from the crisis situation. It allows for self- and team assessment, identification of areas for improvement, and reflection on outcomes as well as the opportunity to defuse emotions when dealing with volatile situations.

Treatment algorithms

The AHA uses treatment algorithms as educational tools for learning ACLS. Algorithms are flowcharts that can serve as memory tools for carrying out the steps involved in different emergency situations.

It's important to remember that real-life patient care rarely corresponds exactly to any particular algorithm. Therefore, algorithms provide a useful guide but can't replace a flexible, thorough understanding of patient care. (For specific algorithms, see Chapter 8, *Treatment algorithms.*)

Using treatment algorithms can help you recall which steps to take in an emergency situation.

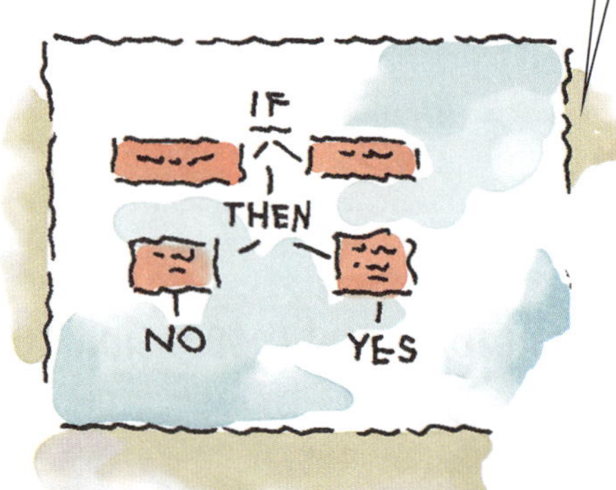

Quick quiz

1. The link in the chain of survival that's most likely to improve the patient's survival rate is:
- A. immediate recognition and activation.
- B. early CPR.
- C. rapid defibrillation.
- D. effective ACLS.

Answer: C. When performed correctly, rapid defibrillation is the link in the chain of survival that's the most important to patient survival because it's ultimately the only way to reverse cardiac arrest resulting from VF/VT. However, all links in the chain are important for successful resuscitation.

2. When confronted with a possible cardiac arrest, which action is important to perform immediately after establishing unresponsiveness?
- A. Call for help and activate the EMS.
- B. Clear the area.
- C. Notify the family.
- D. Call the practitioner.

Answer: A. The step that is important to perform prior to initiating compressions (after assessing unresponsiveness), is calling for help and activating the emergency response team.

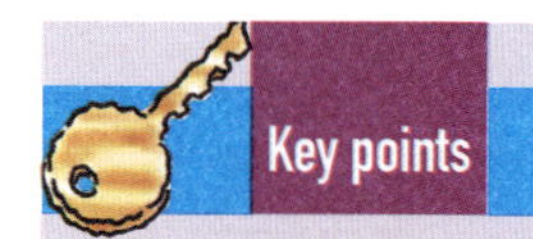

Summary points
- Understanding the chain of survival helps initiate and carry out resuscitation efforts quickly.
- The BLS and ACLS surveys are essential components of resuscitation.
- Incorporation of a team approach decreases stress in an emergency situation and promotes cohesive care.

3. ACLS treatment algorithms are:
- A. mathematical equations used in ACLS.
- B. ACLS educational tools.
- C. flowcharts to guide ACLS treatment.
- D. the second link in the chain of survival.

Answer: C. Treatment algorithms are flowcharts that guide ACLS treatment. They're designed to be a memory tool; however, they aren't absolute because every patient needs to be assessed according to their response to treatment and individual circumstances.

4. Determining a differential diagnosis is part of the:
- A. BLS survey.
- B. ACLS survey.
- C. patient history.
- D. discharge summary.

Answer: B. A differential diagnosis should be discussed as part of the ACLS survey utilizing review of the "H's and T's."

5. Effective communication among team members is key during which component of the team approach?
- A. Entry
- B. Maintenance
- C. Resuscitation
- D. Transfer

Answer: C. Effective communication is key during the resuscitation component. The team members should use closed-loop and clear communication throughout the resuscitation event.

6. After establishing unresponsiveness and assessing ineffective breathing, compressions begin:
- A. at a ratio of 15 to 30 compressions to two breaths.
- B. at a ratio of 30 to 100 compressions to one breath.
- C. at a rate of at least 100 to 120/minute interrupted by pauses for ventilations.
- D. at a rate of at least 100/minute continuously without interruption for ventilation.

Answer: C. After establishing unresponsiveness and ineffective breathing, deliver compressions at a rate of at least 100 to 120/minute interrupted by pauses for ventilation.

Scoring

☆☆☆ If you answered all six questions correctly, outstanding! Your chain of survival is strong.

☆☆ If you answered four or five questions correctly, great job! You're primarily on the right track.

☆ If you answered fewer than four questions correctly, good effort! With a bit more study, you'll master the ABCs of ACLS in no time.

Suggested references

American Heart Association. (2020). *Highlights of the 2020 American Heart Association guidelines update for CPR and ECC*. American Heart Association.

American Heart Association. (2020). *Advanced cardiovascular life support provider manual*, E-book edition.

Villanueva-Reiakvam, S. (2014). *The art of debriefing*. [Online]. Retrieved from http://cdn2.hubspot.net/hub/210798/file-460911360-pdf/CCNL/art-of-debriefing.pdf?t=1460400212009, on October 1, 2022.

Chapter 3

Recognizing cardiac arrhythmias

Just the facts

In this chapter, you'll learn:

- normal cardiac conduction
- application of cardiac rhythm monitoring devices
- methods to analyze and interpret cardiac rhythms
- characteristics of cardiac arrhythmias
- symptoms and treatment of cardiac arrhythmias

The importance of interpretation

An essential component of advanced cardiovascular life support (ACLS) is the rapid recognition of cardiac arrhythmias. Frequently, identification of an arrhythmia is what triggers an ACLS response, especially in the hospital setting. Accurate analysis and interpretation of a cardiac arrhythmia guides appropriate treatment and may help prevent hemodynamic deterioration.

Understanding cardiac conduction

The cardiovascular system contains specialized pacemaker cells that enable the heart to generate a precise rhythm. These cells have four unique characteristics:

- automaticity—the ability to spontaneously initiate an electrical impulse
- conductivity—the ability to transmit the impulse to the next cell
- contractility—the ability to shorten the fibers in the heart when receiving the impulse
- excitability—the ability to respond to an electrical stimulus

Cardiac conduction begins in the sinoatrial (SA) node and proceeds through the cardiac conduction system. (See *Cardiac conduction system*.)

Cardiac conduction system

With normal conduction, each electrical impulse initiates in the sinoatrial (SA) node and travels through the atria along the internodal and interatrial tracts. The impulse slows momentarily as it passes through the atrioventricular (AV) junction to the bundle of His. Then it descends the left and right bundle branches and finally down the Purkinje fibers.

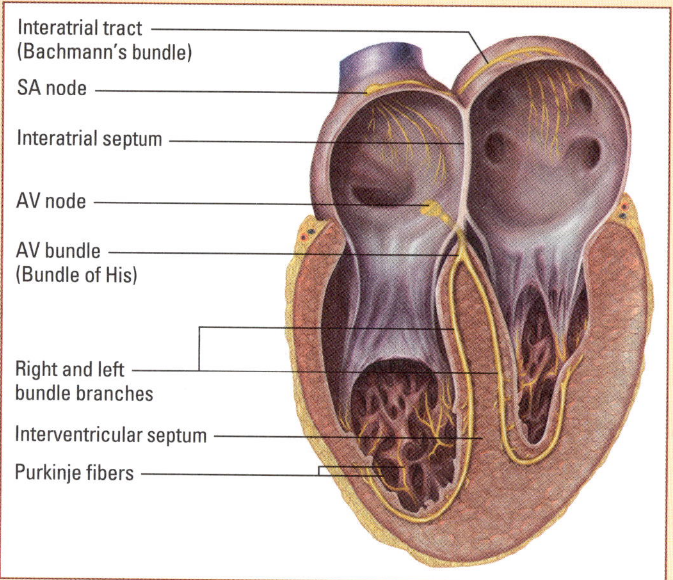

Sinoatrial node

The SA node is the heart's natural pacemaker. It's located on the endocardial surface of the right atrium near the superior vena cava. When the SA node fires, it sends an impulse throughout the right and left atria that results in an atrial contraction. Normally, the SA node generates an impulse 60 to 100 times/minute.

Atrioventricular node

The atrioventricular (AV) node slows impulse conduction between the atria and the ventricles. Situated low in the septal wall of the right atrium, this "resistor" node provides time for the contracting atria to fill the ventricles with blood before the lower chambers contract.

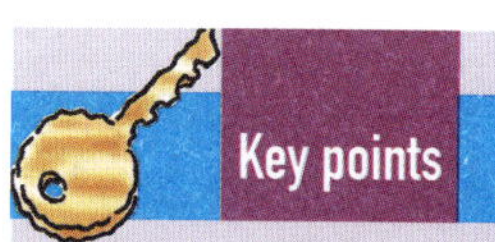

Cardiac conduction
- SA node—normal pacemaker
- AV node—impulse conduction
- AV node will generate impulse if SA node fails.
- Ventricles will generate impulse if SA and AV nodes fail.

From the AV node to the myocardium

The impulse from the AV node travels to the bundle of His (modified muscle fibers), branching off to the right and left bundle branches. Then it travels to the distal portions of the bundle branches called the *Purkinje fibers*. These fibers fan across the surface of the ventricles from the endocardium to the myocardium. As the impulse spreads, it signals the blood-filled ventricles to contract.

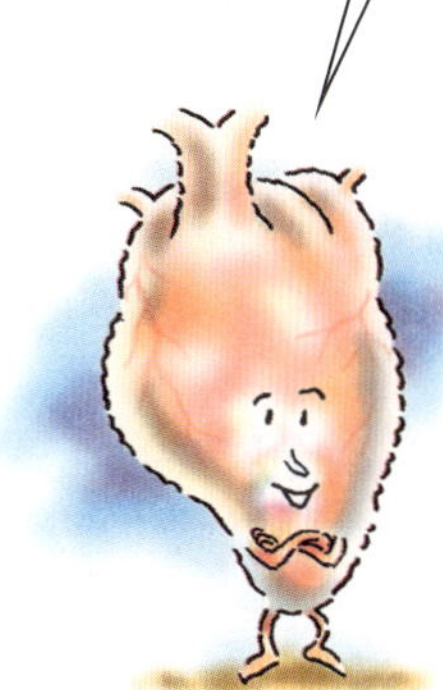

Safety mechanisms

The conduction system has two built-in safety mechanisms. If the SA node fails to fire, the AV node will generate an impulse 40 to 60 times/minute. If the SA node and AV node both fail, the ventricles can generate their own impulse 20 to 40 times/minute.

Abnormal impulses

Abnormal impulse conduction results from disturbances in automaticity, conduction, or both.

It's automatic

Automaticity can increase or decrease the heart rate. For example, increased automaticity of pacemaker cells below the SA node commonly causes tachycardia. Likewise, decreased automaticity of cells in the SA node can cause bradycardia or an escape rhythm.

Conduction junction

Conduction may occur too quickly, as in Wolff-Parkinson-White (WPW) syndrome, or too slowly, as in AV block. Atrial tachycardia with a 4:1 block (this is when there are 4 P waves for every one QRS complex; see *You'll want to get this complex*) is an example of a combined automaticity and conduction disturbance.

Monitoring cardiac rhythms

An electrocardiogram (ECG) is used to monitor the precise sequence of electrical events in the cardiac cycle. There are two types of ECG recordings: the 12-lead and the single lead, commonly known as a *rhythm strip*.

You'll want to get this complex

An ECG tracing reflects the electrical events occurring in the cardiac cycle. Each waveform consists of five components, labeled with the letters P, Q, R, S, and T. The middle three letters—Q, R, and S—are collectively referred to as the *QRS complex*. (See *ECG waveform components*.)

Typically, you identify cardiac arrhythmias by recognizing their effects on the ECG waveform. However, ECG interpretation doesn't replace the need for keen assessment skills. Always remember that ECG findings should correlate with the patient's physical condition.

ECG waveform components

An ECG waveform has three basic components: the P wave, the QRS complex, and the T wave. These elements can be further divided into the PR interval, J point, ST segment, U wave, and QT interval.

P wave and PR interval

The P wave represents atrial depolarization. The PR interval represents the time it takes an impulse to travel from the atria through the AV nodes and the bundle of His. The PR interval measures from the beginning of the P wave to the beginning of the QRS complex.

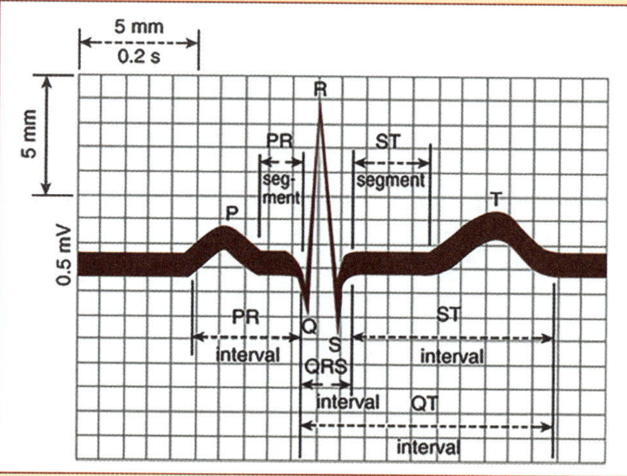

(Rhoades, R. A., & Bell, D. R. (2017). *Medical Physiology* (5th ed., Figure 12-7). Philadelphia: Wolters Kluwer Health.)

J point and ST segment

The J point marks the end of the QRS complex and also indicates the beginning of the ST segment. It is the inflection (angle) as the S wave begins its upstroke. The ST segment represents part of ventricular repolarization; it's measured from the end of the S wave to the beginning of the T wave.

QRS complex

The QRS complex represents ventricular depolarization (the time it takes for the impulse to travel through the bundle branches to the Purkinje fibers).

The Q wave appears as the first negative deflection in the QRS complex; the R wave as the first positive deflection. The S wave appears as the second negative deflection or the first negative deflection after the R wave.

T wave and U wave

The T wave represents ventricular repolarization and usually follows the same deflection pattern as the P wave. The U wave follows the T wave; however, because the U wave reflects a problem, it isn't seen in most patients.

QT interval

The QT interval represents ventricular depolarization and repolarization. It extends from the beginning of the QRS complex to the end of the T wave.

Applying monitoring devices

An ECG monitor is a tool that provides continuous information about the heart's electrical activity. Electrodes applied to the patient's chest pick up the heart's electrical activity and display the waveform on the monitor.

Commonly monitored leads include the three bipolar leads—I, II, and, III—and MCL_1 and MCL_6, which are modified versions of leads V_1 and V_6. You may use a three-, four-, or five-electrode system for cardiac monitoring. (See *Using a five-leadwire system*.)

Technique matters

To ensure accurate lead monitoring, you must apply the electrodes correctly. Follow these steps for accurate lead placement:

- Clip dense hair at each site.
- Prepare the skin by briskly rubbing each site until the skin reddens using the rough patch on the back of the electrode or a dry gauze pad.
- Remove the backing from the electrodes and apply one to each prepared site by pressing it against the patient's skin (the electrode gel should be moist in order to conduct properly).

Peak technique

Using a five-leadwire system

This illustration shows the correct placement of electrodes for a five-leadwire system. The chest electrode shown is located in the V_1 position, but you can place it in any of the chest lead positions. Each lead's color is included in the key.

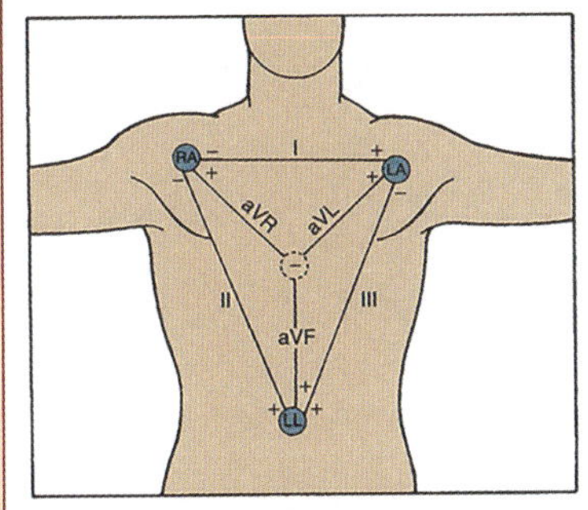

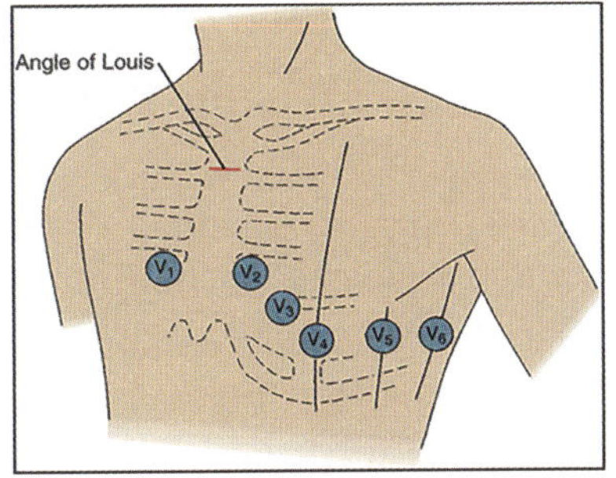

(Reproduced from Badescu, G. C., Sherman, B., Zaidan, J. R., et al. (2013). Atlas of electrocardiography. In: Barash PG, Cullen BF, Stoelting RK, eds. *Clinical Anesthesia* (7th ed., p. 1701). Philadelphia, PA: Wolters Kluwer Health.)

- Attach leadwires or cable connections by clipping them to the electrodes. (If you're using a snap-on leadwire, attach it to the electrode before placing the electrode on the patient's chest to prevent patient discomfort.)
- Turn on the monitor.
- Select the lead you wish to view following the monitor's instructions.

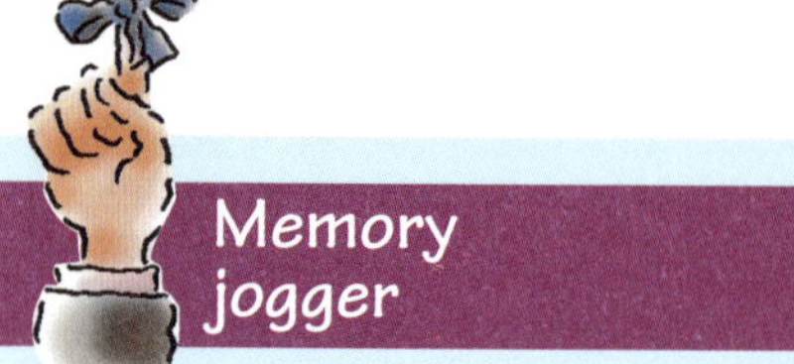

To help you remember where to place electrodes in a five-electrode configuration, think of the phrase "White, upper right." Then think of snow over trees (white above green), and smoke over fire (black above red). And, of course, chocolate (brown electrode) lies close to the heart!

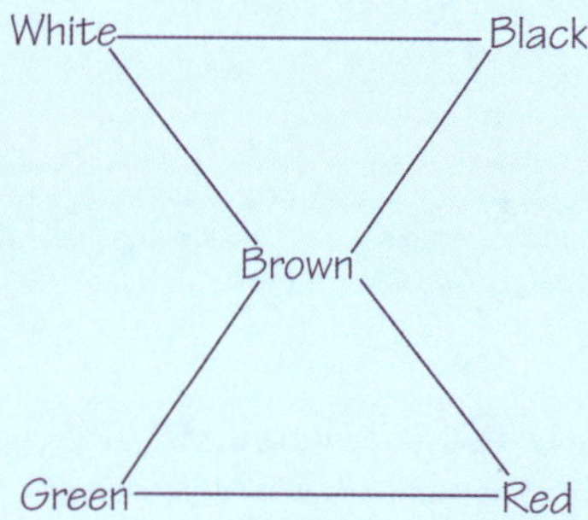

Interpreting rhythm strips: An eight-step method

You can learn to analyze and interpret ECGs systematically and correctly by using this eight-step method. First, scan the entire strip and identify the waveform components. Then follow these steps.

Step 1: Determine the rhythm

To determine the heart's atrial and ventricular rhythms, use either the paper-and-pencil method or the calipers method. (See *Methods of measuring rhythm.*) Then ask yourself, "Is the rhythm regular or irregular?"

Peak technique

Methods of measuring rhythm

You can use either of the following methods to determine atrial and ventricular rhythm.

Paper-and-pencil method

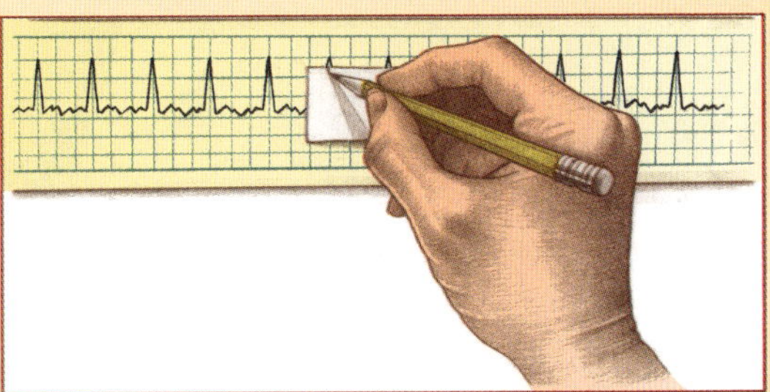

Place the electrocardiogram (ECG) strip on a flat surface. Then position the straight edge of a piece of paper along the strip's baseline. Move the paper up slightly so the straight edge is near the peak of the R wave. With a pencil, mark the paper at the R waves of two consecutive QRS complexes, as shown. This is the R-R interval.

Next, move the paper across the strip and line up those two marks with succeeding R-R intervals. If the distance for each R-R interval is the same, the ventricular rhythm is regular. If the distance varies, the rhythm is irregular.

Use the same method to measure the distance between the P waves (the P-P interval) and determine whether the atrial rhythm is regular or irregular.

Calipers method

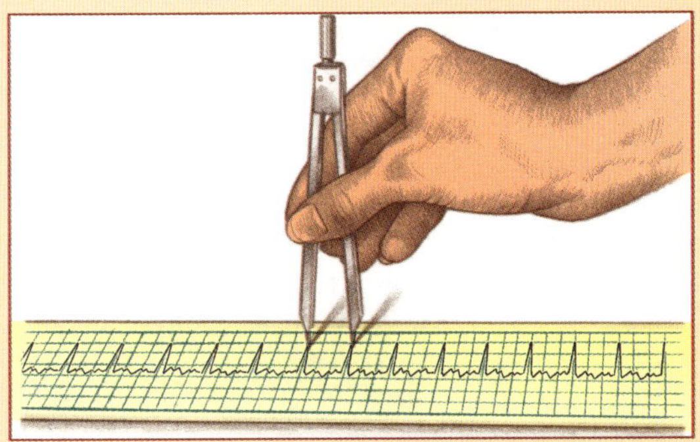

With the ECG strip on a flat surface, place one point of the calipers on the peak of the R wave of two consecutive QRS complexes. Then adjust the legs and place the other point on the peak of the next R wave, as shown. This distance is the R-R interval.

Next, pivot the first point of the calipers toward the third R wave and note whether it falls on the peak of that wave. Check succeeding R-R intervals in the same way. If they're all the same distance, the ventricular rhythm is regular. If the distance varies, the rhythm is irregular.

Using the same method, measure the P-P intervals to determine whether the atrial rhythm is regular or irregular.

Step 2: Determine the rate

Next, calculate the heart's atrial and ventricular rates, using the times 10 method, the 1,500 method, or the sequence method. (See *Calculating heart rate.*)

Peak technique

Calculating heart rate

You can use one of three methods—the times 10 method, the 1,500 method, or the sequence method—to determine atrial and ventricular heart rates from an electrocardiogram waveform.

Times 10 method

The simplest, quickest, and most common technique, the times 10 method is particularly useful if the patient's heart rhythm is irregular. First, obtain a rhythm strip. Then locate the small markings at the top of the strip. Each marking represents 3 seconds. Count the number of P waves (to determine atrial rate) or R waves (to determine ventricular rate) over a 6-second time period (two 3-second markings). Multiply by 10.

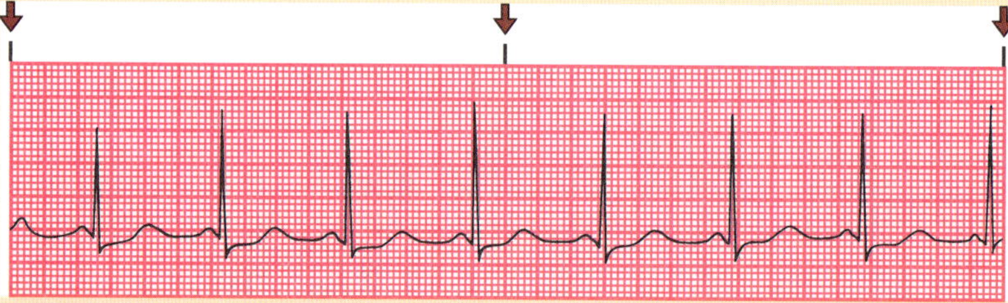

1,500 method

Use the 1,500 method only if the patient's heart rhythm is regular. First, identify two consecutive P waves on the rhythm strip. Next, select identical points in each wave and count the number of small squares between the points. Then divide 1,500 by the number of small squares counted (1,500 small squares equal 1 minute) to get the atrial rate. To calculate the ventricular rate, use the same procedure but with two consecutive R waves instead of P waves.

Sequence method

The sequence method gives you an estimated heart rate. First, find a P wave that peaks on a heavy black line. Assign the following numbers to the next six heavy black lines: 300, 150, 100, 75, 60, and 50, respectively.

Then find the next P wave peak and estimate the atrial rate based on the number assigned to the nearest heavy black line. Estimate the ventricular rate following the same procedure but use the R wave instead of the P wave.

Determine if the rate is within normal limits (60 to 100 beats/minute). Next, determine if the atrial (P-P interval) rate and ventricular (R-R interval) rate are continually the same measurement. Then determine if they're associated with each other.

Step 3: Evaluate the P wave

Look at the rhythm strip and answer these questions:

- Are P waves present?
- Do the P waves have a normal shape (upright and rounded)?
- Are the P waves similar in size and shape?
- Do all the P waves point in the same direction? Are they all upright, inverted, or diphasic?
- Do the P waves and QRS complexes have a one-to-one relationship? In other words, is there a P wave for every QRS complex?

Step 4: Determine the duration of the PR interval

Measure the PR interval of several complexes. (Normal duration is 0.12 to 0.20 seconds.) Then, determine if the PR interval is constant.

Step 5: Determine the duration of the QRS complex

Look at the rhythm strip again and answer these questions:

- Are all the QRS complexes the same size and shape?
- What's the duration of the QRS complex? (Normal duration is 0.06 to 0.10 seconds.)
- Are all the QRS complexes the same distance from the T waves that follow them?
- Do all the QRS complexes point in the same direction?
- Do any QRS complexes appear different from the others on the strip? (If so, measure and describe each one individually.)

Step 6: Evaluate the T wave

Examine the strip once more and answer these questions:

- Are T waves present?
- Do all the T waves have the same size and shape?
- Could a P wave be hidden in a T wave?
- Do the T waves point in the same direction as the QRS complexes?

Step 7: Determine the duration of the QT interval

Measure the QT interval. Note whether the duration of the QT interval falls within normal limits (0.36 to 0.44 seconds, or 9 to 11 small squares).

Step 8: Evaluate other components

Finally, observe other components on the ECG strip, including ectopic or aberrantly conducted beats and other abnormalities. Check the ST segment for any abnormalities, such as elevation above or depression below the isoelectric line, and look for a U wave. Note your findings.

Recognizing normal sinus rhythm

Before you can recognize an arrhythmia, you must be able to recognize a normal sinus rhythm (NSR). NSR is a heart rhythm that starts in the SA node and progresses to the ventricles through a normal conduction pathway—from the SA node to the atria and AV node, through the bundle of His to the bundle branches, and on to the Purkinje fibers. NSR is the standard against which all other rhythms are compared.

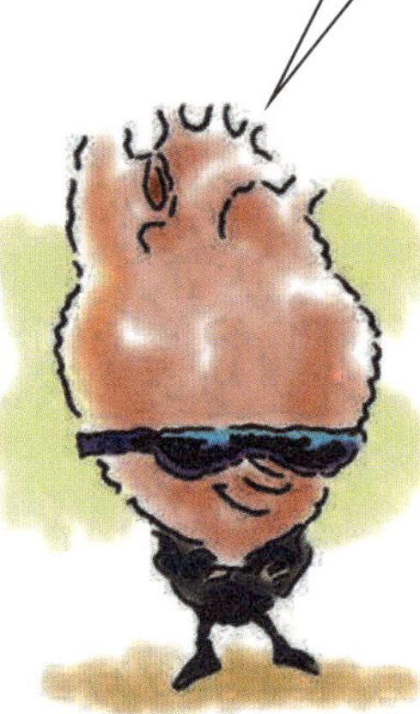

I'm so proud of myself! My normal sinus rhythm is a model of classic cardiac conduction.

What the ECG tells you

- *Rhythm:* atrial and ventricular rhythms are regular.
- *Rate:* atrial and ventricular rates are 60 to 100 beats/minute.
- *P wave:* P waves are similar in size and shape (upright and rounded); P wave precedes every QRS complex.
- *PR interval:* PR interval is within normal limits (0.12 to 0.20 seconds).
- *QRS complex:* QRS complex is within normal limits (0.06 to 0.10 seconds).
- *T wave:* T wave is normally shaped (upright and rounded in lead II).
- *QT interval:* QT interval is within normal limits (0.36 to 0.44 seconds).

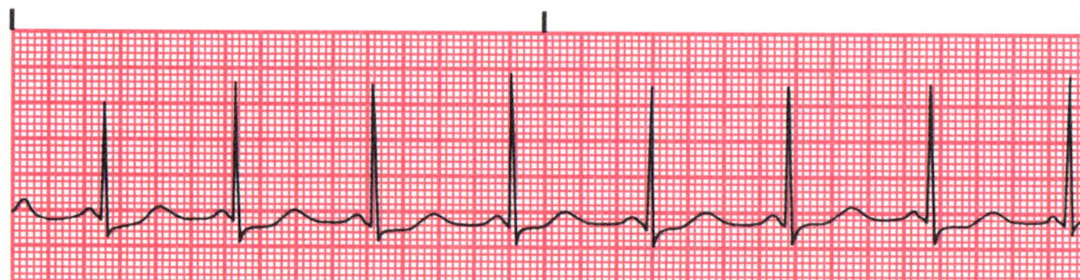

Recognizing sinus bradycardia

Bradycardia is defined as a heart rate less than 60 beats/minute. Sinus bradycardia is a sinus rate below 60 beats/minute with all impulses coming from the SA node. This arrhythmia's significance depends on the amount of cardiac output that occurs with each beat.

What the ECG tells you

- *Rhythm:* Atrial and ventricular rhythms are regular.
- *Rate:* Atrial and ventricular rates are less than 60 beats/minute.
- *P wave:* Normal size and configuration; P wave precedes each QRS complex.
- *PR interval:* Within normal limits and constant.

- *QRS complex:* Normal duration and configuration.
- *T wave:* Normal size and configuration.
- *QT interval:* Within normal limits but may be prolonged.

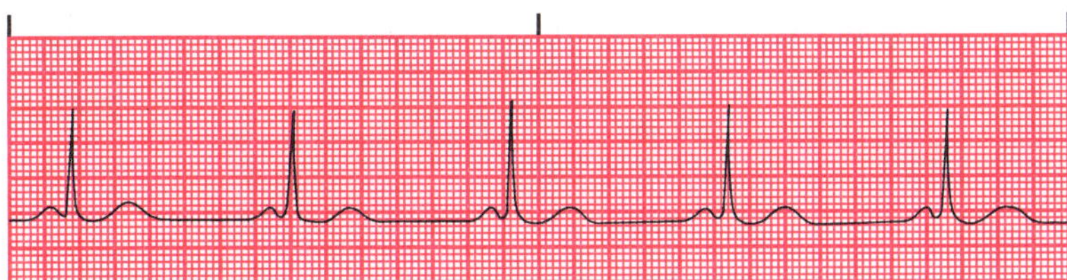

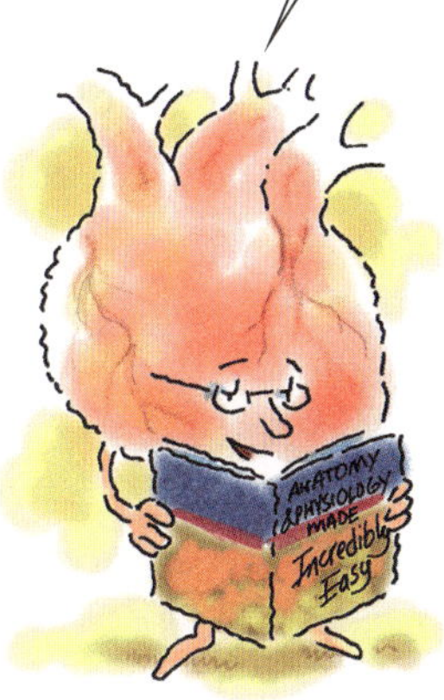

What causes it

- A well-conditioned heart (in athletic people)
- Hyperkalemia
- Increased intracranial pressure
- Increased vagal tone that accompanies straining at stool, vomiting, intubation, mechanical ventilation, sick sinus syndrome, hypothyroidism, or hard physical exertion
- Possible result of inferior MI involving the right coronary artery, which supplies blood to the SA node
- Drugs such as beta-adrenergic blockers, sympatholytic drugs, digoxin, or morphine

What to look for

- Possibly asymptomatic
- Fatigue, light-headedness, syncope, and palpitations
- Chest pain and premature beats (if heart disease exists and coronary blood flow is decreased)

How it's treated

- If the patient normally has a low heart rate, treatment may not be needed. Bradycardia is only treated if heart rate is typically less than 50 and the patient is symptomatic.
  - Identify the underlying factors and treat them (e.g., hypoxia, blood pressure, and fluid load. If possible, get a 12-lead ECG)
- Administer oxygen as required to maintain saturation of peripheral oxygen (SPO2) of 94%.
- Administer atropine if the patient is hemodynamically unstable (use cautiously in patients with acute myocardial ischemia or MI because atropine may cause excessive increases in heart rate, worsening ischemia, or increase of the infarction zone).
- If atropine is ineffective, prepare to apply a transcutaneous pacemaker or administer epinephrine or dopamine infusions
- Obtain expert consultation as transvenous pacing or a permanent pacemaker may be indicated.

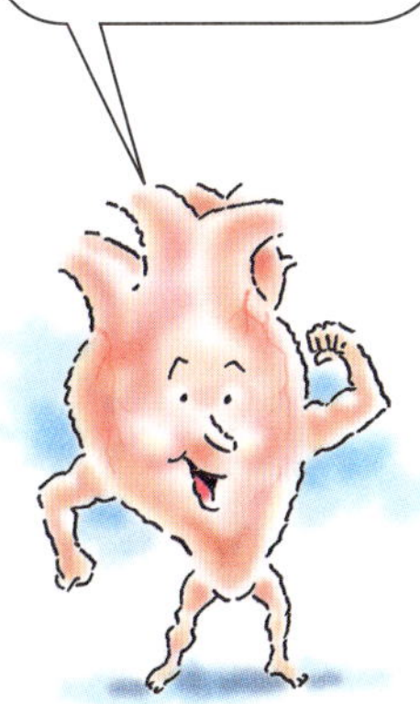

Recognizing premature complexes

Premature complexes involve the early discharge of an electrical impulse. They are common and often require no treatment. Premature complexes include premature atrial contractions (PACs) and premature ventricular contractions (PVCs). The common complaint with premature beats is that the patient is feeling "palpitations."

Premature atrial contractions

Originating outside the SA node, PACs usually arise from an irritable focus in the atria that supersedes the SA node as the pacemaker for one or more beats. PACs can occur in groups of two or every other beat (bigeminy).

A PAC is usually followed by a pause as the SA node is reset, which may be noncompensatory, compensatory, or longer than compensatory. Commonly, the pause is noncompensatory. PACs may also be blocked, with only an early P wave present. The most common cause of a pause is a blocked PAC.

Precipitous PACs

PACs may precipitate a more serious arrhythmia, such as atrial flutter or atrial fibrillation, in patients with heart disease. If PACs occur with an acute MI, they may signal heart failure or an electrolyte imbalance.

What the ECG tells you

- *Rhythm:* Atrial and ventricular rhythms are irregular as a result of the PACs, but the underlying rhythm may be regular.
- *Rate:* Atrial and ventricular rates vary with the underlying rhythm.
- *P wave:* Premature and abnormally shaped; possibly lost in the previous T wave.
- *PR interval:* Usually within normal limits; may be shortened or slightly prolonged for the ectopic beat, depending on where the ectopic focus originates.
- *QRS complex:* Duration and configuration are usually normal. If no QRS complex follows the P wave, a nonconducted PAC has occurred. With nonconducted PACs, the P wave is seen in a distorted T wave.
- *T wave:* Usually has a normal configuration; however, if the P wave is hidden in the T wave, the T wave may be distorted.
- *QT interval:* Usually within normal limits.

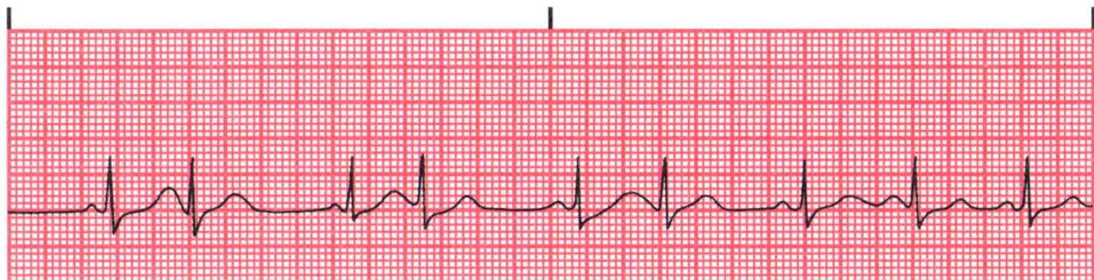

What causes it

- Acute respiratory failure; hypoxia
- Heart failure
- Drugs that prolong the SA node's absolute refractory period, such as digoxin, quinidine, and procainamide
- Excessive use of caffeine, tobacco, recreational drugs, and alcohol
- Ischemic heart disease
- Stress, fatigue, and overeating

What to look for

- Possibly no symptoms
- Irregular pulse
- Complaint of palpitations

How it's treated

- Typically, no treatment is necessary.
- Oxygen therapy, if indicated (oxygen saturation less than 94%).
- Elimination of known causes, such as caffeine, tobacco, recreational drugs, and alcohol
- Treatment of known cause

Premature ventricular contractions

PVCs are ectopic beats that originate low in the ventricles and occur earlier than expected. PVCs may occur singly, in pairs, in threes, or in fours; in many cases, they're followed by a compensatory pause. PVCs that occur every other beat are known as *bigeminy;* those that occur every third beat are known as *trigeminy*. Those that occur every fourth beat are known as *quadrigeminy*. Two PVCs that occur together are called a *couplet*.

PVCs may be unifocal, arising from the same ectopic focus, or they may be multifocal, arising from different ventricular sites or from one site with changing patterns of conduction. (See *When PVCs spell danger*.)

Are you serious?

The significance of PVCs depends on how well the ventricles function and how long the arrhythmia lasts. Cardiac output diminishes because of insufficient ventricular filling time.

Generally, PVCs are more serious if they occur in a patient with heart disease. In an ischemic or damaged heart, PVCs are more likely to develop into ventricular tachycardia, flutter, or fibrillation.

What the ECG tells you

- *Rhythm:* Atrial and ventricular rhythms are irregular during PVCs; the underlying rhythm may be regular.
- *Rate:* Atrial and ventricular rates reflect the underlying rhythm.
- *P wave:* Usually absent in the ectopic beat; however, it may appear after the QRS complex with retrograde conduction to the atria. Usually normal if present in the underlying rhythm.
- *PR interval:* Unmeasurable, except in the underlying rhythm.
- *QRS complex:* Occurs earlier than expected; duration exceeds 0.12 second; bizarre configuration.
- *T wave:* Occurs in direction opposite QRS complex. A horizontal baseline, called a *compensatory pause,* may follow the T wave. (A compensatory pause exists if the P-P interval encompassing the PVC has twice the duration of a normal sinus beat's P-P interval.)
- *QT interval:* Not usually measured.

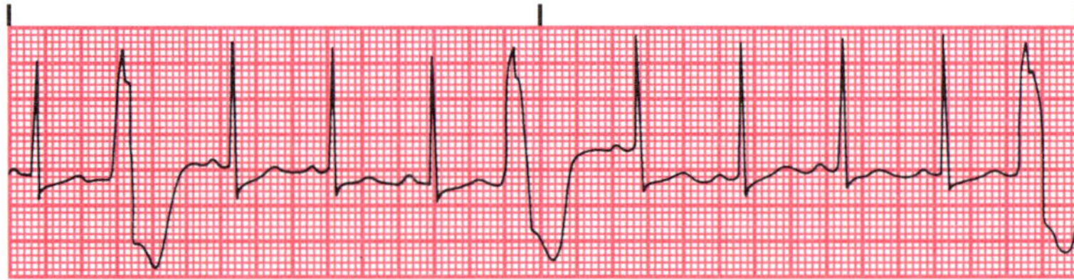

What causes it

- Caffeine, tobacco, and alcohol ingestion
- Stimulant drugs, such as amphetamines or cocaine
- Digoxin toxicity
- Exercise
- Electrolyte imbalances, especially involving potassium
- Hypoxia
- History of hypertension
- Myocardial irritation by pacemaker electrodes or pulmonary artery catheter
- Myocardial ischemia and infarction
- Cardiomyopathy
- Valvular heart disease

- Heart muscle inflammation (such as myocarditis) or injury (such as cardiac contusion)
- Sympathomimetic drugs (such as epinephrine and isoproterenol [Isuprel])
- Antiarrhythmics (proarrhythmic effect)

When PVCs spell danger

Here are some examples of dangerous patterns that occur with premature ventricular contractions (PVCs).

Multiple PVCs

Two PVCs in a row are called a *pair,* or couplet (see shaded areas). A pair can produce ventricular tachycardia because the second contraction usually meets refractory tissue. A salvo (three or more PVCs in a row) is considered a run of ventricular tachycardia.

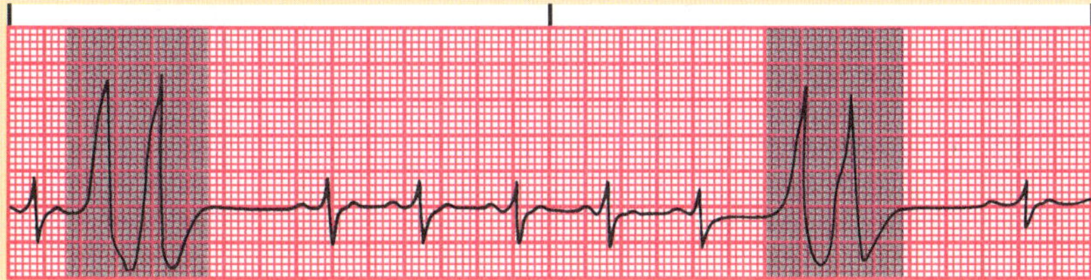

Multifocal PVCs

PVCs that look different from one another and arise from different sites or from the same site with abnormal conduction (see shaded areas) are called *mutlifocal* or *multiform PVCs.* Multifocal PVCs may indicate severe heart disease or digoxin toxicity.

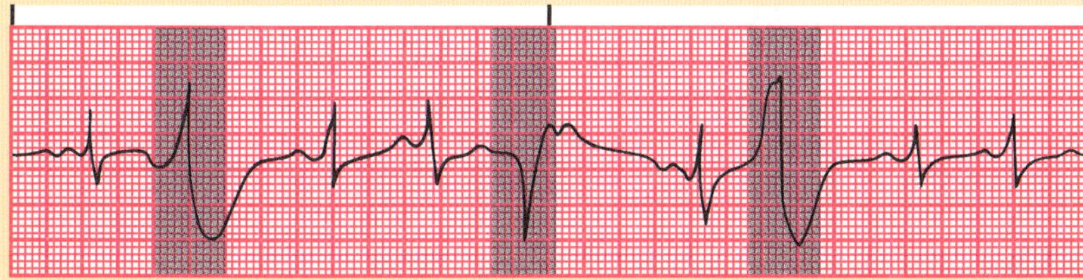

Bigeminy and trigeminy

PVCs that occur every other beat (bigeminy) or every third beat (trigeminy) can cause ventricular tachycardia or ventricular fibrillation (see shaded areas).

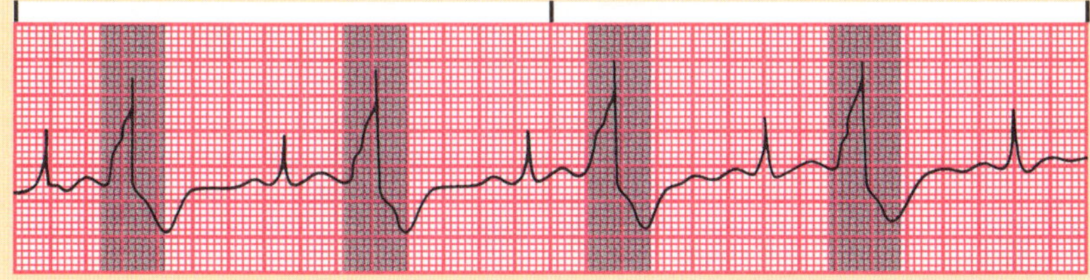

(*continued*)

When PVCs spell danger *(continued)*

R-on-T phenomenon

In R-on-T phenomenon, the PVC occurs so early that it falls on the T wave of the preceding beat (see shaded areas). Ventricular tachycardia or ventricular fibrillation may occur because the cells haven't fully repolarized.

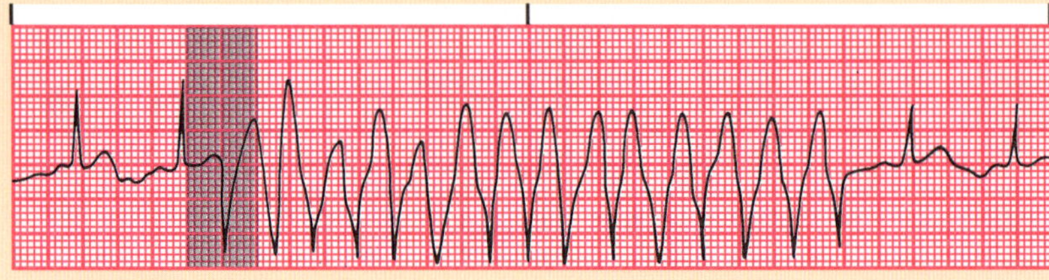

What to look for

- Possibly no symptoms
- A longer than normal pause immediately after the premature beat
- Signs of decreased cardiac output if PVCs are frequent, such as hypotension, altered mental status, and signs of shock or ischemic chest discomfort
- Palpitations

How it's treated

- Identify and correct underlying cause, if possible.
- Administer oxygen, if indicated.
- Correct electrolyte imbalances, if present.
- Consider adenosine if narrow complex regular and monomorphic. Administer amiodarone, procainamide, or sotalol if the patient is symptomatic. Lidocaine may be administered as an alternative drug.

Recognizing narrow complex tachycardias

Narrow complex tachycardias are arrhythmias that involve an accelerated heart rate and a narrow QRS complex. They include sinus tachycardia, atrial fibrillation, atrial flutter, atrial tachycardia, multifocal atrial tachycardia (MAT), WPW syndrome, and junctional tachycardia.

Sinus tachycardia

Sinus tachycardia involves the accelerated firing of the SA node beyond its normal discharge rate, resulting in a heart rate of 100 to 150 beats/minute. The rate rarely exceeds 160 beats/minute, except during strenuous exercise.

Pesty tachy may persist

Persistent sinus tachycardia, especially with acute myocardial infarction (MI), may lead to ischemia and myocardial damage by raising oxygen requirements.

What the ECG tells you

- *Rhythm:* Atrial and ventricular rhythms are regular.
- *Rate:* Atrial and ventricular rates are greater than 100 beats/minute (usually between 100 and 150 beats/minute).
- *P wave:* Normal size and configuration; P wave precedes each QRS complex.
- *PR interval:* Within normal limits and constant.
- *QRS complex:* Normal duration and configuration.
- *T wave:* Normal size and configuration.
- *QT interval:* Within normal limits but commonly shortened.

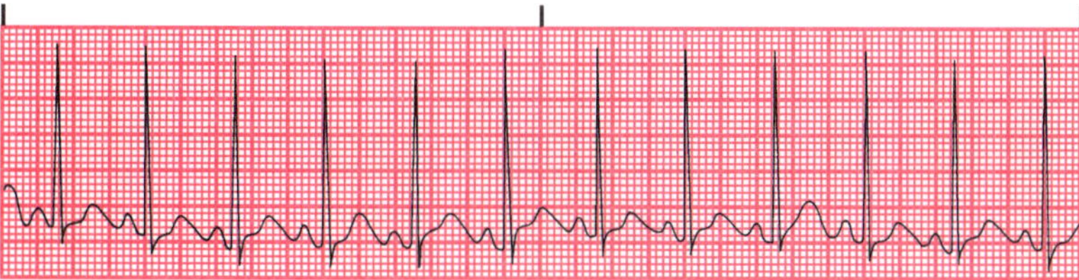

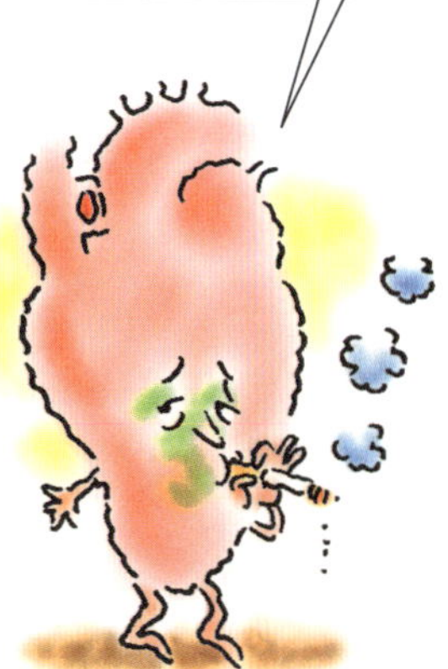

What causes it

- Caffeine, nicotine, alcohol ingestion, and recreational drug use
- Drugs such as digoxin (Lanoxin), adrenergics, anticholinergics, and antiarrhythmics
- Hyperthyroidism and severe hypothyroidism (rare)
- Normal cardiac response to demand for increased oxygen during exercise, fever, stress, pain, and dehydration
- Any occurrence that decreases vagal tone and increases sympathetic tone
- Inflammatory response after MI (In acute MI, it may be one of the first signs of heart failure, cardiogenic shock, pulmonary embolism, or infarct extension.)

What to look for

- Usually no symptoms
- Rapid, regular pulse 100 to 150 beats/minute
- Palpitations or angina caused by increased myocardial oxygen consumption and reduced coronary blood flow

How it's treated

- Treatment aims to correct the underlying cause.
- If the patient is symptomatic, a nondihydropyridine calcium channel blocker such as verapamil or diltiazem or a beta-adrenergic blocker such as metoprolol (Lopressor) may be given.

Atrial fibrillation

Atrial fibrillation, usually called *A-fib,* is defined as chaotic, asynchronous, electrical activity in atrial tissue. It stems from the firing of a number of impulses in reentry pathways. Atrial fibrillation results in a loss of "atrial kick," which is the effective force of contraction of the atrium that increases blood flow to the ventricle. The ectopic impulses may fire at a rate of 400 to 600 times/minute, causing the atria to quiver instead of contract. Afib with an excessively rapid heart rate is called "Afib with RVR (rapid ventricular response)."

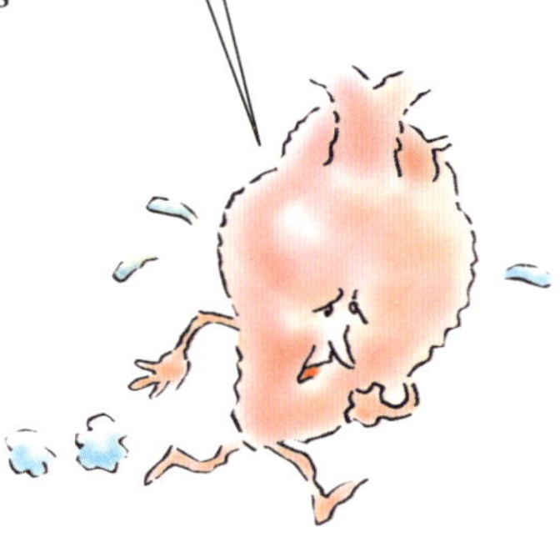

On impulse

The ventricles respond only to those impulses that make it through the AV node. On an ECG, atrial activity is no longer represented by P waves but by erratic baseline waves called *fibrillatory waves*, or *f waves*. This rhythm may be either persistent or paroxysmal (occurring in bursts). It can be preceded by or the result of PACs. The patient may develop an atrial rhythm that frequently varies between a fibrillatory line and flutter waves. This is called *A-fib/flutter*.

What the ECG tells you

- *Rhythm:* Atrial and ventricular rhythms are grossly irregular.
- *Rate:* The atrial rate (almost indiscernible) usually exceeds 400 beats/minute. The ventricular rate usually varies from 40 to 250 beats/minute.
- *P wave:* Absent. Erratic baseline f waves appear instead. These chaotic f waves represent atrial tetanization from rapid atrial depolarizations.
- *PR interval:* Indiscernible.
- *QRS complex:* Duration and configuration are usually normal.
- *QT interval:* Unmeasurable.

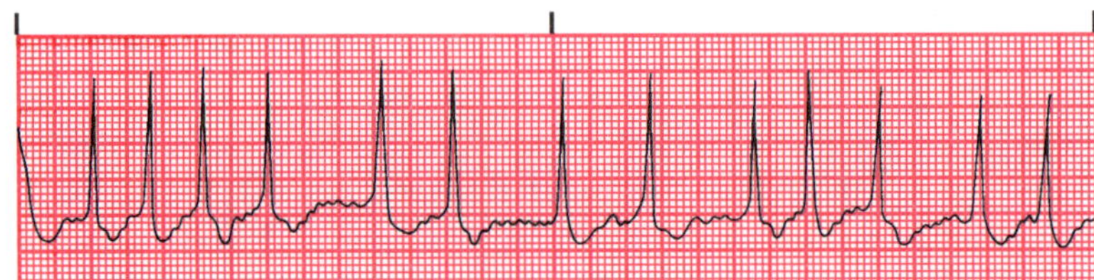

What causes it

- Inflammation, valvular disorders (especially mitral stenosis), hypertension, MI, coronary artery disease (CAD), heart failure, cardiomyopathy, and pericarditis
- Thyrotoxicosis
- Chronic obstructive pulmonary disease (COPD)
- Drugs such as digoxin (Lanoxin)
- Cardiac surgery
- Occasional increased sympathetic activity from exercise

What to look for

- Irregular pulse rhythm with a normal or rapid rate ("palpitations"); peripheral pulse commonly slower than apical pulse
- Signs and symptoms of decreased cardiac output (if ventricular rate is rapid)

How it's treated

- If the patient is hemodynamically unstable (systolic blood pressure below 90), perform synchronized cardioversion immediately (120 to 200 joules biphasic or 200 joules monophasic). If using monophasic energy, start at 200 joules and increase in a stepwise fashion as indicated.
- For patients with a rapid rate, consult an expert practitioner and administer a beta-adrenergic blocker, such as metoprolol IV, or a calcium channel blocker, such as diltiazem (Cardizem), to control the ventricular rate and attempt to convert the rhythm.
- There are two approaches to treating A fib rate control or rhythm control. Medications depend on which option is used. Beta blockers and calcium channel blockers are used for rate control. Amiodarone is an example of a medication used for rhythm control (Knight, 2022).
- Consider anticoagulants when deciding how quickly to convert atrial fibrillation that has been present longer than 48 hours because rapid conversion may cause blood clots to flow into the cardiovascular system.

Atrial flutter

Atrial flutter is characterized by an atrial rate of 250 to 400 beats/minute, although it's generally about 300 beats/minute. Originating in a single atrial focus, this rhythm results from reentry and, possibly, increased automaticity.

Fast flutter, slow kick

The significance of atrial flutter depends on the acceleration of the ventricular rate. The faster the ventricular rate, the more dangerous the arrhythmia. Like atrial fibrillation, atrial flutter results in a loss of atrial kick. Even a small rise in the ventricular rate can cause angina, syncope, hypotension, heart failure, and pulmonary edema. Atrial fibrillation may appear intermittently.

What the ECG tells you

- *Rhythm:* Atrial rhythm is regular. Ventricular rhythm depends on the AV conduction pattern; it is usually regular, although cycles may alternate. An irregular pattern may signal atrial fibrillation or indicate a block.
- *Rate:* Atrial rate is 250 to 400 beats/minute. Ventricular rate depends on the degree of AV block; usually it's 60 to 100 beats/minute but it may accelerate to 125 to 150 beats/minute.
- *P wave:* Saw-toothed or picket fence appearance (called *flutter waves*).
- *PR interval:* Unmeasurable.
- *QRS complex:* Duration is usually within normal limits but the complex may be widened if flutter waves are buried within.
- *T wave:* Not identifiable.
- *QT interval:* Unmeasurable.

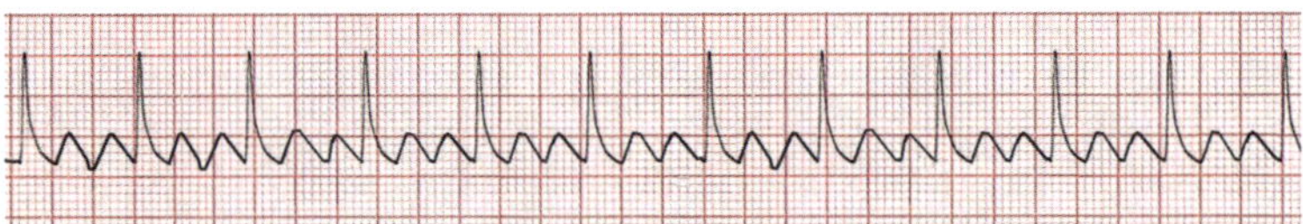

(Reproduced with permission from Donnelly-Moreno, L. A., & Moseley, B. (2021). *Timby's Introductory Medical-Surgical Nursing* (13th ed., Fig. 26-4). Philadelphia: Wolters Kluwer Health.)

In patients with atrial flutter, even a small increase in ventricular rate can cause angina, syncope, hypotension, heart failure, and pulmonary edema.

What causes it

- Acute or chronic cardiac disorder, mitral or tricuspid valve disorder, cor pulmonale, and cardiac inflammation such as pericarditis
- MI (transient complication)
- Lung disease and sleep apnea
- Drugs such as digoxin (Lanoxin)
- Hyperthyroidism
- Alcoholism
- Cardiac surgery

What to look for

- Absence of symptoms or palpitations
- Complaints can include palpitations, light-headedness, and shortness of breath

- Cardiac, cerebral, and peripheral vascular effects (if ventricular filling and coronary artery blood flow are compromised)

How it's treated

- If the patient is hemodynamically unstable, perform synchronized cardioversion immediately, beginning with 50 to 100 joules of biphasic or monophasic energy. Increase energy in a stepwise fashion if the initial shock fails.
- For patients with a rapid rate, consult an expert practitioner and administer a beta-adrenergic blocker, such as esmolol IV, or a calcium channel blocker, such as diltiazem, to control ventricular rate.
- Follow the orders of the practitioner for rhythm control.
- Consider anticoagulants when deciding how quickly to convert atrial flutter that has been present longer than 48 hours because rapid conversion may cause blood clots.

Atrial tachycardia

In atrial tachycardia, also known as supraventricular tachycardia (SVT), the atrial rhythm is ectopic and the atrial rate ranges from 150 to 250 beats/minute. Benign in a healthy person, this arrhythmia can be dangerous in a patient with an existing cardiac disorder.

What the ECG tells you

- *Rhythm:* Atrial and ventricular rhythms are regular.
- *Rate:* The atrial rate is characterized by three or more successive ectopic atrial beats at a rate of 150 to 250 beats/minute. The rate rarely exceeds 250 beats/minute. The ventricular rate depends on the AV conduction ratio.
- *P wave:* Usually upright, the P wave may be aberrant or hidden in the previous T wave. If visible, it precedes each QRS complex.
- *PR interval:* May be unmeasurable if the P wave can't be distinguished from the preceding T wave.
- *QRS complex:* Duration and configuration are usually normal.
- *T wave:* Usually distinguishable but may be distorted by the P wave.
- *QT interval:* Usually within normal limits but may be shortened because of the rapid rate.

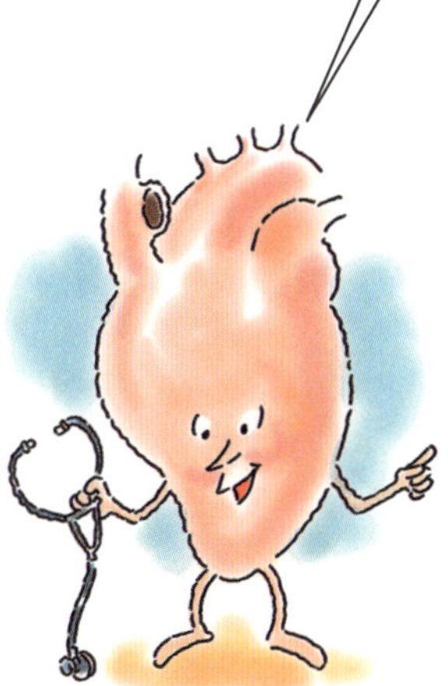

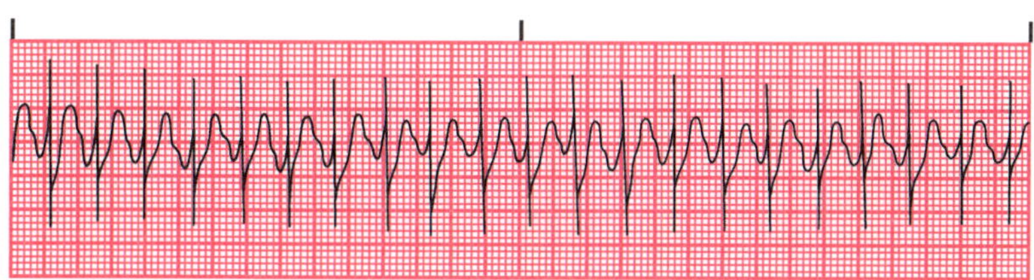

What causes it

- Digoxin toxicity
- Primary cardiac disorders, such as MI, cardiomyopathy, pericarditis, valvular heart disease, and WPW syndrome
- Secondary cardiac problems, such as hyperthyroidism, cor pulmonale, and systemic hypertension
- COPD
- In healthy people, physical or psychological stress, hypoxia, hypokalemia, excessive use of caffeine or other stimulants, and marijuana use

What to look for

- Rapid apical or peripheral pulse rates, palpitations
- Signs and symptoms of decreased cardiac output, such as hypotension, syncope, and blurred vision

How it's treated

- Attempt vagal stimulation.
- Administer adenosine (Adenocard).
- If the patient is hemodynamically unstable, perform synchronized cardioversion immediately (initially, 50 to 100 joules of biphasic or monophasic energy).

Multifocal atrial tachycardia

MAT results from the extreme rapid firing of multifocal ectopic sites. Very rare in healthy people, this arrhythmia is usually found in acutely ill patients with pulmonary disease or elevated atrial pressures.

What the ECG tells you

- *Rhythm:* Atrial and ventricular rhythms are irregular.
- *Rate:* Atrial and ventricular rates range from 100 to 250 beats/minute.
- *P wave:* Configuration varies, usually with at least three unique P waves.
- *PR interval:* Varies.
- *QRS complex:* Duration and configuration are usually normal but may become aberrant if the arrhythmia persists.
- *T wave:* Usually distorted.
- *QT interval:* May be indiscernible.

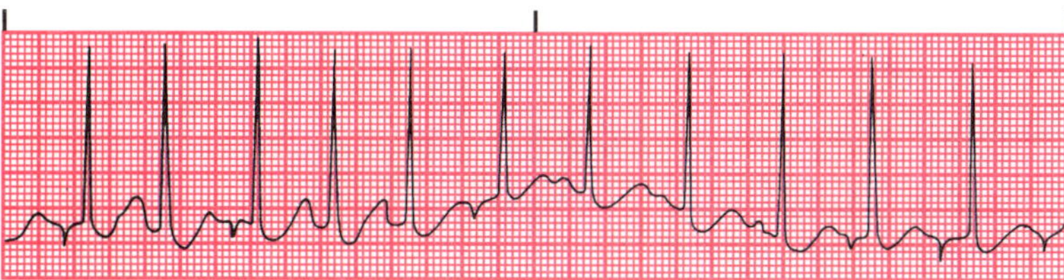

What causes it

- Atrial distention from elevated pulmonary pressure (usually seen in patients with COPD)

What to look for

- Palpitations
- Rapid apical or peripheral pulse rates
- Signs and symptoms of decreased cardiac output, such as blurred vision, syncope, and hypotension
- Symptoms are typically masked by underlying disease processes. (Buxton, 2022)

How it's treated

- First, distinguish MAT from atrial fibrillation, with an ECG, because both may cause an irregular rhythm.
- Administer oxygen to maintain pulse oximetry (POX) of 94%.
- For a patient with a rapid rate, consult an expert practitioner and administer a calcium channel blocker (verapamil [Calan] or diltiazem) or a beta-adrenergic blocker metoprolol (use cautiously in patients with pulmonary disease).
- Treat the underlying problem first, such as an electrolyte inbalance.
- MAT is *not* responsive to cardioversion.

Wolff-Parkinson-White syndrome

Seen mostly in young children and adults ages 20 to 35, WPW syndrome occurs when an anomalous atrial bypass tract (bundle of Kent) develops outside the AV junction, which connects the atria and ventricles. This pathway can conduct impulses either to the ventricles or to the atria. With retrograde conduction, reentry can arise, resulting in reentrant tachycardia.

The delta wave is the hallmark of WPW syndrome. The syndrome may cause abrupt episodes of premature SVT, atrial fibrillation, and atrial flutter with a rate as fast as 300 beats/minute.

No tachy, no problem

WPW syndrome is usually considered insignificant if tachycardia doesn't occur or if the patient has no associated cardiac disease. When tachycardia does occur in WPW syndrome, decreased cardiac output may develop.

What the ECG tells you

- *Rhythm:* Atrial and ventricular rhythms are regular.
- *Rate:* Atrial and ventricular rates are within normal limits, except when SVT occurs.
- *P wave:* Normal in size and configuration.
- *PR interval:* Short (less than 0.12 seconds).
- *QRS complex:* Duration greater than 0.10 second; beginning of the QRS complex may be slurred, producing a delta wave.
- *ST segment:* Usually normal but may go in a direction opposite the QRS complex.
- *QT interval:* Usually within normal limits.
- *T wave:* Usually normal but may be deflected in a direction opposite the QRS complex.

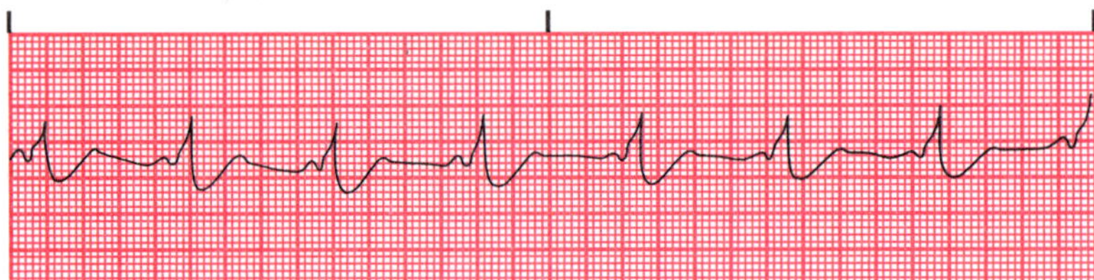

What causes it

- WPW syndrome is congenital in origin.

What to look for

- Usually no symptoms
- If tachyarrhythmias develop with a high ventricular response, palpitations, sudden onset of chest pain, shortness of breath, and possibly syncope, or (rarely) sudden cardiac arrest

How it's treated

- If the patient is hemodynamically unstable, perform synchronized cardioversion immediately (initially 50 to 100 joules of biphasic or monophasic energy).
- For patients with atrial fibrillation and WPW syndrome, consult a expert practitioner and prepare for synchronized cardioversion or to administer procainamide.
- Consider anticoagulants when deciding how quickly to convert atrial fibrillation with WPW syndrome that has been present longer than 48 hours, because rapid conversion may cause blood clots.

Junctional tachycardia

Considered an SVT, junctional tachycardia is characterized by three or more premature junctional contractions in a row. This happens when an irritable focus from the AV junction has enhanced automaticity and overrides the SA node's function as the heart's pacemaker. The atria depolarize by retrograde conduction, and conduction through the ventricles is normal. Usually, the heart rate measures between 100 and 200 beats/minute.

Well, that depends

The significance of junctional tachycardia depends on the rate, the underlying cause, and the severity of the accompanying cardiac disease. At higher ventricular rates, junctional tachycardia may compromise cardiac output by affecting ventricular filling.

What the ECG tells you

- *Rhythm:* Atrial and ventricular rhythms are usually regular. The atrial rhythm may be difficult to determine if the P wave is absent or hidden in the QRS complex or preceding T wave.
- *Rate:* Atrial and ventricular rates exceed 100 beats/minute (usually between 100 and 200 beats/minute). Atrial rate may be difficult to determine if the P wave is hidden in the QRS complex or if it precedes the T wave.
- *P wave:* Usually inverted; it may occur before or after the QRS complex or be hidden in the QRS complex.
- *PR interval:* If the P wave precedes the QRS complex, the PR interval is shortened (less than 0.12 second); otherwise, the PR interval can't be measured.
- *QRS complex:* Duration within normal limits; usually normal configuration.
- *T wave:* Usually normal configuration but may be abnormal if the P wave is hidden in the T wave. Fast rate may make the T wave indiscernible.
- *QT interval:* Usually within normal limits.

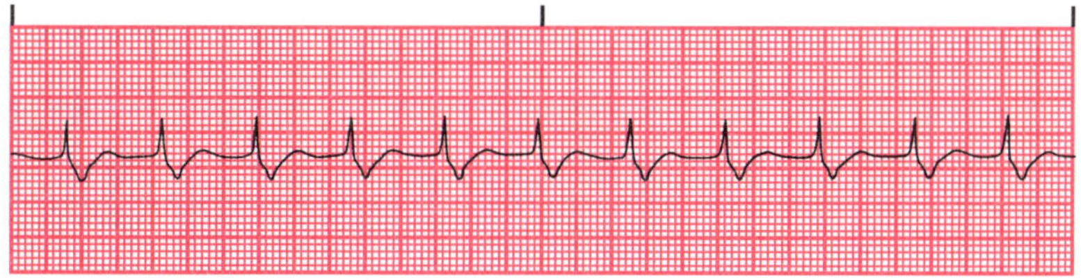

What causes it

- Digoxin toxicity
- Cardiomyopathy
- Enhanced automaticity
- Hypoxia
- Inferior wall MI and ischemia
- Myocarditis
- Vagal stimulation
- Valve replacement surgery

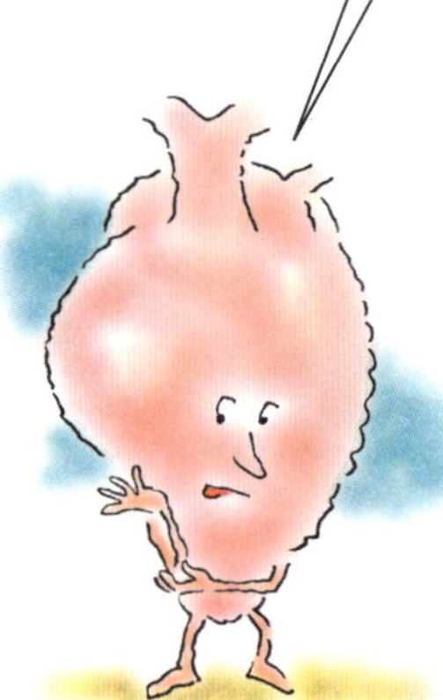

What to look for

- Pulse rate greater than 100 beats/minute
- Usually no symptoms if the patient can compensate
- Possibly signs and symptoms of decreased cardiac output if compensation is poor

How it's treated

- Consult an expert practitioner.
- Discontinue digoxin therapy.
- Administer beta-adrenergic blockers or calcium channel blockers to control rate.

Recognizing atrioventricular blocks

AV blocks result from interruption in the conduction of impulses between the atria and the ventricles. They can be partial, total, or involve only a delay of conduction. Blocks can occur at the AV node, bundle of His, or bundle branches.

You can classify AV blocks as first-, second-, or third-degree.
AV BLOCK
AV BL OC K

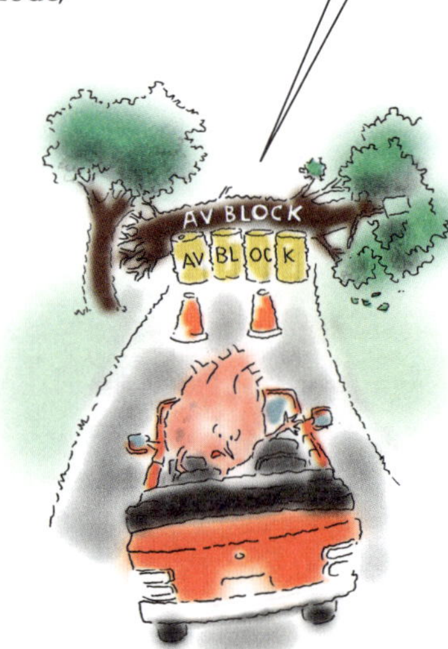

Three degrees of separation

The clinical effect depends on how many impulses are completely blocked, how slow the ventricular rate is, and how the block affects the heart. Blocks with slow rates can decrease cardiac output. AV blocks are classified as first-, second-, or third-degree.

First-degree AV block

A first-degree AV block occurs when impulses from the atria are consistently delayed during conduction through the AV node. It can be temporary and is the least dangerous of the AV blocks; however, it can progress to a more severe block.

What the ECG tells you

- *Rhythm:* Atrial and ventricular rhythms are regular.
- *Rate:* Atrial and ventricular rates are the same and within normal limits.
- *P wave:* Normal size and configuration.
- *PR interval:* Prolonged (exceeding 0.20 second) but constant. (If you see an exceptionally long PR interval, look for hidden P waves; these may indicate a second-degree AV block.)
- *QRS complex:* Duration usually remains within normal limits if the conduction delay occurs in the AV node. If the QRS duration exceeds 0.12 second, the conduction delay may be in the His-Purkinje fibers.
- *T wave:* Normal size and configuration unless the QRS complex is prolonged.
- *QT interval:* Usually within normal limits.

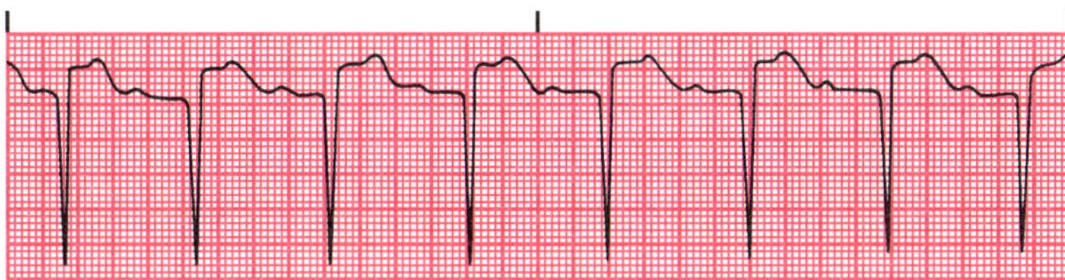

What causes it

- Toxicity from drugs, such as digoxin, propranolol, verapamil, or procainamide
- Chronic degenerative disease of the conduction system and inferior wall MI
- Hypokalemia and hyperkalemia
- Hypothermia
- Hypothyroidism
- Lyme carditis, some muscular dystrophy, and Lenègre disease

What to look for

- Usually asymptomatic (however, the patient's peripheral pulse rate will be normal or slow with a regular rhythm)
- Signs and symptoms of decreased cardiac output, such as hypotension, syncope, and blurred vision, if the patient has a slow rate

How it's treated

- Correct the underlying cause.
- Monitor for worsening heart block, especially if myocardial damage is present.

Second-degree AV block (type I)

In type I (Wenckebach or Mobitz I) second-degree AV block, diseased tissues in the AV node delay conduction of impulses to the ventricles. There is a progressive delay in the atrial/ventricular conduction causing the P wave to fail to conduct a ventricular response. The cycle then repeats. Usually distinguished by group beating, type I second-degree AV block is referred to as the *footprints of Wenckebach*.

Type I second-degree AV block is usually transient. An asymptomatic patient has a good prognosis; however, the block may progress to a more serious type.

What the ECG tells you

- *Rhythm:* Atrial rhythm is regular, whereas ventricular rhythm is irregular. The R-R interval shortens progressively until a P wave appears without a QRS complex; the cycle then repeats.
- *Rate:* The atrial rate exceeds the ventricular rate, but both usually remain within normal limits.
- *P wave:* Normal size and configuration.
- *PR interval:* Typically progressively longer (only slightly) with each cycle until a P wave appears without a QRS complex; the PR interval after the nonconducted beat is shorter than the interval preceding it.
- *QRS complex:* Duration usually remains within normal limits because the block commonly lies above the bundle of His; the complex is absent periodically.
- *T wave:* Normal size and configuration but its deflection may be opposite that of the QRS complex.
- *QT interval:* Usually within normal limits.

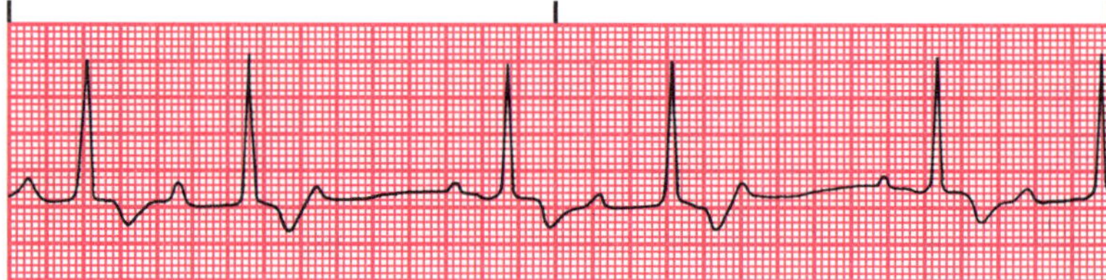

What causes it

- CAD
- Inferior wall MI
- Myocarditis
- Endocarditis
- Hyperkalemia
- Hypervagotonia

- Cardiac surgery
- Digoxin toxicity and use of beta-adrenergic blockers, calcium channel blockers, quinidine, or procainamide

What to look for

- Usually asymptomatic
- Possibly a first heart sound that becomes progressively softer with intermittent pauses
- Hypotension or syncope (if ventricular rate is low)

How it's treated

- For most patients, treat the underlying cause.
- If hemodynamically symptomatic bradycardia is present, prepare to administer atropine.
- If atropine fails to increase the heart rate, transcutaneous pacing is indicated (although rare).

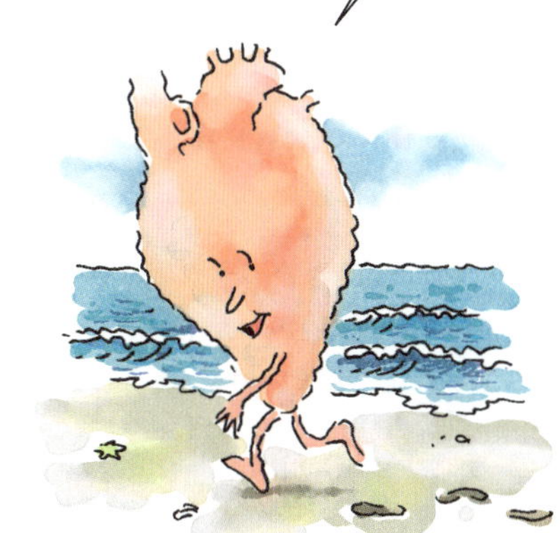

Second-degree AV block (type II)

Produced by a conduction disturbance, delay or interruption in the His-Purkinje fibers, a type II (Mobitz II) second-degree AV block causes an intermittent conduction delay or block. On the ECG, you won't see any warning before a beat is dropped as you would with type I second-degree AV block.

Don't drop the beat

In type II second-degree AV block, the PR and R-R intervals remain constant before the dropped beat. The arrhythmia frequently progresses to third-degree, or complete, heart block.

What the ECG tells you

- *Rhythm:* The atrial rhythm is regular. The ventricular rhythm can be regular or irregular. Pauses correspond to the dropped beat. If the block is intermittent, the rhythm is often irregular; if the block stays constant (for example, 2:1 or 3:1), the rhythm is regular.
- *Rate:* The atrial rate is usually within normal limits. The ventricular rate, slower than the atrial rate, may be within normal limits.
- *P wave:* Normal size and configuration but some P waves aren't followed by a QRS complex.
- *PR interval:* Within normal limits or prolonged but always constant for the conducted beats.
- *QRS complex:* Duration is within normal limits if the block occurs at the bundle of His; prolonged if it occurs below the bundle of His. The complex is absent periodically.

- *T wave:* Usually normal size and configuration.
- *QT interval:* Usually within normal limits.

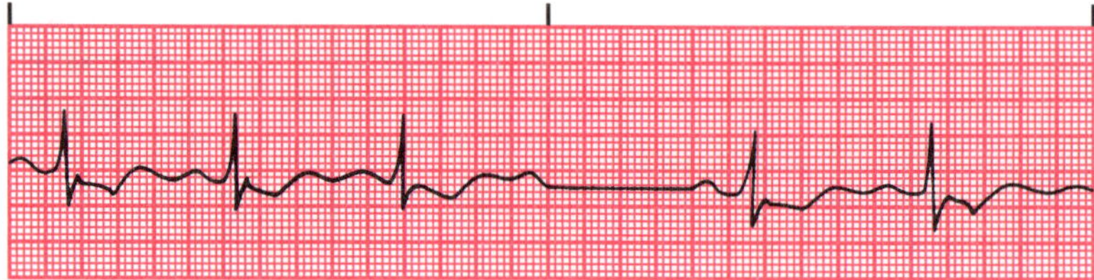

What causes it

- Acute anterior wall MI
- Degenerative changes in the conduction system
- Severe CAD
- Acute myocarditis
- Lyme disease
- Cardiac surgery
- Medications such as beta blockers, calcium channel blockers, digoxin, and some antiarrhtmics

What to look for

- Normal or slow peripheral pulse rate
- Signs and symptoms of decreased cardiac output (if pulse rate is slow)

How it's treated

- If the patient is asymptomatic, immediate treatment usually isn't needed.
- Identify and treat underlying problems.
- Administer oxygen, if indicated.
- If hemodynamically symptomatic bradycardia is present, atropine should not be given as this is usually infranodal cause. Dopamine or epinephrine are better choices.
- Transcutaneous or transvenous pacemaker may be needed. Permanent pacemaker insertion may be necessary.

Third-degree AV block

When all supraventricular impulses are prevented from reaching the ventricles, creating a dissociation of atrial and ventricular activity, the patient has third-degree AV block, also known as *complete heart block.* Just how significant the block is depends on the patient's response to any decline in ventricular rate and the stability of the escape rhythm.

Some rhythms are better than others

Junctional escape rhythms are typically stable and may produce adequate cardiac output. However, ventricular escape rhythms are slower and less stable, posing a risk for intermittent or permanent ventricular standstill.

What the ECG tells you

- *Rhythm:* Atrial and ventricular rhythms are regular but aren't related.
- *Rate:* Atrial rate, which is usually within normal limits, exceeds ventricular rate. A ventricular escape rhythm ranges from 20 to 40 beats/minute. A junctional escape rhythm usually ranges from 40 to 60 beats/minute.
- *P wave:* Normal size and configuration.
- *PR interval:* Not applicable or measurable because the atria and ventricles beat independently (AV dissociation).
- *QRS complex:* Configuration depends on where the ventricular beat originates. A high AV junctional pacemaker produces a narrow QRS complex; a ventricular pacemaker produces a wide, bizarre QRS complex.
- *T wave:* Normal size and configuration unless the QRS complex originates in the ventricle.
- *QT interval:* May be within normal limits.

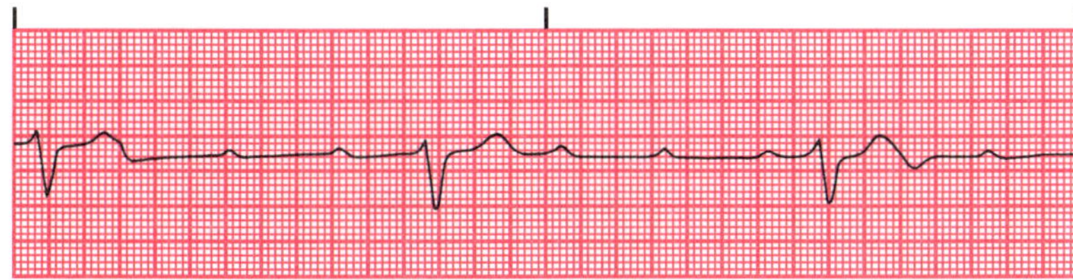

What causes it

- Digoxin toxicity
- Drugs such as beta-adrenergic blockers, calcium channel blockers, antiarrhythmics, digoxin
- Anterior or inferior wall MI
- Hypoxia
- Hyperkalemia
- Severe hypothyroidism
- Cardiac catheterization
- Infections such as Lyme disease and COVID-19, rheumatic fever
- Cardiac surgery
- Congenital heart defect
- Degenerative changes in the myocardial system

What to look for

- Slow peripheral pulse rate, usually less than 40 beats/minute, but a regular rhythm
- Signs and symptoms of decreased cardiac output, such as decreased blood pressure or altered LOC, if the patient has a slow peripheral pulse rate

How it's treated

- Discontinuation of any causative medications or underlying problems.
- Administer oxygen as required to maintain SPO2 at 94%.
- If hemodynamically symptomatic bradycardia is present, atropine may be given as a temporary measure.
- A transcutaneous pacemaker should be applied and on stand-by in case the patient becomes hemodynamically unstable. A transvenous pacemaker may need to be inserted until a permanent pacemaker can be implanted.

Recognizing ventricular rhythms

Ventricular rhythms occur when the AV and SA nodes fail and the ventricle takes over as the heart's pacemaker. Ventricular rhythms are arrhythmias that display a wide QRS complex and are often rapid. They include idioventricular rhythm, monomorphic ventricular tachycardia, polymorphic ventricular tachycardia, torsades de pointes, and ventricular fibrillation.

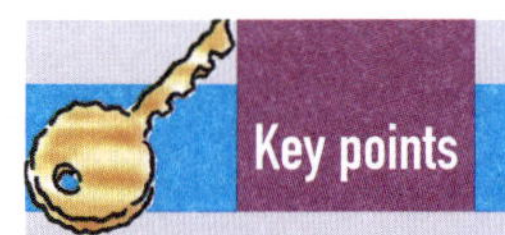

Surviving cardiac arrest
Early identification and treatment of ventricular tachycardias greatly increase a patient's chances for successful resuscitation. The highest survival rates are reported among patients of all ages who have had:
- a witnessed arrest.
- an initial rhythm of pulseless ventricular tachycardia or ventricular fibrillation.
- early defibrillation.
- early, high-quality chest compressions.

Idioventricular rhythm

An idioventricular rhythm is a wide complex that results from a failure of the higher pacemakers of the SA and AV nodes. It's an escape rhythm originating in the Purkinje fibers at a rate of 10 to 40 beats/minute. It is also called as "escape rhythm." If the rate is 50 to 120 beats/minute, it is called "accelerated idioventricular rhythm."

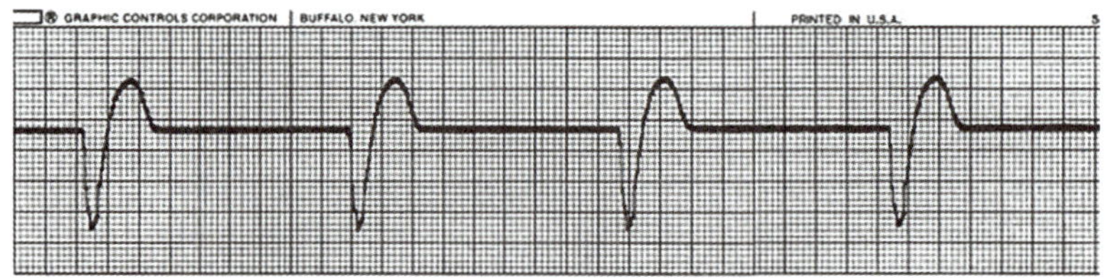

What the ECG tells you

- *Rhythm:* Atrial rhythm is unmeasurable. Ventricular rhythm is usually regular.
- *Rate:* Atrial rate is unmeasurable. Ventricular rate is 20 to 40 beats/minute: accelerated idioventricular is ≥50 beats/minute.
- *P wave:* Absent.
- *PR interval:* Unmeasurable.
- *QRS complex:* Duration greater than 0.12 second and often greater than 0.16 second. Bizarre appearance, usually with increased amplitude.
- *T wave:* Occurs in opposite direction of QRS complex.
- *QT interval:* Unmeasurable.

What causes it

- Reperfusion of coronary arteries
- Acute MI
- Hypoxia
- Severe acidosis or hyperkalemia
- Drugs such as digoxin

What to look for

- Palpitations, dizziness, chest pain, and shortness of breath (if the patient is conscious)
- Signs and symptoms of low cardiac output, such as decreased blood pressure or syncope
- Loss of consciousness and circulatory collapse

How it's treated

- Identify and treat the underlying cause. If the patient is hemodynamically stable, consider administering atropine, dopamine or epinephrine. Also utilizing a temporary pacemaker should be considered if the heart rate remains low.
- Consult an expert practitioner.
- If the patient is pulseless, use go pulseless electrical activity (PEA) algorithm.

Monomorphic ventricular tachycardia

Three or more PVCs that occur in succession at a rate of more than 100 beats/minute is considered ventricular tachycardia. Monomorphic ventricular tachycardia is the most common form of ventricular tachycardia. In this potential life-threatening arrhythmia, all the QRS complexes have the same morphology, indicating that they originate from the same location in the ventricles. The arrhythmia may be paroxysmal or sustained and the patient may or may not have a pulse.

Taking the plunge

Because atrial and ventricular activities are dissociated and ventricular filling time is short, cardiac output may drop sharply. Monomorphic ventricular tachycardia may lead to ventricular fibrillation.

What the ECG tells you

- *Rhythm:* Atrial rhythm is unmeasurable. Ventricular rhythm is usually regular but may be slightly irregular.
- *Rate:* Atrial rate is unmeasurable. Ventricular rate is usually rapid (100 to 250 beats/minute).
- *P wave:* Usually absent; may be obscured by and is dissociated from the QRS complex. Retrograde P waves may be present.
- *PR interval:* Unmeasurable.
- *QRS complex:* Duration greater than 0.12 second; bizarre appearance, usually with increased amplitude.
- *T wave:* Occurs in opposite direction of QRS complex.
- *QT interval:* Unmeasurable.

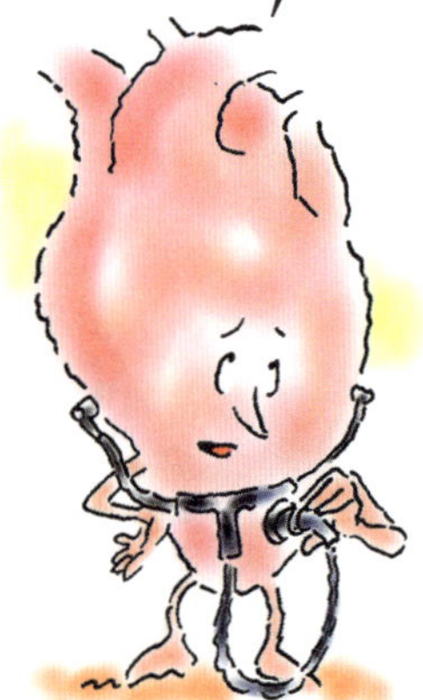

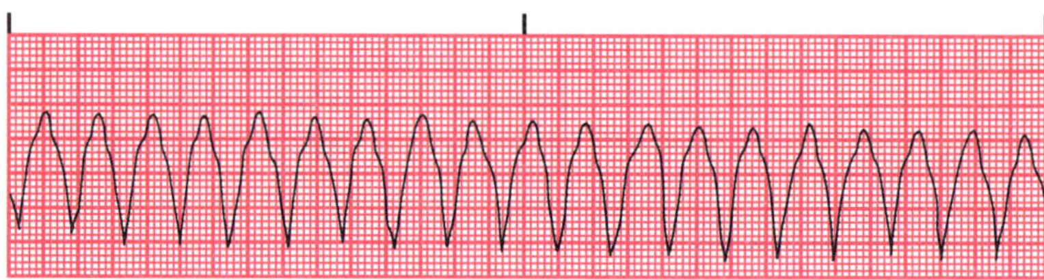

What causes it

- Most commonly, ischemic heart disease, including acute MI, cardiomyopathy, CAD, and CHF
- Hypoxia
- Recreational drug toxicity
- Electrolyte imbalance
- Autoimmune disorders
- Mitral valve prolapse
- Pulmonary embolism
- Rheumatic heart disease
- Sleep apnea

What to look for

- Palpitations, dizziness, chest pain, and shortness of breath (if the patient is conscious)

- Signs and symptoms of low cardiac output, such as decreased blood pressure or syncope
- Loss of consciousness and circulatory collapse

How it's treated

- Identify and treat the underlying cause. If the patient is hemodynamically stable, consider administering adenosine (may help distinguish a wide-complex SVT from ventricular tachycardia [VT]). If adenosine is ineffective, administer amiodarone, procainamide, or sotalol.
- Consider consulting an expert practitioner.
- If the patient is hemodynamically unstable, prepare for immediate synchronized cardioversion (initially, 100 joules of monophasic or biphasic energy; if no response, increase joules in a stepwise fashion.).
- If pulseless VT is present, initiate cardiopulmonary resuscitation (CPR), follow Cardiac Arrest Algorithm (found in Chapter 8).

Polymorphic ventricular tachycardia

Polymorphic ventricular tachycardia is a form of VT in which the QRS complex morphology is unstable, continually varying because the site of origin changes throughout the ventricle. Polymorphic ventricular tachycardia is associated with a poorer prognosis than monomorphic ventricular tachycardia.

What the ECG tells you

- *Rhythm:* Atrial rhythm is unmeasurable. Ventricular rhythm is irregular.
- *Rate:* Atrial rate is unmeasurable. Ventricular rate is usually rapid (100 to 250 beats/minute).
- *P wave:* Absent.
- *PR interval:* Unmeasurable.
- *QRS complex:* Duration varies but is greater than 0.12 second; bizarre appearance, possibly with increased amplitude.
- *T wave:* Abnormal morphology.
- *QT interval:* Unmeasurable.

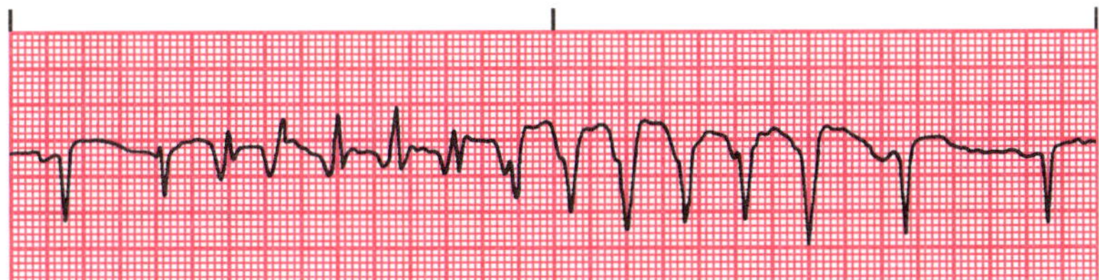

What causes it

- Acute MI
- CAD
- Electrolyte imbalance (especially involving potassium and magnesium)
- Heart failure

What to look for

- Palpitations, dizziness, chest pain, and shortness of breath (if the patient is conscious)
- Signs and symptoms of low cardiac output, such as decreased blood pressure or syncope
- Loss of consciousness and circulatory collapse

How it's treated

- If the patient is stable and has a pulse, consider an antiarrhythmic such as amiodarone.
- Consider consulting an expert practitioner.
- If the patient is pulseless, initiate cardiopulmonary resuscitation (CPR), follow the Cardiac Arrest Algorithm (found in Chapter 8).

Torsades de pointes

A life-threatening arrhythmia, torsades de pointes (or simply "torsades") is a polymorphic ventricular tachycardia characterized by prolonged QT intervals and QRS polarity that seems to spiral around the isoelectric line. Any condition that causes a prolonged QT interval can also cause torsades de pointes. Torsades may be paroxysmal, starting and stopping suddenly.

Although sinus rhythm sometimes resumes spontaneously, torsades de pointes usually degenerates into ventricular fibrillation.

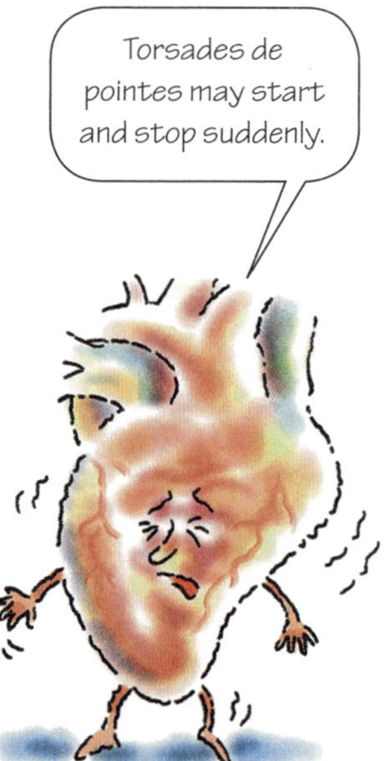

What the ECG tells you

- *Rhythm:* Atrial rhythm can't be determined. Ventricular rhythm is regular or irregular.
- *Rate:* Atrial rate can't be determined. Ventricular rate is 150 to 250 beats/minute.
- *P wave:* Not identifiable because it's buried in the QRS complex.
- *PR interval:* Not applicable because the P wave can't be identified.

- *QRS complex:* Usually wide with a phasic variation in its electrical polarity, shown by complexes that point downward for several beats and then turn upward for several beats and vice versa.
- *T wave:* Not discernible.
- *QT interval:* Prolonged (indicating delayed ventricular repolarization).

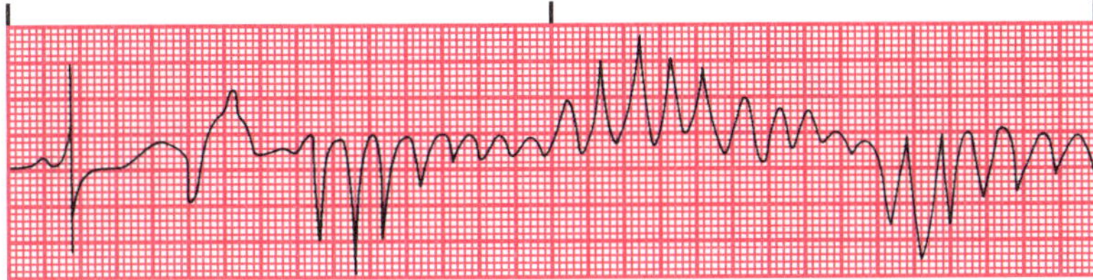

What causes it

- AV block
- Drug toxicity (particularly sotalol, quinidine [Novoquinidin], procainamide, and related antiarrhythmics such as disopyramide [Norpace])
- Electrolyte imbalance (hypokalemia and hypomagnesemia)
- Hereditary QT prolongation syndrome
- Myocardial ischemia
- Psychotropic drugs (phenothiazines, lithium carbonate [Lithobid] and tricyclic antidepressants)
- Anthracycline chemotherapeutic drugs (doxorubicin hydrochloride and daunomycin hydrochloride [Cerubidine])
- SA node disease that results in profound bradycardia
- History of Takotsubo cardiomyopathy

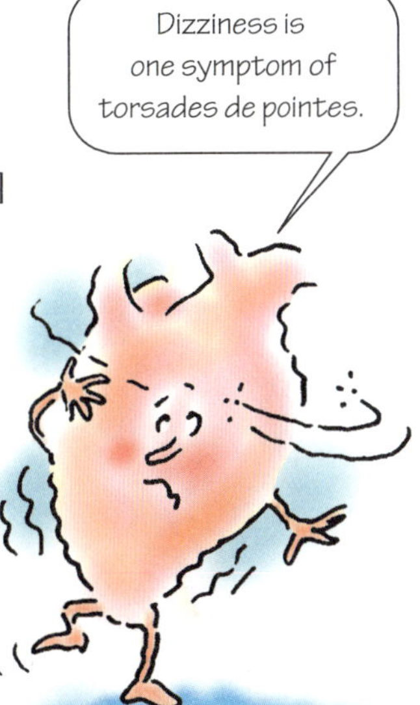

What to look for

- Palpitations, dizziness, chest pain, and shortness of breath (if the patient is conscious)
- Rapidly occurring signs or symptoms of low cardiac output, such as hypotension and altered level of consciousness (LOC)
- If rapid and prolonged torsades, loss of consciousness, pulse, and respirations

How it's treated

- If the patient is stable, correct the electrolyte imbalance, if present. Magnesium isoproterenol is used for torsades de pointes that continues after magnesium has been given. Overdrive pacing may be necessary.
- If a specific drug is causing torsades, discontinue it.

- If torsades is associated with cardiac arrest, consider giving magnesium sulfate.
- If the patient has no pulse, initiate CPR and follow the Cardiac Arrest Algorithm (found in Chapter 8).

Ventricular fibrillation

Commonly called *V-fib,* ventricular fibrillation is a chaotic pattern of electrical activity in the ventricles in which electrical impulses arise from many different foci. It produces no effective muscular contraction and no cardiac output.

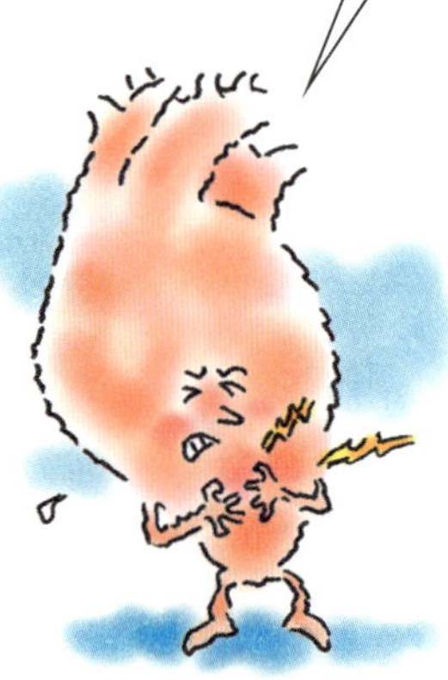

Of coarse

Coarse fibrillation indicates more electrical activity in the ventricles than fine fibrillation. The fibrillatory waves become finer as acidosis and hypoxemia develop. If fibrillation continues, it eventually leads to asystole. Ventricular fibrillation causes most sudden cardiac deaths in people who aren't hospitalized.

What the ECG tells you

- *Rhythm:* Atrial rhythm is unmeasurable. Ventricular rhythm has no pattern or regularity.
- *Rate:* Atrial and ventricular rates are unmeasurable.
- *P wave:* Absent.
- *PR interval:* Unmeasurable.
- *QRS complex:* Duration unmeasurable.
- *T wave:* Unmeasurable.
- *QT interval:* Unmeasurable.

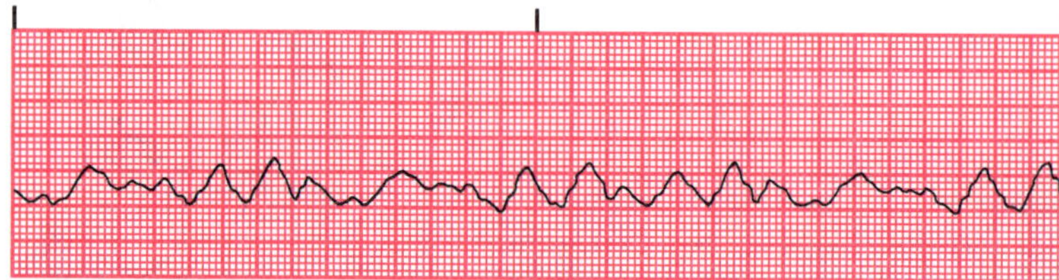

What causes it

- Myocardial ischemia
- Acute MI
- Untreated VT
- Underlying heart disease
- Hypoxia
- Acid-base imbalance
- Electric shock

- Severe hypothermia
- Electrolyte imbalances, such as hypokalemia, hyperkalemia, and hypercalcemia
- Use of illegal drugs (cocaine or methamphetamines)

What to look for

- Absent pulse, heart sounds, and blood pressure
- Dilated pupils
- Loss of consciousness
- Rapid development of cyanosis
- Seizures (occasional)

How it's treated

- Perform CPR until a defibrillator or an automated external defibrillator is available. Then perform defibrillation (120 to 200 joules of biphasic energy or 360 joules of monophasic energy).
- Immediately resume CPR for 2 minutes, assess heart rhythm and if V-fib continues defibrillate again, immediately resume CPR, and administer epinephrine.
- Continue CPR and defibrillation cycles and consider antiarrhythmics such as amiodarone. If the patient is hypomagnesemic, administer magnesium.

Recognizing pulseless electrical activity and asystole

PEA and asystole are both an absence of a perfusing heartbeat and require immediate treatment.

PEA

In PEA, formerly known as *electromechanical dissociation,* isolated electrical activity occurs sporadically without any evidence of effective myocardial contraction. Typically, a flat line tracing occurs within a few minutes, indicating asystole. PEA may be caused by clinical conditions that can be reversed when identified quickly and treated appropriately.

What the ECG tells you

- *Rhythm:* Atrial and ventricular rhythms are the same as the underlying rhythm. They eventually become irregular as the rate slows.
- *Rate:* Atrial rate reflects the underlying rhythm. Ventricular rate also reflects the underlying rhythm but gradually decreases.

- *P wave:* Same as the underlying rhythm but gradually flattens and disappears.
- *PR interval:* Same as the underlying rhythm but eventually disappears as the P wave disappears.
- *QRS complex:* Same as the underlying rhythm but eventually becomes progressively wider.
- *T wave:* Same as the underlying rhythm but eventually becomes indiscernible.
- *QT interval:* Same as the underlying rhythm but eventually becomes indiscernible.

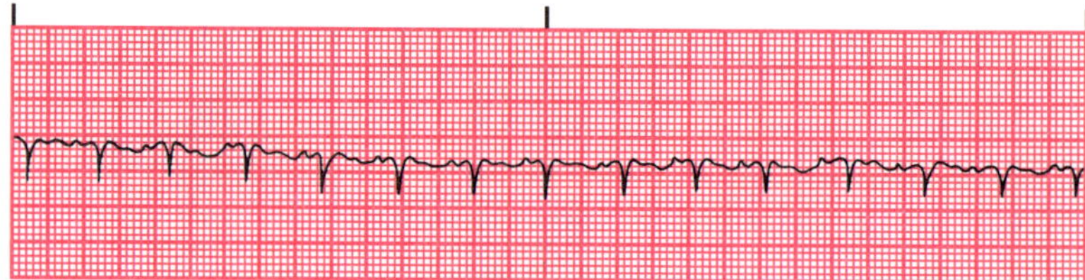

What causes it

- Failure in the calcium transport mechanism
- Extensive myocardial damage, such as rupture of the left ventricular wall or massive MI
- Additional causes (see *The Five H's and T's*)

What to look for

- Apnea and sudden loss of consciousness
- Absence of pulse
- Cardiac rhythm change

How it's treated

- Begin high-quality CPR immediately, and check rhythm every 2 minutes. Establish an airway and IV or intraosseous access with minimal CPR interruption. Monitor airway with continuous waveform capnography.
- Administer epinephrine every 3 to 5 minutes.
- Identify the possible cause of PEA and treat accordingly, if possible. The patient may need volume infusion for hypovolemia from hemorrhage; pericardiocentesis for cardiac tamponade; needle decompression or chest tube insertion for tension pneumothorax; surgery or thrombolytic therapy for massive pulmonary embolism; or ventilation for hypoxemia.

The Five H's and T's

Five H's
- Hypothermia
- Hypovolemia
- Hypoxia
- Hydrogen ion accumulation (acidosis)
- Hyperkalemia or hypokalemia

Five T's
- Tension pneumothorax
- Toxins (overdose)
- Thrombosis (pulmonary)
- Thrombosis (cardiac)
- Tamponade (cardiac)

Asystole

Asystole refers to the total absence of ventricular activity. Some activity may be evident in the atria, but atrial impulses aren't conducted to the ventricles. Without ventricular electrical activity, ventricular contraction doesn't occur. As a result, no cardiac output or perfusion occurs. The ECG waveform is almost a flat line. Asystole may be caused by clinical conditions that can be reversed when identified quickly and treated appropriately.

Asystole is associated with a low rate of survival, even with resuscitation.

Asystole by any other name

It's important to distinguish asystole from fine ventricular fibrillation, which may mimic it. Make sure that you place all ECG leads properly; otherwise, the resulting waveform may also resemble asystole.

What the ECG tells you

- *Rhythm:* Atrial rhythm is indiscernible. No ventricular rhythm is present.
- *Rate:* Atrial rate is indiscernible. No ventricular rate is present.
- *P wave:* May or may not be present.
- *PR interval:* Unmeasurable.
- *QRS complex:* Absent or occasional escape beats.
- *T wave:* Absent.
- *QT interval:* Unmeasurable.

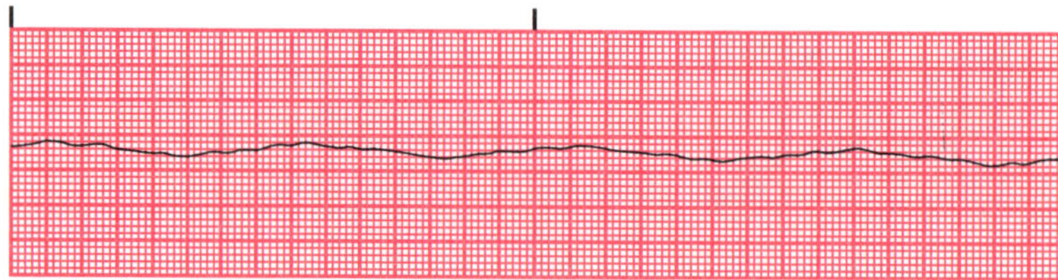

What causes it

- Severe metabolic deficit
- Acute respiratory failure
- Extensive myocardial damage, possibly from myocardial ischemia, MI, or ruptured ventricular aneurysm
- **Additional causes** (see *The Five H's and T's*)

What to look for

- Loss of consciousness
- Absence of peripheral pulses, blood pressure, and respirations
- Absence of cardiac rhythm on the cardiac monitor

How it's treated

- Confirm that the patient is in asystole by checking for a pulse and verifying the rhythm in another lead, along with checking lead and cable connections.
- Begin high-quality CPR and establish a patent airway and IV or intraosseous access with minimal CPR interruption.
- Identify and treat reversible causes.
- Administer epinephrine every 3 to 5 minutes.

Quick quiz

1. Identify the characteristics and interpret the rhythm strip below.

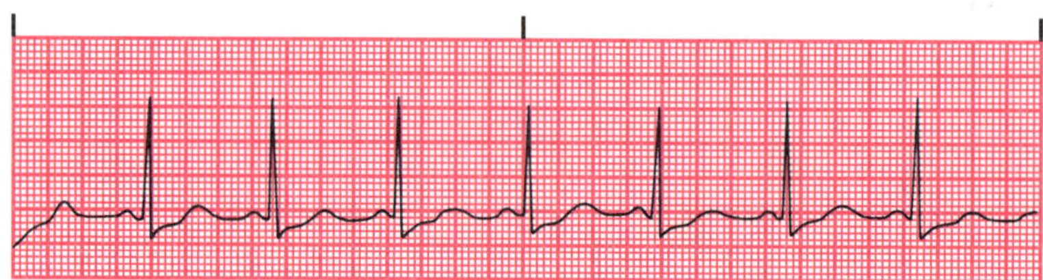

Rhythm: ____________________

Rate: ____________________

P wave: ____________________

PR interval: ___________________

QRS complex: ___________________

T wave: ___________________

QT interval: ___________________

Interpretation: ___________________

Answer:

Rhythm: Atrial and ventricular rhythms are both regular.

Rate: Atrial and ventricular rates are both 79 beats/minute.

P wave: Normal size and configurations.

PR interval: 0.12 seconds.

QRS complex: 0.08 seconds; normal size and configuration.

QT interval: 0.44 seconds.

Interpretation: Normal sinus rhythm.

2. A telemetry patient shows sinus bradycardia at a rate of 40 beats/minute on the cardiac monitor. Which signs or symptoms might the patient display that indicates hemodynamic instability?

A. High blood pressure
B. Chest pain and dyspnea
C. Facial flushing and ataxia
D. No perceptible symptoms

Answer: B. A patient with hemodynamically symptomatic bradycardia suffers from low cardiac output, which may produce chest pain and dyspnea. The patient may also have crackles, an S_3 heart sound, and a sudden onset of confusion.

3. A patient with supraventricular tachycardia (rate = 225; rhythm = regular) is diaphoretic, complains of chest pain, and has a blood pressure of 80/50. The recommended treatment for this patient is:

A. CPR.
B. defibrillation.
C. synchronized cardioversion.
D. pacemaker.

Answer: C. Synchronized cardioversion at 50 to 100 joules is the recommended treatment for the patient who is hemodynamically unstable.

4. The preferred treatment for symptomatic third-degree AV block is:

A. atropine.
B. a pacemaker.
C. epinephrine.
D. dopamine.

Answer: B. Use of either a transcutaneous or transvenous pacemaker is recommended for symptomatic third-degree AV block until a permanent pacemaker can be inserted.

5. In the strip that follows, the ventricular rhythm is irregular, the ventricular rate is 130 beats/minute, the P wave is absent, the PR interval and QT interval aren't measurable, the QRS complex is wide and bizarre with varying duration, and the T wave is opposite the QRS complex. You would interpret this rhythm as:

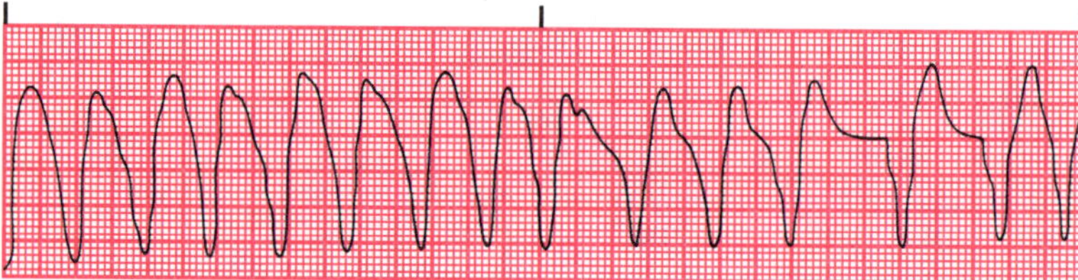

A. ventricular fibrillation.
B. ventricular tachycardia.
C. idioventricular rhythm.
D. sinus bradycardia.

Answer: B. This strip shows ventricular tachycardia: the rhythm is irregular, the rate is from 100 to 200 beats/minute, the P wave is absent, the PR and QT intervals are unmeasurable, the QRS complex is wide and bizarre, and the T wave is opposite the QRS complex. The patient must be checked to see if the patient has a pulse.

Scoring

☆☆☆ If you answered all five questions correctly, brilliant! You're really in rhythm with arrhythmias.

☆☆ If you answered four questions correctly, super job! At this junction, you're doing fine.

☆ If you answered fewer than four questions correctly, not to worry! A quick review will help you get the beat.

Suggested references

Buxton, A. (2022). *Multifocal atrial tachycardia*. Retrieved from UpToDate: https://www.uptodate.com/contents/multifocalatrial-tachycardia?search=multifocal%20atrial%20tachycardia&source=search_result&selectedTitle=1~29&usage_type=default&display_rank=1#H754616.

Foth, C., Gangwani, M., & Alvey, H. (2021). *Ventricular tachycardia*. Retrieved from National Library of Medicine.

Knight, B. P. (2022). *Control of ventricular rate in atrial fibrillation: Pharmacologic therapy*. Retrieved from UpToDate: https://www.uptodate.com/contents/control-of-ventricular-rate-in-atrial-fibrillation-pharmacologic-therapy?topicRef=1022&source=see_link#H7

Phang. R., & Prutkins, J. (2022). *Overview of atrial flutter.* Retrieved from UpToDate: https://www.uptodate.com/contents/overview-of-atrial-flutter?search=Atrial%20flutter&source=search_result&selectedTitle=1~150&usage_type=default&display_rank=1#H2

Protrainings, LLC. (2022). *Atrial flutter.* Retrieved from ProACLS.com: https://www.proacls.com/training/video/atrial-flutter

Reading, J. (2020). *Demystifying the 12 Lead ECG!*. Retrieved from Nurseyourownway.com: https://nurseyourownway.com/2016/04/20/demystifying-the-12-lead-ecg/

Sauer, W. H. (2022). *First-degree atrioventricular block.* Retrieved from UpToDate: https://www.uptodate.com/contents/firstdegree-atrioventricular-block?search=fist%20degree%20AV%20block&source=search_result&selectedTitle=2~150&usage_type=default&display_rank=2#H2724240708

Sauer, W. H. (2022). *Second-degree atrioventricular block: Mobitz type I (Wenckebach Block)*. Retrieved from UpToDate: https://www.uptodate.com/contents/second-degree-atrioventricular-block-mobitz-type-i-wenckebach-block?search=Second%20degree%20AV%20block&source=search_result&selectedTitle=2~150&usage_type=default&display_rank=2#H8022855

Sauer, W. H. (2022). *Second-degree atrioventricular block: Mobitz type II.* Retrieved from UpToDate: https://www.uptodate.com/contents/second-degree-atrioventricular-block-mobitz-type-ii?search=Second%20degree%20AV%20block%20Mobitz%20type%20II&source=search_result&selectedTitle=1~56&usage_type=default&display_rank=1#H125048228

Chapter 4

Airway management

Just the facts

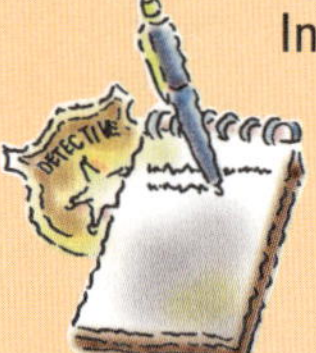

In this chapter, you'll learn:

- anatomy of the respiratory system
- effective techniques to open the airway
- use of airway, ventilation, and barrier devices
- use of oxygen administration devices

Respiratory system basics

The major function of the respiratory system is gas exchange. Air enters the body on inhalation and travels through respiratory passages to the lungs. Oxygen in the lungs replaces carbon dioxide in the blood, and the carbon dioxide is expelled from the body on exhalation. (See *A close look at the respiratory system.*)

I need to exchange this carbon dioxide for oxygen, please.
No problem! That's our business. Now, we'll just need to see your receipt...
RETURNS & EXCHANGES
CO2

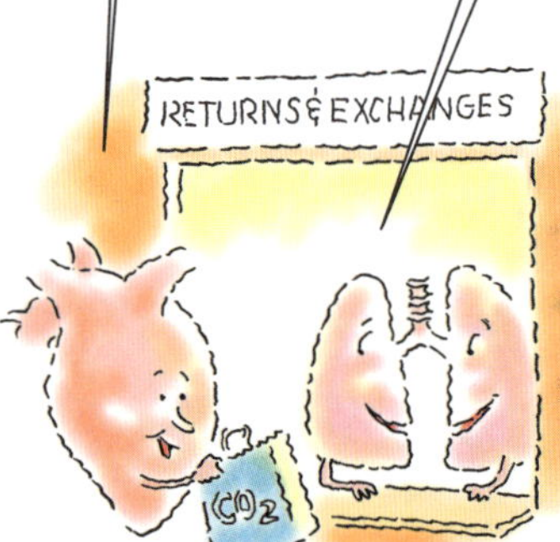

No interruptions, please

When respiratory function is interrupted, the whole body becomes compromised. Brain damage occurs within 5 minutes, and brain cell death occurs within 10 minutes. Therefore, maintaining a patent airway and adequate gas exchange are vital to advanced cardiovascular life support (ACLS) success.

Conducting airways

The conducting airways allow air into and out of the lungs. Conducting airways include the upper and lower airways.

You take the high road...

The upper airway consists of the nose, mouth, pharynx, and larynx. These structures allow air to flow into and out of the lungs. They warm, humidify, and filter inspired air and protect the lower airway from foreign matter.

A close look at the respiratory system

Get to know the basic structures and functions of the respiratory system so you can perform a comprehensive respiratory assessment and identify abnormalities. The major structures of the upper and lower airways are illustrated below. The pulmonary airway is shown in more detail in the inset.

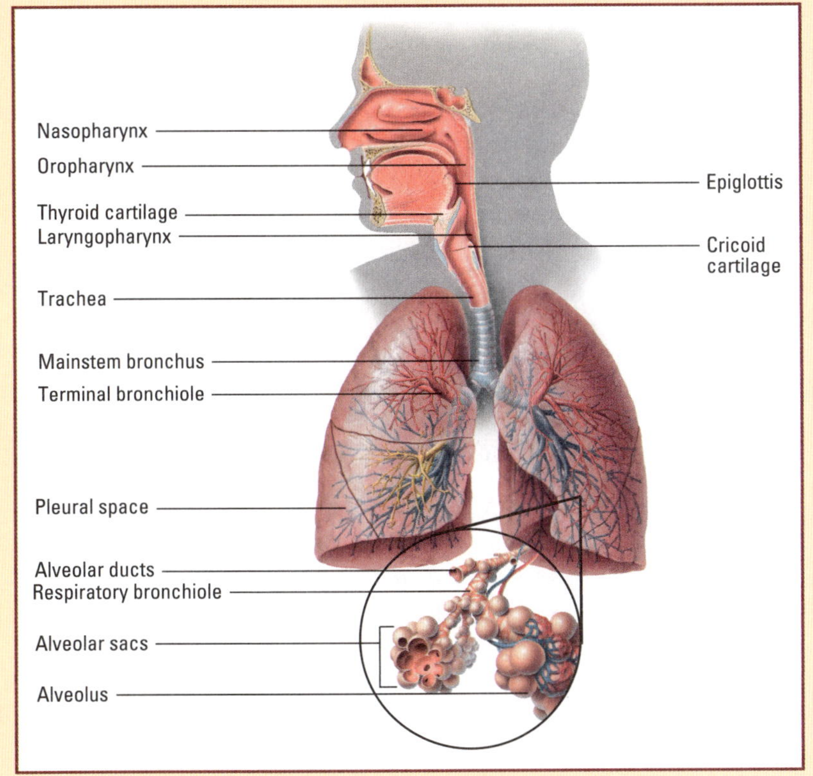

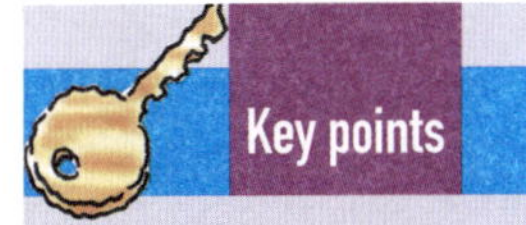

Basics of conducting airways

- The upper airway consists of the nose, mouth, pharynx, and larynx.
- The upper airway warms, humidifies, and filters inspired air.
- The lower airway consists of the trachea, right and left mainstem bronchi, five secondary bronchi, and bronchioles.
- The lower airways facilitate gas exchange.
- Upper and lower airway obstruction occurs when a structure becomes partially or totally blocked.

Upper airway obstruction occurs when the nose, mouth, pharynx, or larynx becomes partially or totally blocked. Upper airway obstruction can be caused by the tongue, food, edema, secretions, trauma, tumors, or foreign objects.

. . . And I'll take the low road

The lower airway consists of the trachea, right and left mainstem bronchi, five secondary bronchi, and bronchioles. These structures facilitate gas exchange. Each bronchiole descends from a lobule and contains terminal bronchioles, alveolar ducts, and alveoli. Terminal bronchioles are anatomic dead spaces because they don't participate in gas exchange. Conversely, the alveoli are the chief units of gas exchange.

The lower airway can become partially or totally blocked as a result of inflammation, secretions, blood, tumors, foreign bodies, or trauma.

Airway management steps

Steps in airway management include proper positioning and manual techniques to open the patient's airway. Without an open (or patent) airway, attempts to ventilate and oxygenate the patient will fail. Proper positioning of both yourself and the patient is key to ensuring correct assessment and establishment of a patent airway.

Proper positioning

When you approach a patient in possible cardiopulmonary compromise, the first step in airway management is proper positioning of both yourself and the patient. Without proper positioning, it's difficult to assess the patient's breathing and ensure a patent airway. You should be at the patient's side, at about the level of his upper chest. From this position, you can provide both ventilations and chest compressions effectively.

Supine is superlative

Optimally, place the patient in a supine position on a firm, flat surface. You may find a patient lying face down or on his side. If so, roll the patient so that his head, shoulders, and torso move together. Avoid twisting the patient's body. If you suspect the patient has a neck injury, attempt to keep his head, neck, and spine in alignment and immobile. With the patient in a supine position, you can perform a better assessment.

Opening the airway

A patient's airway can become obstructed or compromised by vomitus, food, edema, his tongue or teeth, saliva, secretions, or a foreign object. The most common cause of airway obstruction is the tongue. Muscle tone decreases when a person is unconscious or unresponsive, which increases the potential for the tongue and epiglottis to obstruct the pharynx.

Assess airway patency. Check to see if the chest rises with inspiration and falls with expiration. Wheezing, suprasternal, supraclavicular, or intracostal retractions, and cyanosis may all point to partial or complete airway obstruction.

Open for business

If the patient is not breathing adequately, open the airway using the head-tilt, chin-lift maneuver, or the jaw-thrust maneuver. Use the head-tilt, chin-lift maneuver to relieve an upper airway obstruction caused by the patient's tongue or epiglottis. (See *Performing the head-tilt, chin-lift maneuver.*) If you suspect a neck injury, use the jaw-thrust maneuver to avoid causing spinal trauma. (See *Performing the jaw-thrust maneuver.*) If the jaw-thrust maneuver isn't effective in opening the airway, use the head-tilt, chin-lift maneuver because opening the airway and providing adequate ventilations is a priority when performing cardiopulmonary resuscitation (CPR).

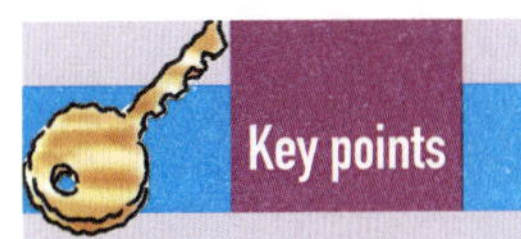

Key points

Opening an airway

- Most common cause of airway obstruction: the tongue.
- Perform the head-tilt, chin-lift maneuver for upper airway obstruction caused by the patient's tongue or epiglottis.
- Perform the jaw-thrust maneuver for patients with suspected neck injury (or if the head-tilt, chin-lift maneuver is unsuccessful).
- Remove a foreign body obstructing the airway of an unconscious patient by performing chest compressions.

Peak technique

Performing the head-tilt, chin-lift maneuver

If the patient doesn't appear to have a neck injury, perform the head-tilt, chin-lift maneuver to open his airway.

First, place your hand closest to the patient's head on his forehead. Then apply firm pressure—firm enough to tilt the patient's head back.

Next, place the fingertips of your other hand under the bony portion of the patient's lower jaw, near his chin. Then lift the patient's chin, making sure to keep his mouth partially open (as shown).

Avoid placing your fingertips on the soft tissue under the patient's chin because this may inadvertently obstruct the airway.

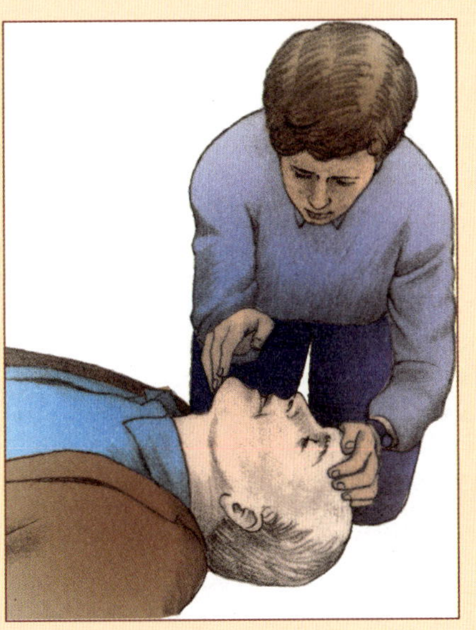

Obstinate obstructions

Suspect possible foreign body airway obstruction if the unconscious patient's chest doesn't rise with attempted ventilations. Check the patient's mouth to see if a foreign body is visible. If so, remove it. If it

Peak technique

Performing the jaw-thrust maneuver

If you suspect a neck injury, or if the head-tilt, chin-lift maneuver is unsuccessful, perform the jaw-thrust maneuver.

Kneel at the patient's head with your elbows on the ground. Rest your thumbs on the patient's lower jaw near the corners of his mouth, pointing your thumbs toward his feet.

Then place your fingertips around the lower jaw. To open the airway, lift the lower jaw with your fingertips (as shown).

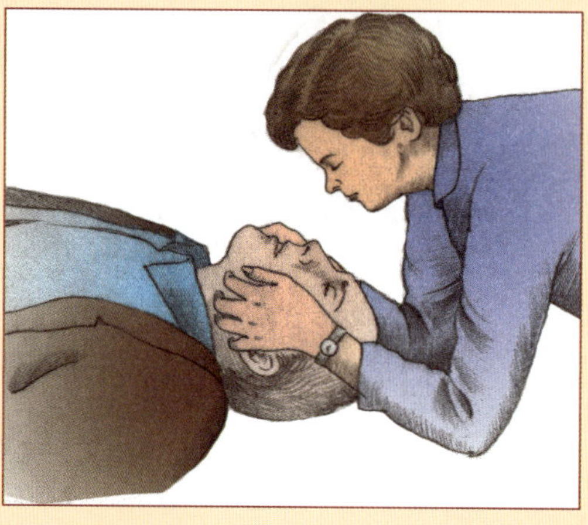

isn't, attempt to dislodge the foreign object by performing chest compressions. Recheck the patient's mouth to see if the foreign body is visible. If so, remove it.

Free and clear

After you open the patient's airway, they may begin breathing spontaneously. If so, deliver supplemental oxygen in the most effective but least invasive manner possible. If spontaneous breathing doesn't resume, initiate rescue breathing using a barrier device or bag valve mask device until an advanced airway can be inserted.

Barrier devices

Barrier devices serve as a physical barrier between you and the patient when providing ventilations. Remember to always follow standard precautions when using barrier devices. Two categories of barrier devices are available: the face shield and pocket face mask.

Face shield

The face shield is a cover that is placed over the patient's mouth. It contains a clear plastic or silicone section to prevent direct contact between you and the patient during mouth-to-mouth ventilation.

What you need

- Face shield
- Gloves

How it's done

To use the face shield:

- Establish a patent airway.
- Place the shield over the patient's mouth and nose with the center opening over their mouth.
- Slowly blow a sufficient volume of air into the center opening to make the patient's chest rise.

What to consider

- Obtaining adequate ventilation with a face shield can be difficult.
- A supplemental oxygen source is necessary as soon as possible to prevent or treat hypoxemia.

Pocket face mask

The pocket face mask (also called *mouth-to-mask*) is used to deliver enriched oxygen to patients with spontaneous, ineffective respirations or to those requiring artificial ventilation. It's made of transparent, moldable plastic that allows visualization so that vomiting can be detected. Its components include an inflatable cushion, an oxygen port, a low-resistance one-way valve, and a disposable filter that prevents contact between you and the patient's mouth. (See *The pocket face mask.*)

Be careful—adequate ventilation is difficult with a face shield.

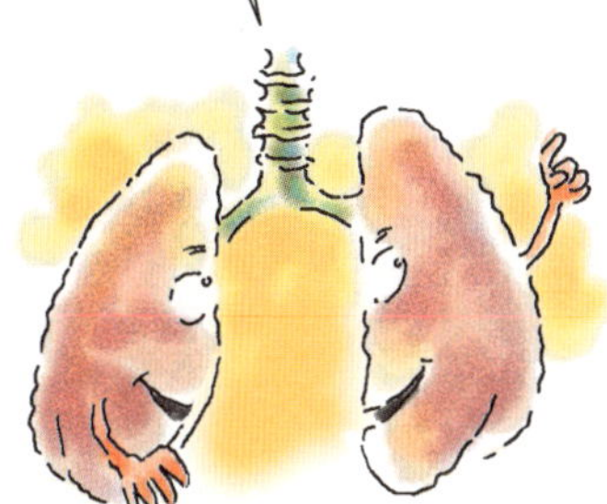

Concentrate on oxygen

The pocket face mask delivers 16% oxygen concentration from your delivered breaths. By connecting the mask to an oxygen source, you can provide a higher oxygen concentration.

What you need

- Pocket face mask
- Supplemental oxygen (optional)
- Gloves

How it's done

To prepare the mask and the patient:

- Establish a patent airway.
- Snap the mask's filter firmly in place; the dome should be popped out.
- Attach the one-way valve to the mask port, directing the exhalation port away from the narrow end.

The pocket face mask

Portable and easy to use, a pocket face mask is a barrier device that allows you to deliver breaths through a one-way valve. Some devices contain an oxygen administration port that allows you to administer supplemental oxygen.

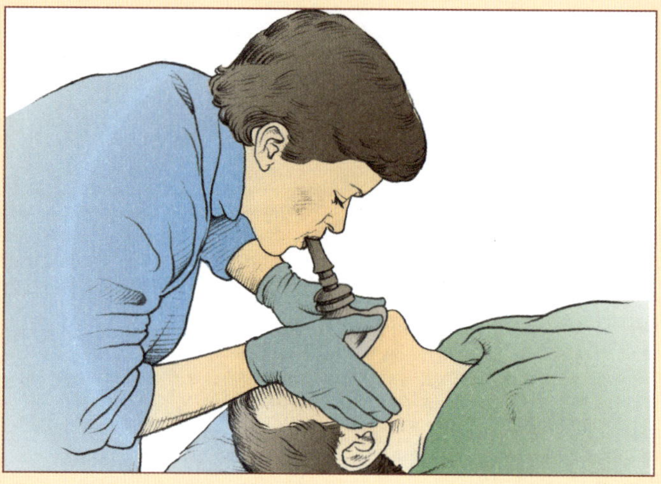

To attach the mask:

- Position the mask on the patient's face with the narrow end at the bridge of the patient's nose and the rounded end between their lower lip and chin.
- Encircle the mask with your thumbs and index fingers, and apply pressure to both sides of the mask with the thumb sides of your hands, forming a tight seal.
- Use your other three fingers to lift the mandible while maintaining head tilt, opening the airway.
- Blow a sufficient volume slowly into the opening of the mask to make the patient's chest rise.
- Remove your mouth, allowing exhalation to occur.
- Apply the oxygen source at a flow rate of 10 to 15 L/minute for 50% to 80% oxygen concentration as soon as possible.

What to consider

- If an adequate seal is not achieved, it can cause inadequate ventilation.
- A supplemental oxygen source is necessary as soon as possible to prevent or treat hypoxemia.

Oxygen administration devices

In a respiratory emergency, supplemental oxygen administration reduces the patient's ventilatory effort. In a cardiac emergency, oxygen therapy helps meet the increased myocardial workload as the heart tries to compensate for hypoxemia. It's particularly important for a patient with a compromised myocardium (as in myocardial infarction or arrhythmia). Oxygen administration devices include the nasal cannula, nonrebreather mask, simple face mask, and Venturi mask.

Nasal cannula

The nasal cannula is the most frequently used low-flow oxygen delivery system for a spontaneously breathing patient who doesn't need precise oxygen concentration. It's composed of flexible plastic tubing with two nasal prongs (about ⅝″ [1.5 cm] long) and an adjustable strap that's comfortable and easy to use.

It isn't the heat, it's the humidity

The nasal cannula provides 24% to 44% humidified oxygen concentration with 1 to 6 L/minute flow rates for patients with minimal or no respiratory distress. Every 1 L/minute increase equals a 4% oxygen concentration increase.

What you need

- Nasal cannula
- Oxygen source

How it's done

Assess the patient for nasal airway patency. Then:

- Attach the cannula tubing to the oxygen source.
- Set the flow rate to the desired flow.
- Check the flow by holding the cannula against your hand.
- Place the cannula tubing behind the patient's ears and the strap under his chin.
- Slide the adjuster to secure the tubing in place.

What to consider

- The nasal cannula is contraindicated for patients with nasal obstructions.
- May not be as effective in patients who are primarily mouth breathers.

- Flow rates greater than 6 L/minute may cause headaches.
- The nasal cannula is easily removed or dislodged.
- Humidity should be added to nasal cannulas and high-flow nasal cannula oxygen delivery.

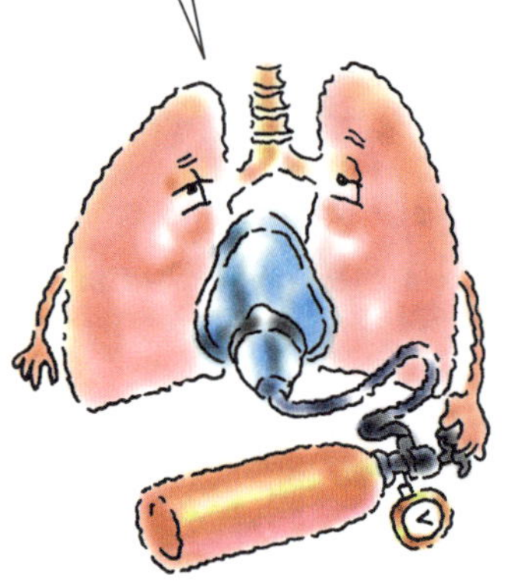

Simple face mask

The simple face mask, also called a *basic face mask,* is a low-flow system that allows oxygen to enter through a bottom port and exit through side holes. The face mask is capable of delivering 44% to 60% humidified oxygen concentrations to a patient with adequate spontaneous respirations. Air is exhaled through holes in the side of the mask.

Simply adjustable

The simple face mask comes in various standard sizes for adults and children with an adjustable strap to assist with proper fit.

What you need

- Simple face mask
- Oxygen source

How it's done

To prepare the mask:

- Attach the tubing to the oxygen source and adjust to the desired flow rate. (The ideal flow rate is 8 to 10 L/minute with a minimum of 5 L/minute.)
- Choose a face mask size that fits from the bridge of the patient's nose to the tip of his chin.

To attach the mask:

- Mold the metal nosepiece to conform to the bridge of the patient's nose.
- Place the elastic strap over the patient's head and adjust the strap so that the mask fits comfortably and securely over his chin, cheeks, and nose to prevent the intake of room air, which dilutes oxygen concentration.

What to consider

- The mask may not fit properly based on individual facial structures, which can cause dilution of the oxygen concentration delivered.
- Air may enter and dilute the oxygen concentration delivered if the mask is improperly placed.
- Depending on the flow rate and the patient's respirations, delivered oxygen concentration may vary.

- The mask must be momentarily removed for the patient to eat, drink, or expectorate.
- Patients on simple face masks are at increased risk for aspiration.

Venturi mask

The Venturi mask is a face mask designed to mix room air with oxygen. It allows you to administer varying percentages of oxygen at a constant concentration of 24% to 50%, regardless of the patient's respiratory rate.

The Venturi mask delivers a mixture of room air and oxygen at varying percentages.
Take a deep breath and join the oxygen movement

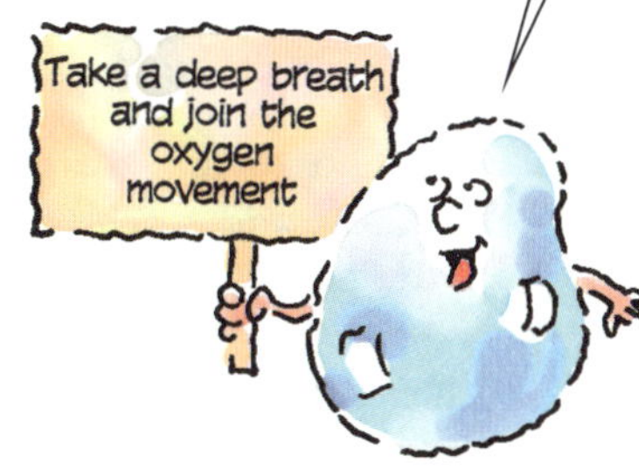

Magnificent mix

The Venturi mask increases the oxygenation of patients with chronic lung disease without drying mucous membranes. A wide-bore flexible tube attaches between the adapters and the mask, allowing inhaled oxygen and room air to mix. The mask has a perforated cuff that allows exhaled air to flow into the atmosphere. Adapters can change the size of the orifice and oxygen flow. (See *Components of the Venturi mask.*)

What you need

- Venturi mask
- Color-coded adapter
- Oxygen source

Components of the Venturi mask

This illustration shows the components of the Venturi mask.

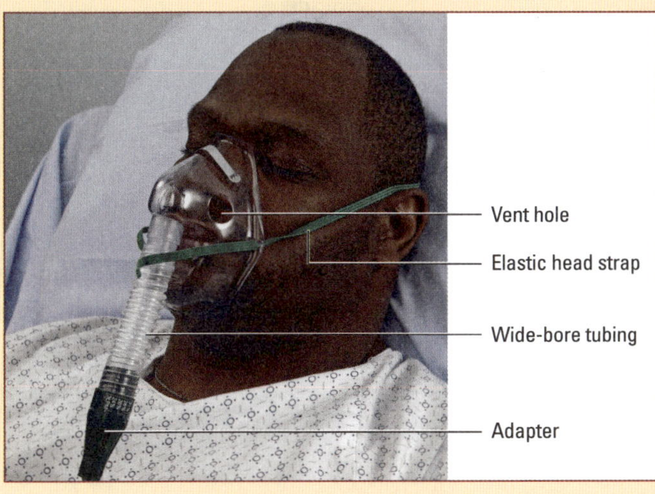

How it's done

To prepare the mask:

- Attach the appropriate color-coded adapter to the flexible tube, and then attach the oxygen source.
- Turn the oxygen flowmeter to the prescribed rate (indicated on adapter).
- Check that flow is occurring.

To attach the mask:

- Position the mask on the patient's face so it is covering the nose and mouth.
- Place the elastic strap over the patient's head and adjust the strap so that the mask fits comfortably and securely over his chin, cheeks, and nose to prevent the intake of room air, which will dilute oxygen concentration.

What to consider

- Maintain a good seal for proper oxygen concentration delivery.
- If intake ports are obstructed, altered oxygen delivery concentration may occur.
- The mask must be momentarily removed for the patient to eat, drink, or expectorate.
- Patients using a venturi mask are at increased risk for aspiration.

Nonrebreather mask

The nonrebreather mask is a face mask with an oxygen reservoir. It provides oxygen concentrations (60% to 100%) to the spontaneously breathing patient.

One-way street

On inhalation, the one-way inspiratory valve opens, directing oxygen from a reservoir bag into the mask. On exhalation, gas exits the mask through the one-way expiratory valves and enters the atmosphere. The patient breathes air only from the reservoir bag. (See *Components of a nonrebreather mask.*)

What you need

- Nonrebreather mask
- Oxygen source

Components of a nonrebreather mask

This illustration shows the components of a nonrebreather mask.

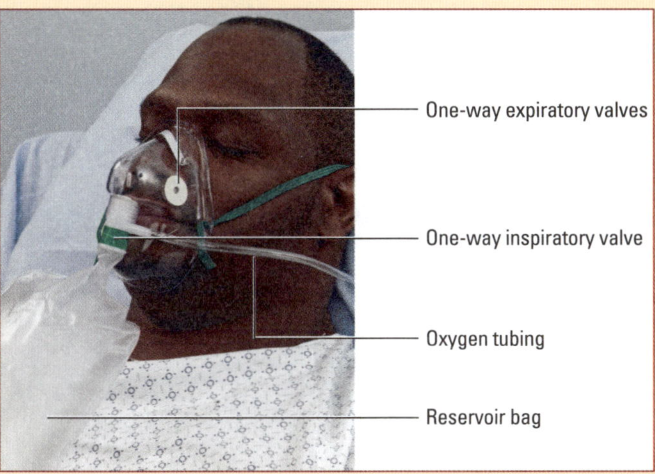

How it's done

To prepare the mask:

- Attach the tubing to the oxygen source and adjust to the desired 12 to 15 L/minute oxygen flow rate.
- Choose a face mask size that fits from the bridge of the patient's nose to the tip of their chin.
- Inflate the reservoir bag by occluding the outlet to the mask.

To attach the mask:

- Mold the metal nosepiece to conform to the bridge of the patient's nose.
- Place the elastic strap over the patient's head, and adjust the strap so that the mask fits comfortably and securely over their chin, cheeks, and nose to prevent the intake of room air, which will dilute oxygen concentration.
- Adjust the oxygen flow so the reservoir bag remains at least two thirds inflated during inspiration and expiration, never completely collapsing.
- Don't allow the reservoir bag to kink.

What to consider

- Oxygen concentration varies depending on the manufacturer's design, patient's respiratory pattern, oxygen flow rate, proper fit of the mask, and removal of the one-way valve from side exhalation ports.

- An inhalation valve malfunction or kink in the bag may cause rebreathing of accumulated carbon dioxide.
- The nonrebreather mask can be uncomfortable and hot.
- The mask must be momentarily removed for the patient to eat, drink, or expectorate.
- Patients on nonrebreather masks are at increased risk for aspiration.

Ventilation devices

Devices used to ventilate patients and help deliver oxygen include the bag valve mask device and automatic transport ventilator (ATV). When in place, these devices can deliver ventilations with room air or supplemental oxygen. Remember to always follow standard precautions when using these devices.

Bag valve mask device

The bag valve mask is an inflatable handheld resuscitation bag with a reservoir and an adapter that can be directly attached to a face mask, endotracheal (ET) tube, or tracheostomy tube. It's used to manually deliver ventilation with room air or supplemental oxygen (if an oxygen source is available) by positive pressure to patients with apnea or inadequate respirations.

Seal of approval

When the bag valve mask device is used with a face mask, it is essential that the mask fits tightly, providing a good seal. If you use a mask with an inflatable rim, it can be molded to facial contours. A tidal volume of 6 to 7 mL/kg with the bag valve mask device should adequately inflate the average adult's lungs while minimizing gastric inflation. Remember, only deliver enough volume to cause chest rise.

What you need

- Gloves (gown and goggles if indicated)
- Pharyngeal suctioning equipment
- bag valve mask device with oxygen reservoir
- Oxygen source
- Nasopharyngeal or oropharyngeal airway

Peak technique

How to use a bag valve mask device

Here's a step-by-step guide for using a bag valve mask device.

Cover the bridge

Place the mask over the patient's face so that the apex of the triangle covers the bridge of their nose and the base lies between his lower lip and chin. Notice the hand in the photo—the practitioner is using the E-C (hand placement) technique to hold the mask to the patient's face (creating a "C" with the thumb and index finger and creating the "E" with the last three fingers of the hand while lifting the patient's jaw).

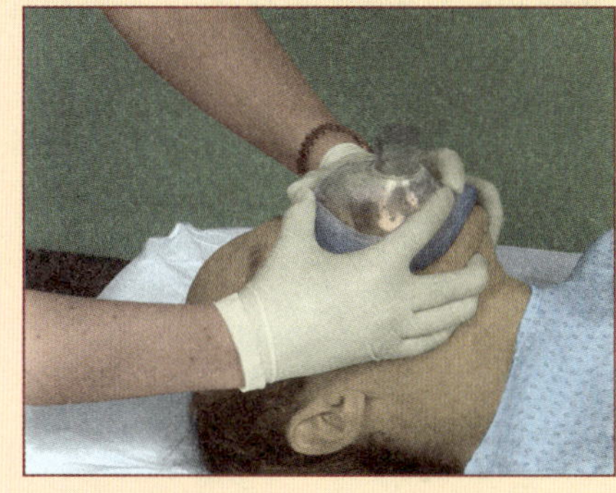

Keep the mouth open

Make sure that the patient's mouth remains open underneath the mask. Attach the bag to the face mask and to the tubing leading to the oxygen source.

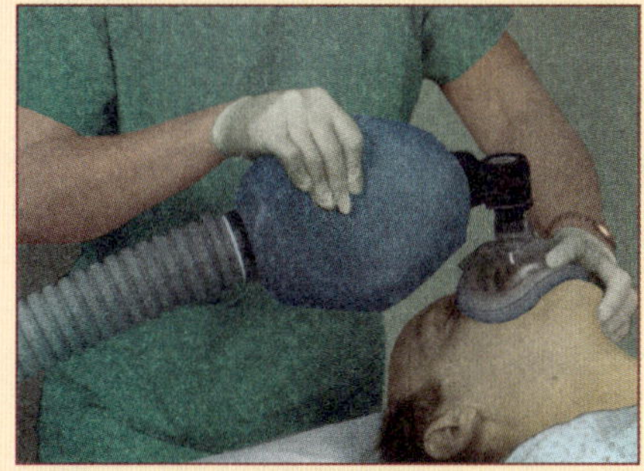

If the patient has a tube

If the patient has a tracheostomy tube or endotracheal tube in place, attach the bag directly to the tube.

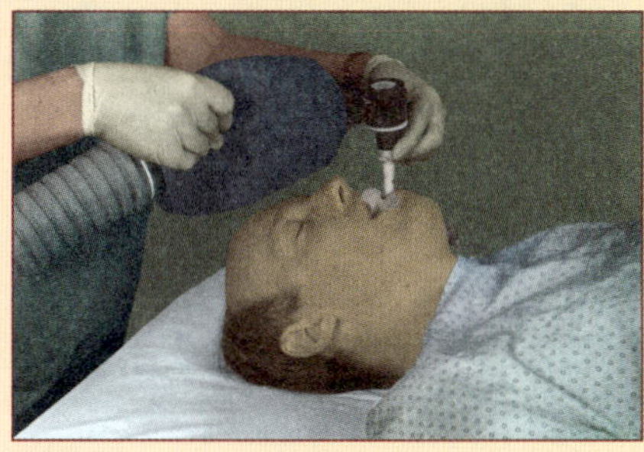

How it's done

To prepare the patient and the device:

- Don gloves (as soon as able).
- Suction the airway to ensure patency.
- Insert a nasopharyngeal or oropharyngeal airway in an unconscious patient, if needed.
- Connect the tubing to the oxygen source, and set the flow rate between 10 and 15 L/minute (this flow rate should yield from 90% to 100% oxygen).

  To use the device:
- Place the narrow end of the mask over the patient's nose while lifting the patient's lower jaw with the fingers of both your hands (the patient's mouth should be open under the mask, and the tip of the patient's chin should be at the rounded end of the mask). Use the E-C (hand placement) technique if two people aren't available for bag valve mask ventilation. (See *How to use a bag valve mask device.*)
- If the patient is intubated, attach the adapter to the ET tube, esophageal-tracheal tube, laryngeal tube, or laryngeal mask (LMA).
- Squeeze the bag with enough volume to result in adequate chest rise.

What to consider

- Inadequate mask seal or improper bag squeeze may result in insufficient ventilations.
- Gastric distention, which can trigger vomiting and aspiration or pneumothorax, may occur with large volume or too rapid bag squeezing.
- During CPR, ventilation rate is based on type of delivery. When using a mask, deliver ventilations at a ratio of 30 compression to 2 ventilations. With an advanced airway, deliver 8 to 10 breaths/minute.

Automatic transport ventilator

The automatic transport ventilator (ATV) provides supplemental oxygen at a constant inspiratory flow rate for an extended time and gives you the freedom to perform other treatments or procedures. It can be used with an ET tube, supraglottic airway, or tracheostomy. Here are the basic types of ATVs:

- Time cycled: stops delivery when a preset time for inspiration expires. The timing mechanism can run on oxygen or electricity, and you set the length of inspiration
- Volume cycled: delivers a preset volume for inspiration, then stops.
- Pressure cycled: stops when a preset airway pressure is met during the inspiratory phase
- Flow cycled: stops when the inspiratory flow rate drops to a preset critical level

What you need

- Gloves and goggles
- ATV
- Oxygen source
- Suction equipment

How it's done

To prepare the ATV:

- Don gloves, and use goggles if indicated.
- Turn the device on, and check that it is functioning properly.
- Use a bag valve mask device to assist ventilation until the equipment is ready. (Keep the bag valve mask device handy in the event that the oxygen supply is diminished.)
- Have suction equipment ready.

To attach the ATV:

- Turn on the unit, and, if necessary, set the tidal volume (4 to 8 mL/kg is the guideline) and rate (8 to 12 breaths/minute).
- Set the peak inspiratory pressure at 60 cm H_2O pressure. (It should have the ability to increase to 80 cm.)
- Lung protective strategies should be applied to all patients requiring an ATV.
- Attach the device to the airway adjunct.
- Observe the patient for adequate chest expansion. (The tidal volume knob can be adjusted for more or less expansion.)

When using an ATV, you must have a reliable oxygen source available.

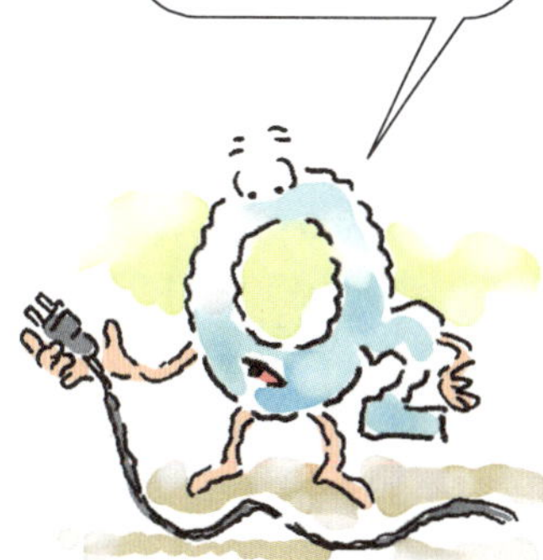

What to consider

- Reliable oxygen source and backup bag valve mask device are necessary.
- Ventilation may stop if the patient fights the equipment, causing increased airway resistance.
- Increased intrathoracic pressure and hypotension caused by decreased blood flow to the heart are possible.
- Increased airway pressure is possible, causing barotrauma to the airway.
- Watch for gastric distention if the patient isn't intubated with an ET tube.

Advanced airway devices

If actions such as the head-tilt, chin-lift maneuver aren't successful in opening the patient's airway, an advanced airway device may need to be inserted. Always follow standard precautions and wear personal protective equipment, as needed, when using airway devices.

Typically, these devices are used for an unconscious patient who has no gag reflex because insertion in a conscious patient would stimulate the gag reflex and increase the risk of aspiration. When it becomes necessary to use an advanced airway device in a conscious patient, administer sedation before insertion.

This invasion saves lives

Advanced airway devices include nasopharyngeal and oropharyngeal airway, the endotracheal (ET) tube, and supraglottic airways (esophageal-tracheal tube airway, laryngeal tube airway, and LMA airway). If the use of these advanced airway devices is unsuccessful or inappropriate, a transtracheal catheter or a surgical cricothyroidotomy may be necessary. These techniques may be explained during ACLS instruction; however, they are considered beyond the scope of practice of most ACLS providers.

During a cardiac arrest, the best device to use to manage the airway depends upon the patient's condition, the provider's experience, the health care facility policies, and the emergency response system available.

Staff training and competency checks are essential components of use of advanced airway devices.

Nasopharyngeal airway

The nasopharyngeal airway is a soft rubber uncuffed tube with a smooth curvature that's inserted through the nose into the oropharynx. When properly positioned, it creates a wide air channel and permits positive pressure ventilation through the trachea.

A semiconscious or conscious patient with an intact gag reflex can tolerate a nasopharyngeal airway. It's useful for maintaining an airway in an adult with poor tongue control, seizures, trismus (tonic contraction of the muscles involved in chewing), or cervical spine injuries.

What you need

- Gloves (gown and goggles if indicated)
- Appropriate size airway
- Water-soluble lubricant

How it's done

Use a nasal tube of the largest diameter size that will fit the patient's nares. Determine the correct size by measuring from the tip of the nose to the tip of the earlobe. The typical sizes are:

- small adult—6 to 7 mm internal diameter (24 to 28 French)
- medium adult—7 to 8 mm internal diameter (28 to 32 French)
- large adult—8 to 9 mm internal diameter (32 to 36 French).

Perform hand hygiene, don gloves, and assess the nares for patency. Place the patient in a supine position, and properly position the airway using the head-tilt, chin-lift maneuver.

Apply a water-soluble lubricant to the distal half of the tube. Then gently insert the tube bevel-side toward the patient's septum. Rotate the tube slightly if resistance occurs but don't force entry.

Peak technique

Inserting a nasopharyngeal airway

First, hold the airway beside the patient's face to make sure it's the proper size (as shown). It should be slightly smaller than the patient's nostril diameter and slightly longer than the distance from the tip of their nose to his earlobe.

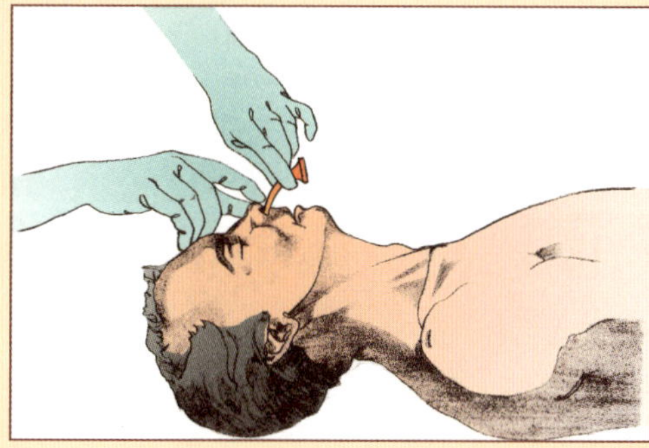

To insert the airway, hyperextend the patient's neck (unless contraindicated). Then push up the tip of their nose, and pass the lubricated airway into his nostril (as shown). Avoid pushing against any resistance to prevent tissue trauma and airway kinking.

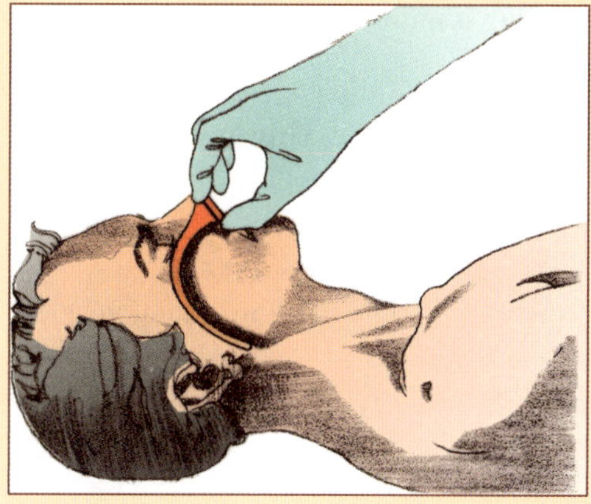

To check for correct airway placement, first close the patient's mouth. Then place your finger in front of the tube's opening to detect air exchange. Also, depress the patient's tongue with a tongue blade and look for the airway tip behind the uvula.

Auscultate the lungs for clear and equal breath sounds after you've inserted the tube. Also be sure to have suction equipment available. (See *Inserting a nasopharyngeal airway*.)

What to consider

- The nasopharyngeal airway may stimulate laryngospasm, gag reflex, and vomiting.
- Improper placement may cause hypoxemia. (If this occurs, check respiration, and provide ventilatory assistance as needed.)
- The nasopharyngeal airway may injure nasal mucosa.
- The nasopharyngeal airway is contraindicated when basilar skull fracture is suspected.

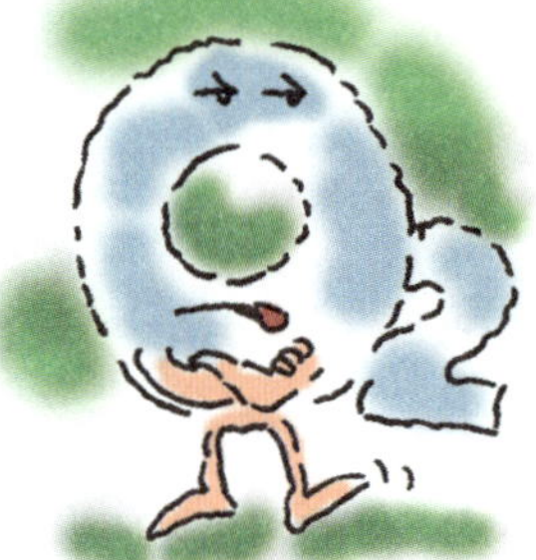

Oropharyngeal airway

The oropharyngeal (or oral) airway is a C-shaped tubular or channeled device made of firm plastic or flexible vinyl (to prevent occlusion by the teeth). It's inserted between the tongue and the posterior wall of the pharynx to lift the base of the tongue off the hypopharynx and establish an open airway.

The oral airway is generally used:

- as a bite block with ET intubation to prevent accidental occlusion of the tube by biting
- to prevent airway occlusion by the tongue in the unconscious patient with spontaneous breathing.

What you need

- Gloves (gown and goggles if indicated)
- Suction and tonsillar (oral suction) catheter
- Appropriate size oropharyngeal airway
- Tongue blade to move the tongue out of the way

How it's done

Perform hand hygiene and don personal protective equipment. Before you begin, place the patient in a supine position, and, if needed, suction the oropharynx area. Determine the appropriate size by measuring from the corner of the mouth to the tip of the earlobe or the bottom angle of the jaw. The typical sizes are:

- small adult—size 3 (80 mm)
- medium adult—size 4 (90 mm)
- large adult—size 5 (100 mm)

To insert the airway using the cross-finger method, turn the airway upside down, and insert it into the patient's mouth. Then turn it 180 degrees into proper position as the end of the airway reaches about the middle of the tongue (one half of the curved part is in the mouth). The flange should rest on the patient's lips, and the end of the airway should be in place between the base of the tongue and the back of the throat. To use the tongue blade technique, open the patient's mouth, and depress their tongue with the blade. Guide the airway over the back of the tongue as you did for the cross-finger technique. Auscultate for breath sounds during ventilation. Clear and equal breath sounds indicate proper ventilation. (See *Inserting an oral airway*.)

Peak technique

Inserting an oral airway

Hyperextend the patient's head, unless this position is contraindicated, before using either the cross-finger or tongue blade insertion method.

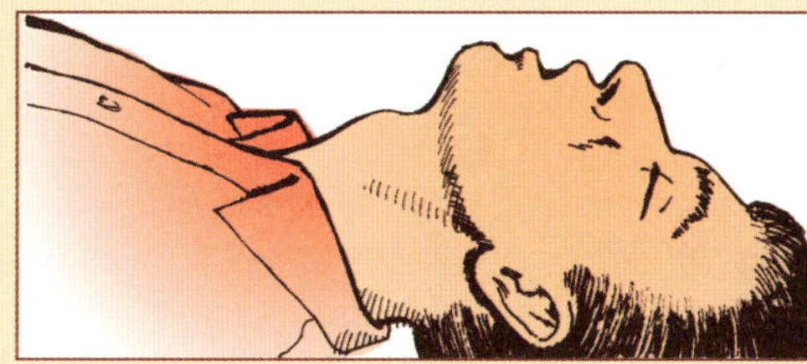

To insert an oral airway using the cross-finger method, place your thumb on the patient's lower teeth and your index finger on their upper teeth. Gently open their mouth by pushing his teeth apart.

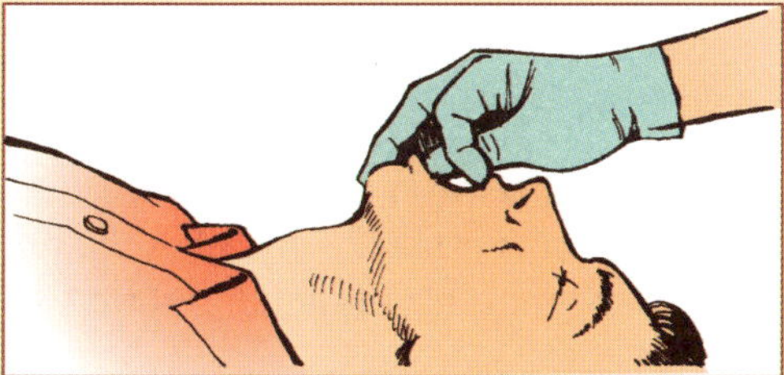

Insert the airway upside down to avoid pushing the tongue toward the pharynx, and slide it over the tongue toward the back of the mouth. As it approaches the posterior wall of the pharynx, rotate the airway so that it points downward.

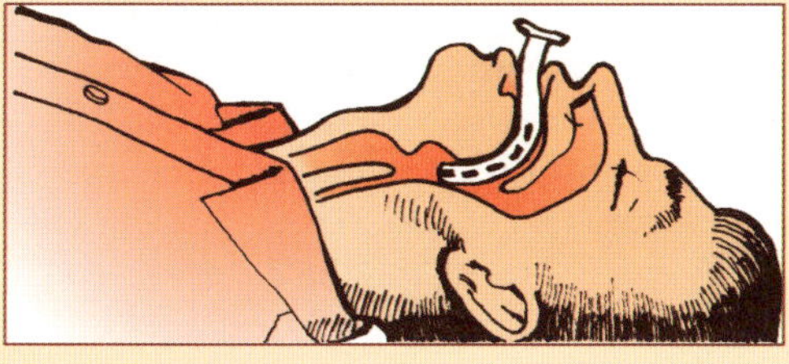

To use the tongue blade technique, open the patient's mouth, and depress their tongue with the blade. Guide the airway over the back of the tongue as you did for the cross-finger technique.

What to consider

- Trauma is possible to the oral mucosa, lips, tongue, or teeth as well.
- Incorrect insertion may airway occlusion due to displacement of the tongue back into the pharynx.
- Elderly patients are at risk for palate injury when an airway is inserted upside down. (Use the tongue blade to pull the tongue to the front and insert the airway right side up into the pharynx, if necessary.)
- Use the oral airway only in unconscious patients because insertion of an oral airway can cause gagging and vomiting or stimulate laryngospasm in the conscious patient.

Be careful when inserting an oral airway in elderly patients because palate injury is possible if the airway is inserted upside down.

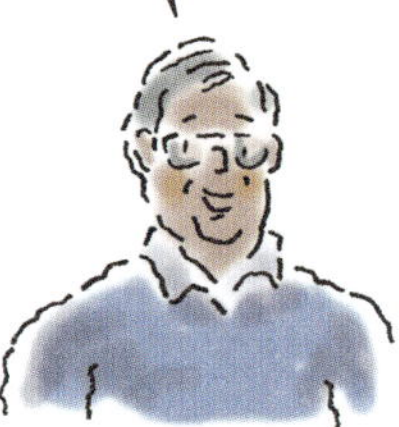

Endotracheal tube

ET intubation involves inserting a tube through the patient's mouth or nose into the trachea to obtain or maintain a patent airway and provide oxygen. In the past, ET intubation was considered the gold standard of advanced airway control. Studies have shown, however, that the rate of complications due to staff inexperience may be unacceptably high. Staff training and regular competency checks are required. This procedure also needs to be within the practitioner's scope of practice.

Ten seconds on the clock

Health care practitioners must be trained in ET tube insertion before performing the procedure. First, you'll ventilate the patient with 100% oxygen via a bag valve mask device. During CPR, chest compressions should be interrupted only for the time required for the intubating provider to visualize the vocal cords and insert the ET tube, ideally in less than 10 seconds.

ET tube insertion should occur in less than 10 seconds.

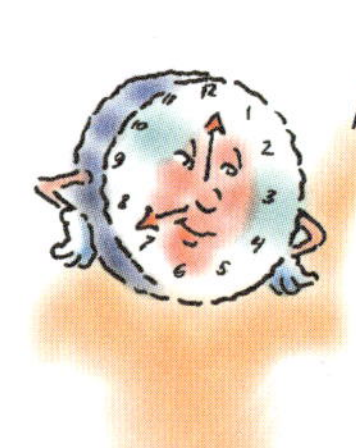

Intubation indications

ET intubation should be performed for a patient who's unable to maintain adequate spontaneous ventilation and oxygenation or has ineffective airway protective reflexes. It's used for patients receiving general anesthesia and in cardiopulmonary arrest and also for those with:

- respiratory distress or failure
- obstructive angioedema (edema involving the deeper layers of the skin, subcutaneous tissue, and mucosa)
- upper airway hemorrhage
- risk of increased intracranial pressure
- laryngeal or upper airway edema
- inability to maintain patent airway
- absent swallowing or gag reflexes

What you need

- Personal protective equipment (gown, gloves, and goggles)
- Sedative, if appropriate
- Laryngoscope, comprised of a handle (where the batteries for the light source are housed) and a blade (curved or straight) with a light bulb
- ET tube of proper size and type (for average adult men, use size 8 mm; for average adult women, use size 7.5 mm), also have available ET tubes that are 0.5 and 1 mm smaller than the selected size for cases in which the initial size you choose is inappropriate for the patient, and tubes with low-pressure cuffs are used in patients older than age 8
- Stylet to facilitate proper tube insertion; plastic-coated for ease of insertion into the tube (may be lubricated with water-soluble lubricant); must end ½″ (1.3 cm) before it reaches the distal end of the tube
- 10-mL syringe to inflate tube cuff
- Magill forceps to assist with tube placement or to remove foreign matter from the airway
- Water-soluble lubricant
- Suction device (both rigid and soft devices should be available)
- Bag valve mask device and oxygen source
- Oral airway or bite block
- Tape or tube holder
- Extra laryngoscope batteries and bulbs
- Equipment to assist with detecting proper placement (stethoscope, capnometer (end-tidal carbon dioxide [ETCO_2] detector) and waveform capnography, if available
- Pulse oximetry to detect oxygen saturation level

How it's done

Begin by assembling the equipment and checking it for proper functioning. Select the proper size and type of blade, either the straight (Miller) blade or the curved (Macintosh) blade, according to the patient's size, anatomy, and practitioner preference. Attach the blade to the laryngoscope and snap it to a right angle to test the light.

Inflate the tube cuff to detect air leaks, and check the tube lumen for patency, keeping it in the sterile wrapper until you use it. Insert the stylet, ensuring that the tip does not protrude out the end, as this may cause injury during ET tube insertion. Ensure functioning suction equipment is available. Next, prepare the patient:

- Assess respiratory status and color. Preoxygenate using a bag valve mask device and 100% oxygen.
- Place the patient's head in the sniffing position to align the airway and visualize the larynx. Suction any secretions from the airway to ensure visualization. Use Magill forceps to remove a foreign body

if present. Remove the patient's dentures, if present. (See *Essential anatomic landmarks.*)

- Administer a pharmacologic agent, if appropriate (such as a sedative to induce sleep and relax the conscious patient and a paralyzing agent to prevent movement, if necessary).
- Perform hand hygiene and put on personal protective equipment. Now begin the procedure to insert the tube:
- Hold the laryngoscope in your left hand.
- Hold the ET tube in your right hand.
- Insert the lubricated blade into the side of the patient's mouth, and advance it midline to the base of their tongue.
- After visualizing the arytenoid cartilage, lift the epiglottis directly with the straight blade or indirectly by inserting the curved blade into the vallecula. (See *Varying technique with blade type* and *Structures seen during direct laryngoscopy.*)
- Expose the larynx by pulling the handle of the laryngoscope in the direction toward which it points (90 degrees to the blade); don't cock the handle (especially with the straight blade) because doing so may fracture teeth.
- Lift forward and upward to expose the glottis.
- Insert the ET tube to the right of the laryngoscope and into the trachea, passing through the vocal cords.

Essential anatomic landmarks

Locate the landmarks shown here when inserting an endotracheal tube through the oral cavity. These landmarks will help you ensure proper tube placement.

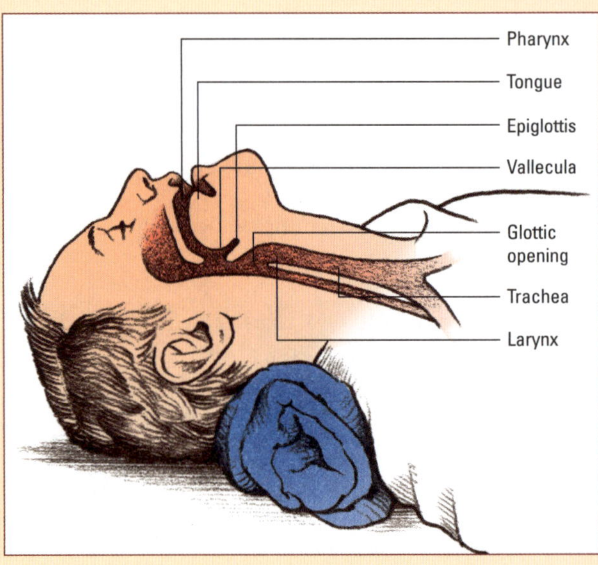

- If you can visualize the arytenoid cartilage but not the glottis, an experienced person, such as a respiratory therapist, can apply cricoid pressure or use a curved stylet to direct the tube anteriorly. (See *Applying cricoid pressure.*) During a cardiac arrest, cricoid pressure shouldn't be used routinely because it can impede ventilation.
- Remove the laryngoscope while holding the tube in place.
- Remove the stylet.
- Look for tube depth marks between the 19- and 23-cm marks at the front teeth.
- Inflate the cuff using the 10-mL syringe.
- Attach the bag valve mask device (with the mask removed), and provide ventilations.
- Insert an oral airway or a bite block, if necessary, to prevent occlusion of the airway caused by the patient biting and occluding the tube.

Now assess for proper placement. Check that:

- the patient's chest rises and falls with each ventilation
- breath sounds are auscultated using a five-point check (left and right anterior chest, left and right midaxillary points, and over the epigastrium)
- capnometer indicates the presence of carbon dioxide (CO_2), confirming that the tube is in the trachea
- continuous waveform capnography confirms ET placement by CO_2 detection (see *Waveform capnography*)

Peak technique

Varying technique with blade type

You need to vary your laryngoscope technique during intubation depending on the type of blade used.

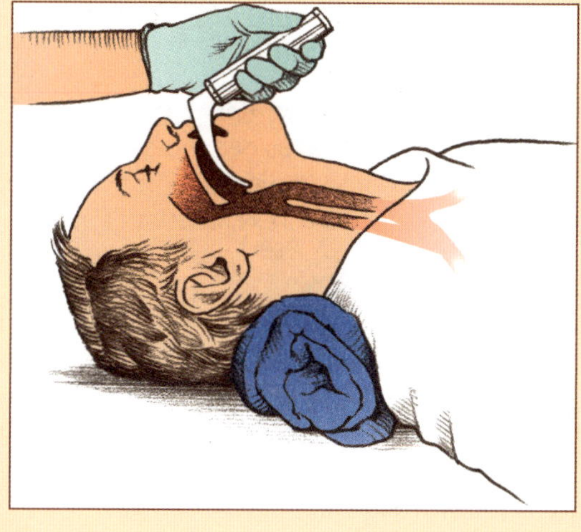

Curved blade

If you use a curved blade, apply upward traction with the tip of the blade in the vallecula. This displaces the epiglottis anteriorly (as shown).

Straight blade

If you use a straight blade, lift the epiglottis anteriorly, exposing the opening of the glottis.

Structures seen during direct laryngoscopy

Locating anatomic structures with a laryngoscope is the key to successful intubation. This illustration shows the anatomic structures of the larynx.

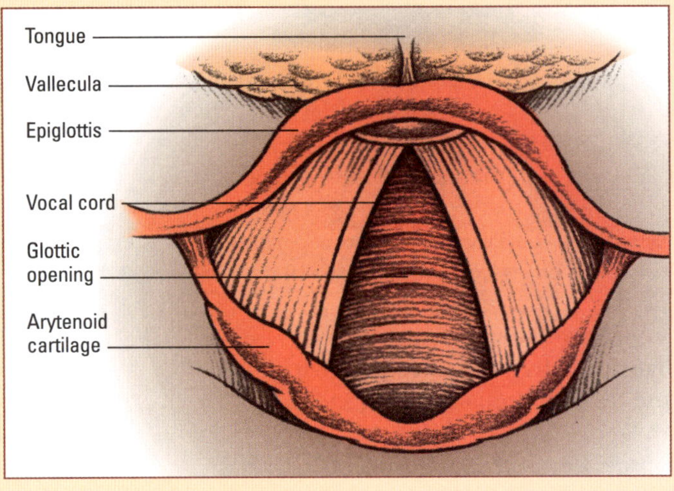

- oxygen saturation is improved using pulse oximetry.
- Obtain a chest X-ray to confirm proper ET placement above the carina.
- Proper tube placement must be determined to ensure adequate oxygenation.

Inflation in moderation

Overinflation of the ET tube balloon can affect its integrity, resulting in an air leak. To check for proper cuff inflation, make sure that no audible leaks are present. If you detect a leak, remove air from the balloon and reinflate. If the leak persists, you must replace the ET tube.

Overinflation can also result in tracheal damage. Too much pressure can injure the tracheal mucosa, which can lead to tracheal necrosis if not corrected. Use a cuff manometer to verify the correct amount of pressure.

Strive for stability

Next, stabilize the ET tube. You may use a commercially produced ET tube holder or tape or ties to secure the tube so that it's immobile. If you use a commercial product, follow the manufacturer's directions. If you use tape:

- Tear about 2′ (60 cm) of tape, split both ends in half about 4″ (10 cm), and place it adhesive-side up on a flat surface.
- Tear another piece of tape about 10″ (25 cm) long, and place it adhesive-side down in the center of the 2″ piece.

- Slide the tape under the patient's neck, and center it.
- Bring the right side of the tape up and wrap the top split end counterclockwise around the tube; secure the bottom split end beneath the lower lip.
- Bring the left side of the tape up and wrap the bottom split piece clockwise around the tube; secure the top split above the patient's upper lip.

If you're using ties:

- Cut about 2′ (60 cm) and place it under the patient's neck.
- Bring both ends up to the tube, and cross them at the bottom of the tube near his lips.
- Bring the ends to the top of the tube, and tie an overhand knot.
- Bring the ends back to the bottom of the tube, tie another overhand knot, and then secure it with a square knot (right over left, left over right).

Reconfirm tube placement after you've finished securing the tube. Following ET intubation, monitor continuous waveform capnography to verify ET tube placement.

Peak technique

Applying cricoid pressure

Also called the Sellick maneuver, the cricoid pressure technique involves applying pressure to the patient's cricoid cartilage, which displaces the trachea posteriorly, compressing the esophagus.

Cricoid pressure may help prevent gastric inflation, reducing the risk of vomiting and aspiration. It's contraindicated in a conscious patient and isn't recommended for routine use during cardiac arrest because improper technique may impede ventilation or interfere with the placement of a supraglottic airway or intubation.

Health care professionals should apply cricoid pressure only when a third rescuer is present.

To apply cricoid pressure:

- Locate the patient's thyroid cartilage with your index finger; then slide your index finger to the base of the thyroid cartilage.
- Palpate the prominent horizontal ring, which is the cricoid cartilage.
- Apply firm but moderate pressure to the cricoid cartilage using the tips of your thumb and index finger (as shown).

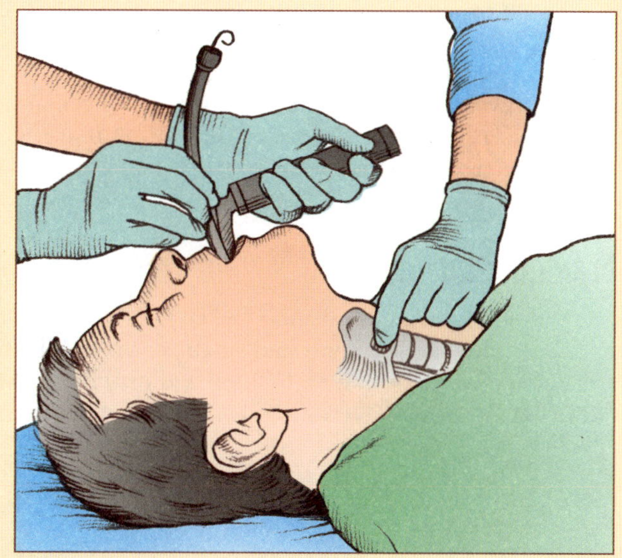

Waveform capnography

Studies of waveform capnography to verify endotracheal (ET) position in victims of cardiac arrest have shown 100% sensitivity and 100% specificity in identifying correct ET tube placement. ET tubes can be easily displaced during such activities as transfer or transport. Continuous waveform capnography is recommended, in addition to clinical assessment, as the most reliable method of confirming and monitoring correct placement of the ET tube.

If waveform capnography isn't immediately available, a capnometer (exhaled carbon dioxide (CO_2) detector), in addition to clinical assessment, can be used as the initial method for confirming correct tube placement. However, studies of exhaled CO_2 detectors indicate that the accuracy of these devices don't exceed that of auscultation and direct visualization of the vocal cords for confirming the tracheal position of an ET tube.

Sock it to secretions

Suction the patient, as necessary, orally and through the ET tube to remove secretions. (See *Open tracheal suctioning*.) After the patient is connected to the ventilator, in-line suctioning is the preferred method of ET suctioning. (See *Closed tracheal suctioning*.)

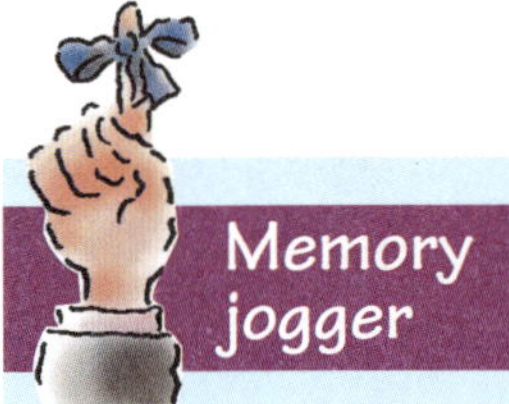

When you perform endotracheal (ET) suctioning, remember EMS:

Explain what's happening to your patient.

Maintain ET tube stability during suctioning.

Stop for respiratory distress immediately.

What to consider

- Practitioners who perform ET intubation need adequate training and frequent experience to reduce the risk of complications, such as oropharyngeal trauma.
- ET intubation isn't an ideal intubation method for patients with suspected cervical spine injury.
- Awake or uncooperative patients may need a short-acting muscle relaxant before ET intubation while you provide oxygenation with a bag valve mask device.

Supraglottic airways

Supraglottic airway devices (SADs) are advanced airways that are inserted via the mouth and sit above the vocal cords. They are easier to insert than an ET tube and may be used for short-term ventilation, such as for surgery patients, or when inserting an ET tube is difficult due to laryngeal edema or injury. Another advantage of using a SAD is that it takes minimal training to have successful insertion. The disadvantage of using SAD is that it is less secure than an ET tube, so it is not ideal for use in patients who require extended ventilation. Types of SADs include the esophageal-tracheal tube airway, the laryngeal-mask airway, and the laryngeal tube airway.

Esophageal-tracheal tube airway

The esophageal-tracheal tube airway consists of a plastic tube with two lumens and a ventilation bag attachment port for each lumen. Proximal and distal balloons help secure the tube and prevent ventilation gases from escaping around the tube. Rings on the proximal tube indicate the depth of the tube's insertion and should be at the level of the patient's teeth. The pharyngeal lumen of the tube has the longer primary port (port #1) at the proximal end, holes along the lumen between the balloons for supraglottic ventilation, and a blind distal end. The tracheoesophageal lumen has the shorter secondary proximal port (port #2), is patent between the balloons, and has an open distal end.

Ease and versatility

The tube may be inserted blindly, usually in prehospital cardiac arrest situations, and may be inserted by those not trained in ET intubation or in place of ET intubation. If used properly, insertion in either the esophagus or trachea provides satisfactory oxygenation. When the tube is inserted blindly, it most commonly enters the esophagus. With esophageal intubation, port #1 of the pharyngeal lumen (blind end) is used to administer ventilations, and port #2 of the tracheoesophageal lumen (open distal end) can then be used to suction gastric contents. If the tube is inserted into the trachea, port #2 of the tracheoesophageal lumen (open distal end) is used to ventilate the patient, similar to using an ET tube.

Peak technique

Open tracheal suctioning

Open tracheal suctioning involves the removal of secretions from the trachea. It's performed by inserting a catheter through the mouth, nose, tracheal stoma, and tracheostomy or endotracheal (ET) tube. This procedure helps maintain a patent airway to promote optimal exchange of oxygen and carbon dioxide and can be performed as frequently as the patient's condition warrants. Tracheal suctioning calls for strict aseptic technique.

What you need

- Oxygen source
- Portable or wall-mounted suction system
- Connecting tube
- Suction catheter kit or a sterile suction catheter, sterile gloves, and a disposable, sterile solution container
- Sterile water or normal saline solution
- Handheld resuscitation bag

How it's done

When preparing to perform tracheal suctioning:

- Perform hand hygiene.
- Check all equipment for proper functioning.
- Attach the suction canister and tubing to the wall or portable system.
- Set the suction between 80 and 100 mm Hg (this amount is adequate to clear the airway without causing tissue trauma); the suction catheter should be one half the diameter of the ET tube.
- Open the suction kit or catheter.
- Fill the sterile container with sterile water or normal saline solution, according to your facility's policy.
- Deliver three to six breaths with the handheld resuscitation bag to preoxygenate the patient (as shown), or set the ventilator on 100% oxygen for suctioning (if available).

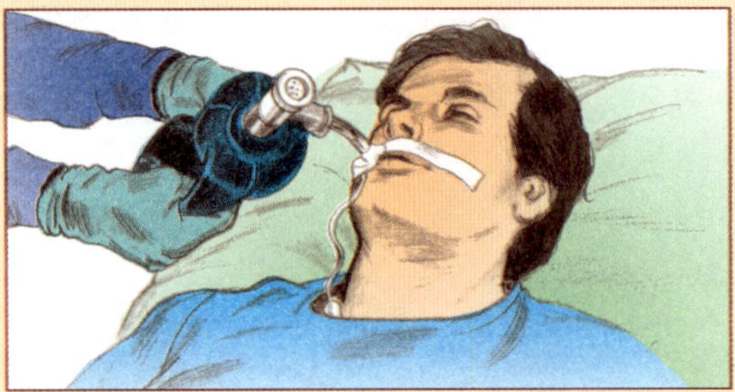

To perform tracheal suctioning:

- Put on sterile gloves.
- Remove the catheter from the kit.
- Manipulate the connecting tubing, and attach the catheter to the tubing (as shown).

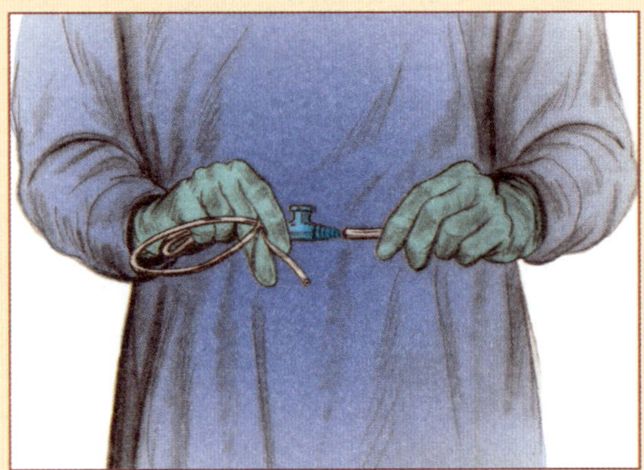

- Hold the catheter with your dominant hand while placing the thumb of your other hand over the control valve (as shown).

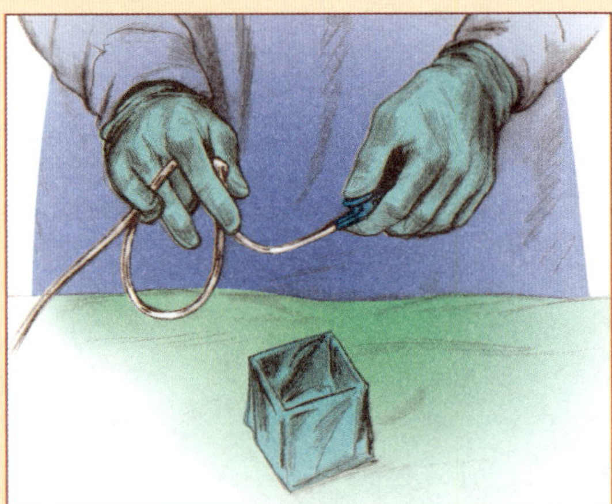

Open tracheal suctioning *(continued)*

- Dip the catheter tip in the sterile solution, and suction a small amount of solution through the catheter (as shown).

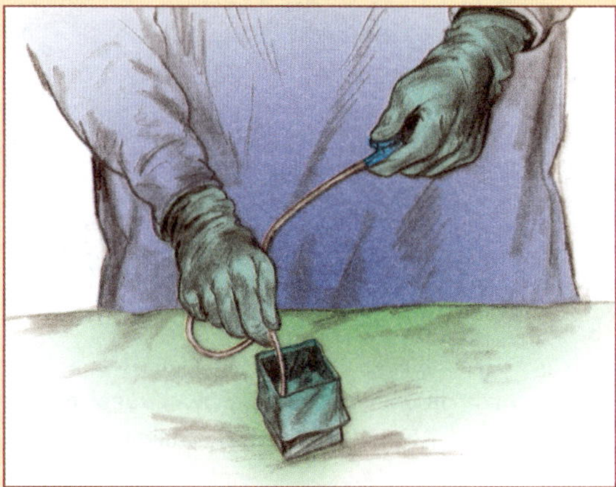

- Disconnect the resuscitation bag or ventilator tubing from the ET tube.
- Place the catheter into the tube without engaging suction, with the ET tube firmly positioned, and gently advance it until you feel resistance.
- Pull the catheter back about 1 cm, slowly rotate and withdraw it, and use your thumb to intermittently occlude the vent (as shown): Suction the patient for no longer than 10 seconds.

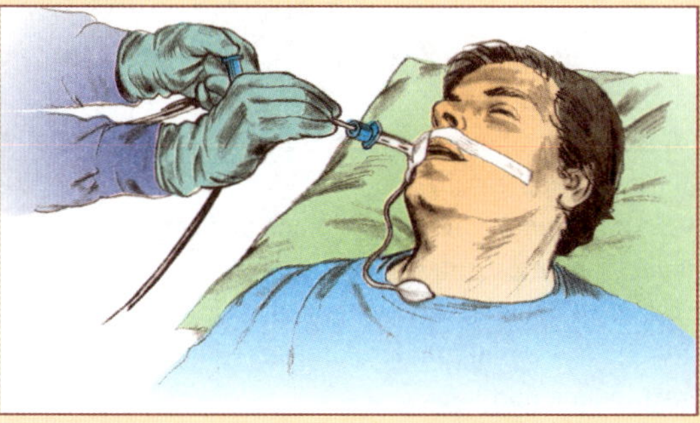

- Deliver breaths with the handheld resuscitation bag between attempts.
- Assess for a patent airway.

After you've finished suctioning:

- Reconnect the patient to the ventilator.
- Clean the catheter and tubing by aspirating sterile saline solution.
- Properly dispose of the catheter and gloves.

What to consider

- Remember to explain to the patient what's occurring, and observe him for signs of anxiety or distress.
- Maintain ET tube stability during suctioning.
- Observe for respiratory distress, and discontinue suctioning if the distress is caused by the procedure.
- Interrupting ventilation causes decreased lung volume, which may cause hypoxemia and lead to cardiac arrest.
- Suctioning of the oral mucosa may stimulate the gag reflex and cause vomiting.
- Prolonged suctioning (more than 15 seconds) may cause hypoxia and can lead to cardiac arrest.
- ET suctioning may cause displacement of the ET tube if it isn't secured properly.
- Suctioning may increase ICP and blood pressure, produce cardiac arrhythmias, or stimulate a vagal response. Monitor the patient closely.
- Suctioning may cause feelings of suffocation in the patient (be sure to reassure him).
- Suctioning may introduce bacterial infection into the airway if performed incorrectly. Maintain aseptic technique.
- Overzealous suctioning or improper technique may cause tracheal trauma.
- Observe for blood in the secretions of patients taking anticoagulants.

Peak technique

Closed tracheal suctioning

The closed tracheal suction system can ease removal of secretions, maintain sterility of the suction catheter, and reduce patient complications. The system consists of a sterile suction catheter in a clear plastic sleeve (as shown). It allows the patient to remain connected to the ventilator during suctioning, as well as decreases the chance of contamination of the catheter by the user.

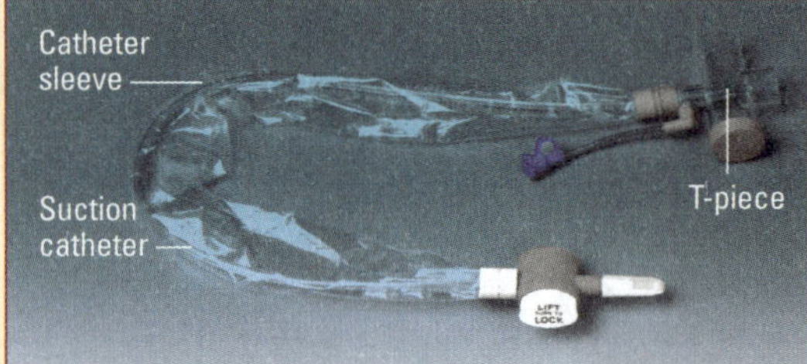

As a result, the patient can maintain the tidal volume, oxygen concentration, and positive end-expiratory pressure delivered by the ventilator while being suctioned. In turn, this reduces the occurrence of suction-induced hypoxemia.

What you need

- Closed suction control valve
- T-piece
- Catheter sleeve (with connections at each end)
- Gloves

How it's done

To perform closed tracheal suctioning, follow these steps:

- Perform hand hygiene.
- Remove the closed suction system from its wrapping; attach the control valve to the connecting tubing.
- Depress the thumb suction control valve, and keep it depressed while setting the suction pressure to the desired level.
- Connect the T-piece to the ventilator breathing circuit, making sure that the irrigation port is closed; then connect the T-piece to the patient's endotracheal or tracheostomy tube (as shown above right).

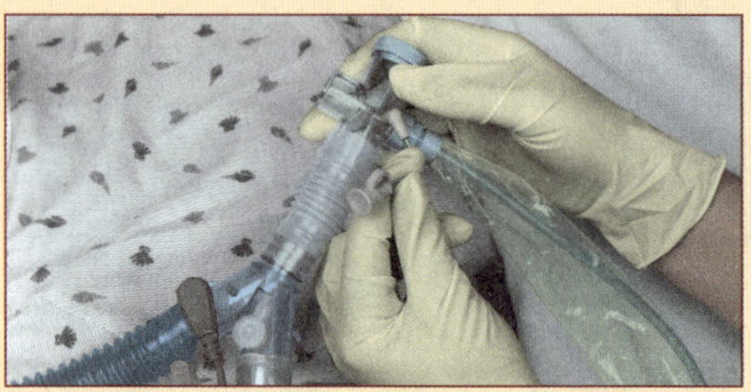

- Advance the catheter through the tube and into the patient's tracheobronchial tree (as shown), keeping one hand on the T-piece parallel to the patient's chin.

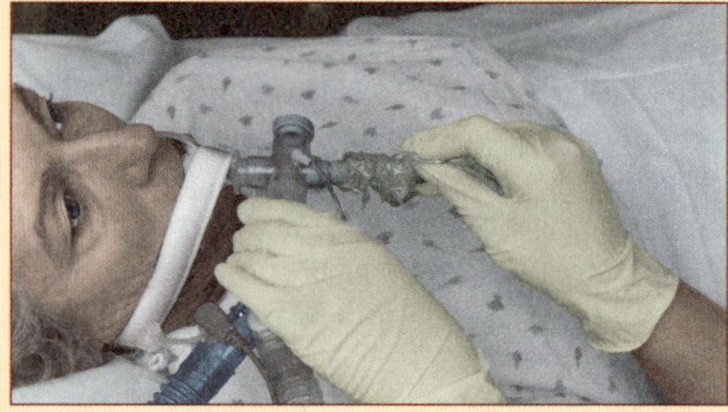

- Gently retract the catheter sleeve as you advance the catheter, if necessary.
- Apply intermittent suction, and withdraw the catheter until it reaches its fully extended length in the sleeve, while continuing to hold the T-piece and control valve. Repeat the procedure as necessary.
- Flush the catheter by maintaining suction while slowly introducing normal saline solution or sterile water into the irrigation port.
- Place the thumb control valve in the off position.
- Dispose of and replace the suction equipment and supplies and change the closed suctioning system, according to your facility's policy.

What you need

- Esophageal-tracheal tube (37 French or 41 French; follow manufacturer's instructions for appropriate size tube based on the patient's height)
- 50-mL syringe to inflate proximal balloon
- 15-mL syringe to inflate distal balloon
- Stethoscope to auscultate for proper position
- Suction device
- Bag valve mask device
- Oropharyngeal or nasopharyngeal airway
- Oxygen source
- Water-soluble lubricant
- Placement confirmation devices (capnometer ($ETCO_2$ detector), continuous waveform capnography if available)
- Personal protective equipment (gown, gloves, and goggles)

How it's done

To prepare, you should first:

- Determine cuff integrity according to the manufacturer's directions.
- Lubricate the tube, as necessary, with water-soluble lubricant.
- Gather all necessary components and accessories.
- Perform hand hygiene, and put on personal protective equipment.
- Inspect the patient's upper airway, and remove any visible obstruction.

To insert the esophageal-tracheal tube:

- Position the patient's head in a neutral position.
- Insert the esophageal-tracheal tube in the same direction as the natural curvature of the pharynx.
- Grasp the tongue and lower jaw between your index finger and thumb, and lift upward.
- Insert the esophageal-tracheal tube gently but firmly until the black rings on the tube are positioned between the patient's teeth.
- Place the proximal cuff between the base of the patient's tongue and his hard palate. (If the tube doesn't insert easily, withdraw it and retry).
- Inflate the large proximal balloon to stop ventilatory gases from exiting through the pharynx to the mouth or nose; inflate the distal cuffs according to the manufacturer's instructions.
- Ventilate through the primary tube (see *Esophageal-tracheal tube airway*).

Placement test

Proper tube placement is essential. After attaching the ventilation bag to the primary port (port #1 located on the pharyngeal lumen), check to see if the tube is in the esophagus by attempting to ventilate the patient. Listen for breath sounds and epigastric insufflation sounds, and look for the chest to rise. If breath sounds are present, the chest rises, and no epigastric insufflation sounds are heard, the tube is probably in the esophagus. Confirm tube placement with a capnometer or waveform capnography if it's available. Secure the tube.

Absence doesn't make the heart grow fonder

If breath sounds are absent and the chest doesn't rise but gastric sounds are heard, the tube may be in the trachea. Immediately switch the ventilation bag to the shorter port #2, which is located on the tracheoesophageal lumen (open distal end), attempt to ventilate, and reassess the patient. If the tube is in the trachea, you will hear breath sounds, the chest will rise, and epigastric insufflation sounds will be absent. Tube placement should be confirmed with a capnometer or waveform capnography if it's available. Secure the tube after placement confirmation.

If both breath and epigastric sounds are absent using either port:

- Immediately deflate both cuffs.
- Withdraw the tube ¾″ to 1¼″ (2 to 3 cm), and then reinflate the cuffs.
- Ventilate and reassess for placement by using the capnometer and waveform capnography.

If breath and epigastric sounds are still absent:

- Immediately deflate the cuffs and extubate.
- Suction as necessary.
- Insert an oropharyngeal or nasopharyngeal airway.
- Hyperventilate.
- Continue ongoing respiratory assessment and treatment.

What to consider

- When used by properly trained health care professionals, the esophageal-tracheal tube delivers ventilation and oxygenation comparable to an ET tube.
- This method is only used as a temporary measure.
- Do not use the esophageal-tracheal tube for responsive patients with an intact gag reflex, patients with known esophageal disease, or patients who have ingested caustic substances.
- Esophageal tears and subcutaneous emphysema are possible because of tube insertion or increased pressure distal to the placed tube during CPR.
- You must remove the esophageal-tracheal tube if the patient regains consciousness or his gag reflex.

Esophageal-tracheal tube airway

The esophageal-tracheal tube is a supraglottic airway that can be used to manage the airway and reduce the risk of aspiration during cardiac arrest. Ventilation and oxygenation compare favorably to endotracheal tube intubation, and training is easier.

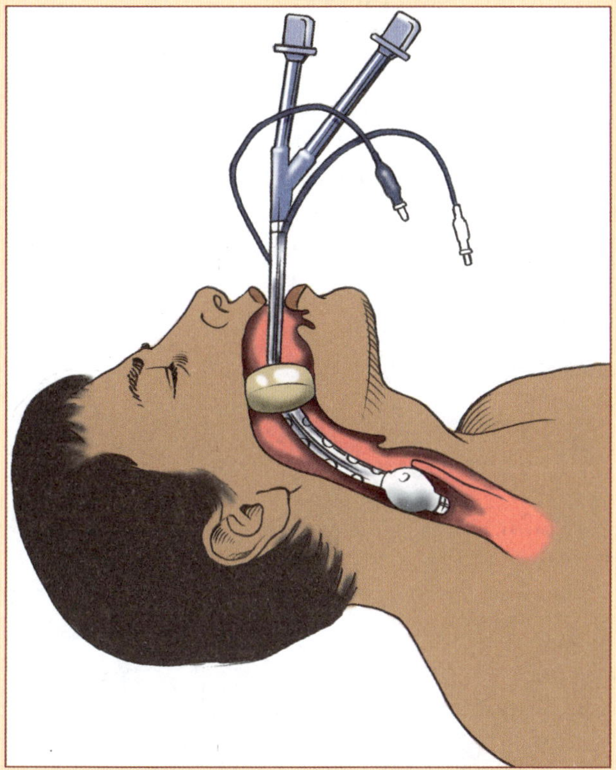

Laryngeal tube airway

The laryngeal tube airway consists of a curved tube with ventilation holes located between two inflatable cuffs. Both cuffs are inflated using a single valve/pilot balloon. The distal cuff is designed to seal the esophagus, while the proximal tube is intended to seal the oropharynx. There is a connector at the proximal tube to connect it to a standard resuscitation bag.

Not so complicated

Like the esophageal-tracheal tube, the laryngeal tube helps prevent aspiration while protecting the patient's airway, and it's more compact and less complicated to insert. During CPR, chest compressions don't have to be interrupted for its insertion. In cardiac arrest situations, the American Heart Association (AHA) has determined that properly trained health care professionals may consider using the laryngeal tube as an alternative to bag valve mask ventilation or ET intubation for airway management.

What you need

- Laryngeal tube of appropriate size according to the patient's height
- 10-mL syringe
- Stethoscope
- Suction device
- Bag valve mask device
- Oropharyngeal or nasopharyngeal airway
- Oxygen source
- Water-soluble lubricant
- Placement confirmation device (capnometer ($ETCO_2$ detector) or waveform capnography)
- Personal protective equipment (gown, gloves, and goggles)

How it's done

To prepare the equipment and patient:

- Assess for contraindications for use.
- Assess the cuff for defects. Inject the recommended amount of air into the inflation port, then deflate.
- Apply a water-based lubricant to the beveled distal tip and posterior aspect of the tube, taking care to avoid introducing lubricant in or near the ventilation openings.
- Perform hand hygiene, and don personal protective equipment.
- Inspect the patient's upper airway, and remove visible obstructions.

  To insert the airway:
- Preoxygenate the patient with a bag valve mask device.
- Place the patient in the "sniffing" position.
- Hold the laryngeal tube at the connector with the dominant hand. With the nondominant hand, hold the mouth open, and apply the chin-lift maneuver, unless contraindicated.

Laryngeal tube airway

The laryngeal tube airway is a type of supraglottic airway that may be used to manage a patient's airway during cardiac arrest situations. It's less complicated to insert than the esophageal-tracheal tube airway and less likely to enter the trachea.

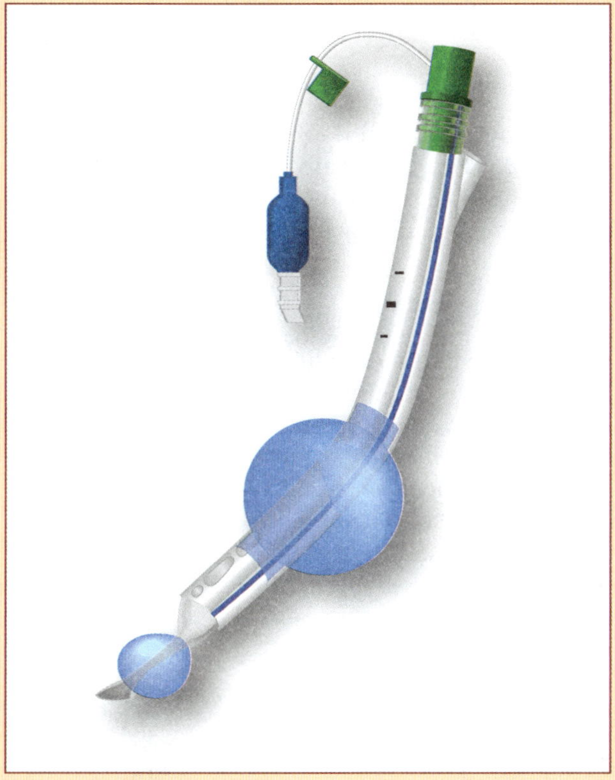

- Introduce the tip into the mouth, with the laryngeal tube rotated laterally 45 to 90 degrees (so that the orientation line is touching the corner of the mouth). Then advance it behind the base of the tongue. Never force the tube into position.
- Rotate the tube back to midline (the orientation line should face the chin).
- Advance the tube until the base of the connector aligns with the teeth or gums. Do not use excessive force.
- Inject the correct amount of air into the cuff according to the manufacturer's specifications.
- Confirm tube placement by auscultation and by capnometer or waveform capnography and then secure the tube.

What to consider

- Don't use a laryngeal tube airway for responsive patients with an intact gag reflex, patients with known esophageal disease, or patients who have ingested caustic substances.
- The laryngeal tube hasn't been proven to fully protect the airway from aspiration due to regurgitation of gastric contents.

Laryngeal mask airway

The LMA is a silicone device that is composed of an airway tube with an elliptical mask and is used to maintain a patent airway in an unconscious patient. It is a temporary airway adjunct that can be used in emergency situations, as well as for temporary airway management, such as during surgery.

When immediacy is needed

The LMA is useful for situations in which endotracheal intubation attempts have failed, bag valve mask ventilation is unsuccessful, and the patient needs immediate airway management. It's simple to use and insert, and may be inserted by nurses, respiratory therapists, and emergency services personnel after receiving adequate training.

For airway management during cardiac arrest, the LMA is an acceptable alternative to bag valve mask or ET ventilation. Occasionally, patients can't be adequately ventilated with the LMA after successful insertion. Make sure an alternative ventilation method is available.

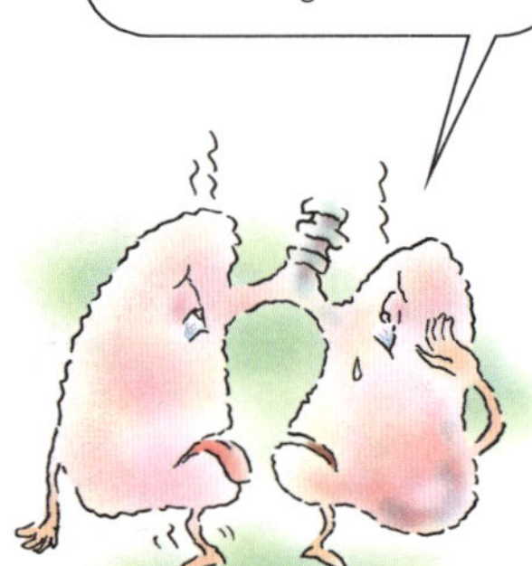

What you need

- LMA of appropriate size with syringe to inflate the cuff
- Stethoscope to auscultate for proper position
- Suction device
- Bag valve mask device
- Oxygen source
- Water-soluble lubricant
- Placement confirmation devices (capnometer ($ETco_2$ detector), continuous waveform capnography if available).
- Personal protective equipment (gown, gloves, and goggles)

How it's done

Before you begin the procedure:

- Perform hand hygiene and put on personal protective equipment.
- Assess the cuff for defects and deflate the cuff.
- Ventilate and oxygenate the patient with a bag valve mask or mouth-to-mask device.
- Place the patient in the sniffing position.

To insert the airway:

Laryngeal mask airway

The laryngeal mask airway doesn't require direct visualization of the vocal cords for insertion so it's easier to insert than an endotracheal tube and provides a more secure and reliable means of ventilation than the face mask.

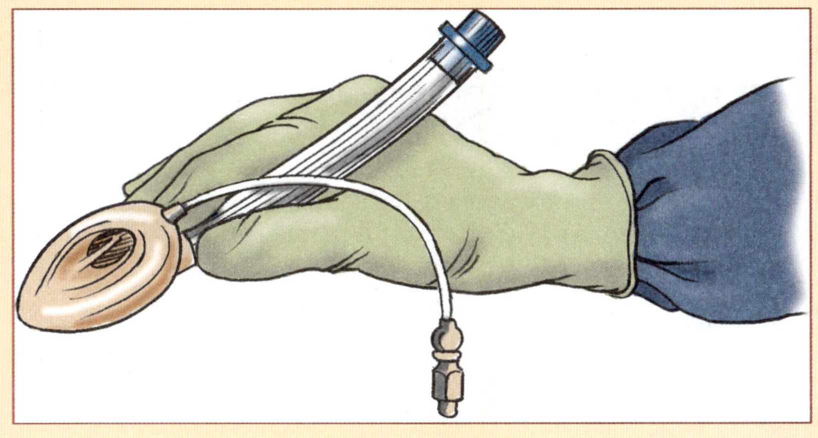

- Press the distal tip of the lubricated, deflated LMA cuff against the hard palate using your index finger to guide the tube over the back of the tongue. (Avoid lubricating the anterior surface of the mask because the lubricant may be aspirated.) (See *Laryngeal mask airway*)
- Gently advance the tube until you feel resistance as the upper esophageal sphincter is engaged.
- Without holding the tube, inflate the cuff with the appropriate amount of air.

The tube will move outward about ⅝″ (1.5 cm), and the cuff will position itself around the laryngeal inlet, resulting in a slight movement of the thyroid and cricoid cartilage. The longitudinal black line on the shaft of the tube should lie in the midline against the upper lip.

In the right place at the right time

Confirm placement using auscultation and a capnometer or waveform capnography. When correctly positioned, the tip of the LMA cuff lies at the base of the hypopharynx against the upper esophageal sphincter, the sides lie in the pyriform fossa, and the upper border of the mask lies at the base of the tongue, pushing it forward.

Once the LMA is correctly placed, ventilate the patient and assess for chest rise. Pulse oximetry should show an increase in oxygenation. If vomiting occurs, leave the LMA in place, immediately tilt the patient's head down, and suction through the LMA.

What to consider

- Consider using the LMA for patients with suspected cervical injury or when you have limited access to the patient.
- The LMA is contraindicated for patients at risk for aspiration and in patients who are morbidly obese or more than 14 weeks pregnant.
- Don't use the LMA if the patient's mouth can't be opened more than ⅝″.

Quick quiz

1. Paramedics are called to the scene of an accident and find an unconscious man lying on the ground. Which is the preferred method for opening the airway of an unconscious patient who may have suffered a neck injury?
   - A. Head-tilt, chin-lift maneuver
   - B. Chin-lift maneuver
   - C. Jaw-thrust, chin-lift maneuver
   - D. Jaw-thrust maneuver

Answer: D. The jaw-thrust maneuver is the preferred method for opening an airway in an unconscious patient if a neck injury is suspected. However, if you're unable to open the airway using this method, use the head-tilt, chin-lift maneuver.

2. After performing ET intubation, you auscultate the patient's chest. You find that breath sounds aren't audible. Based on this finding, you've most likely:
   - A. intubated the esophagus.
   - B. intubated the left mainstem bronchus.
   - C. intubated the right mainstem bronchus.
   - D. wedged the tube against the carina.

Answer: A. If breath sounds aren't audible after ET intubation, you've most likely intubated the patient's esophagus. Remove the tube and oxygenate the patient with 100% oxygen for 1 minute and then reattempt ET intubation.

3. The preferred tidal volume when delivering ventilation with a bag valve mask device is:
   - A. 6 to 7 mL/kg.
   - B. 7 to 10 mL/kg.
   - C. 10 to 15 mL/kg.
   - D. 15 to 20 mL/kg.

Answer: A. A tidal volume of 6 to 7 mL/kg with the bag valve mask device adequately inflates the average person's lungs while minimizing gastric inflation.

4. The most common cause of airway obstruction is:
   A. food.
   B. the tongue.
   C. small toys.
   D. false teeth.

Answer: B. The tongue is the most common cause of airway obstruction. The tongue may slide into the airway as a person's neck muscles relax, causing an obstruction. When a person is unconscious, the tongue loses muscle tone, and the muscles of the lower jaw relax, allowing the tongue to remain in an obstructed position.

5. An ET tube is inserted during the course of resuscitation. What is a reliable method of both confirming and monitoring correct placement of an ET tube?
   A. CO_2 detector
   B. Pulse oximeter
   C. Continuous waveform capnography
   D. Breath sounds

Answer: C. According to the AHA's guidelines, continuous waveform capnography is the most reliable method of confirming and monitoring the correct placement of an ET tube.

Scoring

☆☆☆ If you answered all five questions correctly, excellent! You managed to ace the test.

☆☆ If you answered four questions correctly, good work! You're managing quite well.

☆ If you answered fewer than four questions correctly, don't despair! Take a deep breath and review the chapter to manage a perfect score next time.

Suggested references

American Heart Association (2020). *Advanced cardiovascular life support provider manual*, E-book edition.

Kacmarek, R. M., Stoller, J. K., Heuer, A. J., Chatburn, R. L., & Kallet, R. H. (2017). *Eagan's Fundamentals of Respiratory Care*. Elsevier.

Chapter 5

Electrical therapy

Just the facts

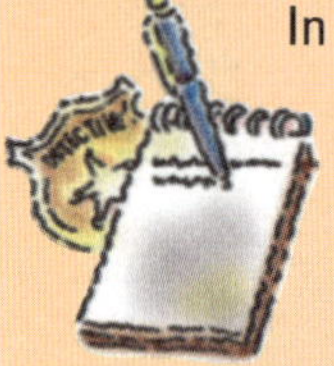

In this chapter, you'll learn:

- the procedure for defibrillation
- the procedure for synchronized cardioversion
- techniques for using pacemakers
- techniques for evaluating pacemaker function

Defibrillation

Defibrillation is the delivery of a large amount of electric current over a brief period of time to stop the fibrillation of the heart. It's the standard treatment for ventricular fibrillation (VF) and pulseless ventricular tachycardia (VT).

A defibrillation shock aims to temporarily depolarize the heart when the rhythm is chaotic or "fibrillating." It does so by completely depolarizing the myocardium, producing a momentary asystole. This provides an opportunity for the heart's natural pacemaker center to restore a normal rhythm.

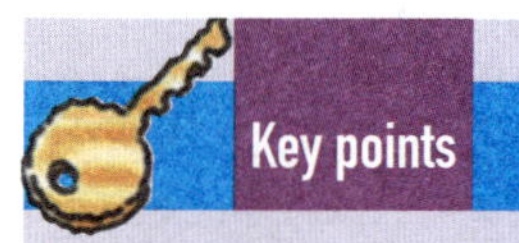

Defibrillation

- Delivery of electric shock to the heart to depolarize irregular heartbeat and allow coordinated electrical and contractile activity to resume
- Treatment for ventricular fibrillation and pulseless ventricular tachycardia
- Early defibrillation most effective for positive outcomes

CPR before and after is better

According to the 2020 American Heart Association (AHA, 2020) *Guidelines for Cardiopulmonary Resuscitation and Emergency Care,* the foundation of successful advanced cardiac life support (ACLS) is high-quality cardiopulmonary resuscitation (CPR) and, for VF or pulseless VT, defibrillation as soon as possible after arrest. For monitored hospital patients, the time from VF to defibrillation should be less than 3 minutes, and CPR should be performed while the defibrillator is readied. This is because high-quality chest compressions help deliver blood to the coronary arteries and brain.

It's also important to perform CPR immediately after defibrillation because the patient may experience a period of asystole or pulseless electrical activity, which CPR may help convert to a perfusing rhythm.

If the patient does have a return of cardiac rhythm, 2 minutes of high-quality compressions will help strengthen the heart and provide additional perfusion to cardiac tissues. Remember, basic CPR can't convert VF to a normal rhythm. The only way to end VF and restore normal cardiac rhythm is by defibrillation.

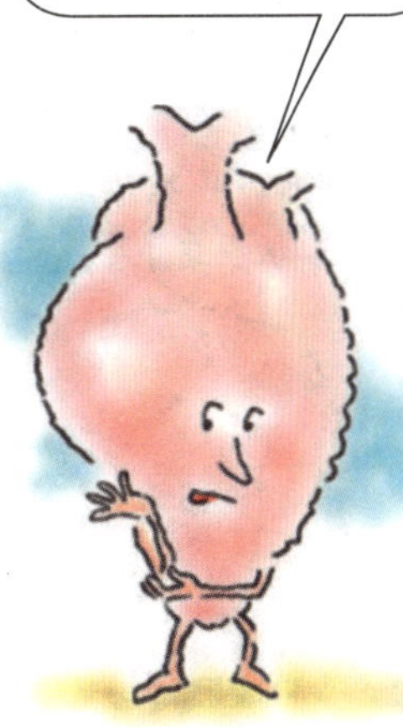

A real need for speed

Defibrillation is significantly more effective when VF is recognized and treated quickly. A study of cardiac arrests in casinos (Wanis, 2007) showed VF survival rates as high as 73% when defibrillation was performed within the first 3 minutes. When defibrillation is performed within the first 5 minutes of cardiac arrest, the survival rate is 50%. Survival rates decrease by 7% to 10% for each minute that a patient is in VF.

When performing defibrillation, you can use either an automated external defibrillator (AED) or a conventional defibrillator.

Automated external defibrillators

The AED is a portable defibrillator with a microcomputer that analyzes a patient's heart rhythm and identifies a shockable rhythm that needs defibrillation. It then gives you step-by-step directions on how to proceed with providing defibrillation to the patient. Some AEDs have the capability of changing languages, also.

Form and function

All AED models have the same basic functions but offer different operating options. For example, all AEDs communicate directions by displaying messages on a screen, giving voice commands, or both. Some AEDs may also simultaneously display a patient's heart rhythm. All devices record your defibrillation attempts, and some may have an integral printer for immediate event documentation. AED adhesive pads have two functions: to transmit the patient's cardiac rhythm and to deliver a shock if indicated. The first step required with any AED is to turn it on!

Two types of AEDs currently exist:

- The fully automated AED, which delivers a shock if VF or Rapid VT is present without operator assistance
- The semiautomated AED, which automatically performs a rhythm analysis once electrode pads are attached; charges automatically if a shock is indicated; then audibly or visually prompts you to press a SHOCK control to deliver the shock (See *Understanding AEDs*.)

Understanding AEDs

Automated external defibrillators (AEDs) vary with the manufacturer, but the basic components for each device are similar. This illustration shows a typical AED and proper electrode pad placement.

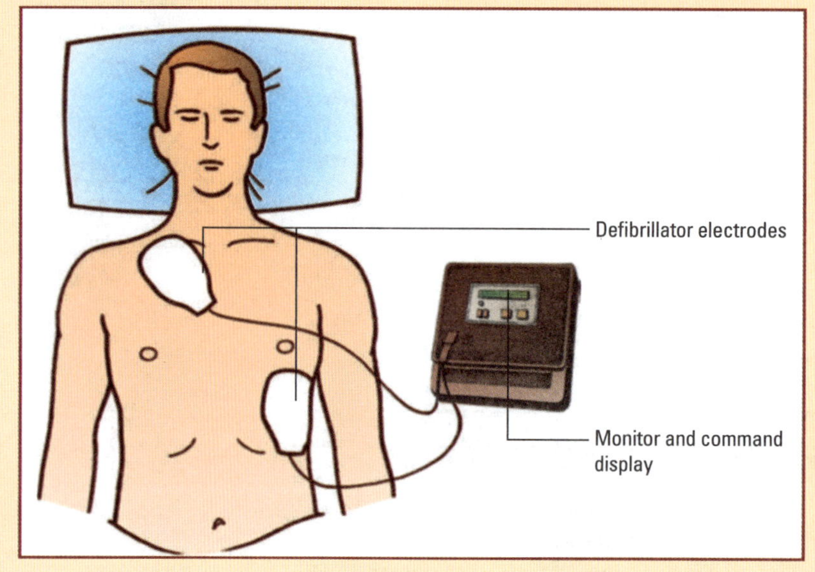

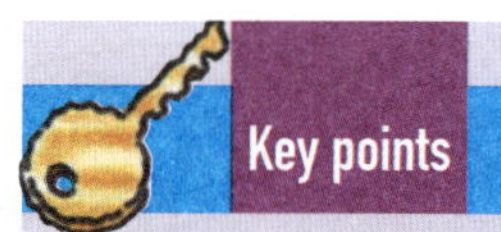

Automated external defibrillators

- Contain cardiac rhythm analysis systems that recognize shockable rhythms
- May be fully or semiautomated
- Used for patients without a pulse
- Easy to use by almost anyone
- Fast speed of operation and delivery
- Hands-free delivery of shock
- Energy level = 200 to 360 joules when using adult electrode pads

With either device, the electrical shock is delivered through two adhesive electrode pads applied to the patient's chest (upper-right sternal border, lower-left ribs over the cardiac apex). The adhesive pads have two functions: to transmit the patient's cardiac rhythm and to deliver a shock if indicated.

How it's done

For a person who has collapsed, is unconscious, and does not have a palpable pulse, initiate CPR immediately and use an AED as soon as it's available.

To perform defibrillation with an AED:

- Check the AED and then call for further assistance.
- Turn the AED on and follow the directions it then provides:
- Open the packets containing adult electrode pads.
- Expose the patient's chest. If the patient's chest is wet, wipe it dry quickly (for better adherence of the adhesive) and then attach the pads.
- Remove the plastic backing film from the electrode pads. Place the pads according to the pictures on the pads.
- Connect the cable to the AED as instructed by the machine. Connection site may have a flashing light to emphasize access site.

How AEDs sense rhythm

The accuracy of the automated external defibrillator (AED) in rhythm analysis is considered very high. A microprocessor analyzes features of the patient's electrocardiogram signal for frequency, amplitude, and integration of frequency and amplitude. A safety filter checks for false signals, such as those deriving from radio transmissions, poor electrode contact, 60-cycle interference, or loose electrodes.

Multiple analyses

At the beginning of the rhythm, the AED makes multiple analysis, or multiple looks each lasting a few seconds. Several analyses must confirm the presence of a shockable rhythm. The fully automated AED will then charge and deliver a shock; the semiautomated AED will signal the operator that a shock is advised and when to deliver the shock.

- Press the ANALYZE button when the machine prompts, or simply follow directions provided by machine, such as "Analyzing rhythm—DO NOT touch the patient." Stop compressions during this time.
- Don't touch or move the patient while the AED is in analysis mode. Analysis takes 5 to 15 seconds, depending on the machine. (See *How AEDs sense rhythm.*)
- Continue to follow directions provided by the AED. If a shock isn't needed, the AED will display or say "No shock advised" and then prompt you to resume CPR starting with chest compressions. If the patient needs a shock, the AED will announce a "charging" message and emit a beep that changes to a steady tone when it is fully charged. Compressions may be performed while the AED is charging.
- When the AED is fully charged and ready to deliver a shock, an automated machine may simply deliver the charge after stating "STAND CLEAR." A semiautomated machine will prompt you to press the SHOCK button by stating "Deliver shock now."
- Make sure no one is touching the patient and call out "STAND CLEAR." Then press the SHOCK button on the AED.
- After you deliver the first shock, immediately resume CPR, performing five cycles (about 2 minutes).

Data entry

- Every 2 minutes, the AED will reanalyze the patient's rhythm and prompt you to deliver another shock if needed. If the AED states "Shock not advised," check the patient for a pulse to determine if compressions need to be resumed. This is also a reminder to switch providers if able.

- When resuscitation is complete, remove the computer memory module or tape from the AED and transcribe it, or prompt the AED to print a rhythm strip with code data for inclusion into the medical record.

What to consider

- The patient can't be touched while the AED analyzes the rhythm and when the shock is being delivered.
- You'll need to modify your actions for patients with implanted pacemakers, implantable cardioverter-defibrillators, transdermal medication patches, and for those being resuscitated around water. (See *Tips for defibrillation in special situation.*)

Tips for defibrillation in special situations

Some situations produce challenges to effective and safe defibrillation. For instance, you must take precautions when defibrillating a patient with an implantable cardioverter-defibrillator (ICD) or pacemaker or for a patient who has a transdermal medication patch in place. You must also be careful when defibrillating a patient who's in contact with water. A hairy patient presents other challenges.

Defibrillating a hairy patient

If the patient has a hairy chest and the pads do not adhere well to the chest, the AED may prompt you to check the pads. Initially press down on the pads to see if that is helpful. If the pads still do not adhere, look for a razor in the AED case, shave the areas for pad placement, and reapply the pads. If there is no razor available, but pediatric pads are in the AED case, place the pediatric pads on the patient, and then quickly pull them off, which will hopefully also pull off enough hair from the chest to allow better pad adherence. Then attempt to apply the adult pads.

Defibrillating a patient with an ICD or pacemaker

If the patient has an ICD or pacemaker that is visible (it looks like a small lump on the chest under the skin), avoid placing the defibrillator paddles or pads directly over the implanted device. Place them at least 1 inch (2.5 cm) away from the device.

Defibrillating a patient with a transdermal medication patch

If the patient has a transdermal medication patch on the chest, such as nitroglycerin, nicotine, analgesics, or hormone replacements, avoid placing electrodes directly on top of it. The patch can block delivery of energy and cause a small burn to the skin. Instead, remove the patch and quickly wipe the area clean before applying the defibrillation pad.

Defibrillating a patient in water

Water is a conductor of electricity and may provide a pathway for energy from the defibrillator to the rescuers treating the patient. If the patient is in free-standing water, move the patient to a dry area and quickly dry their chest before defibrillation.

Conventional defibrillators

Conventional defibrillators are commonly used in most health care facilities. Unlike an AED, they require you to analyze the rhythm, select the energy level to be administered, apply the paddles or "hands-off" pads to the patient's chest, charge the machine, and discharge the current by pressing both paddle buttons simultaneously or by pressing the SHOCK button on the defibrillator.

Two types of conventional defibrillators exist: monophasic and biphasic. (See *Monophasic and biphasic defibrillators.*)

How it's done

To analyze the patient's cardiac rhythm, place the defibrillator pads on the patient's chest. Paddles may be used if "hands-free" pads are not available. Assess the rhythm on the defibrillator monitor. If the display shows VF or VT, and the patient does not have a pulse, defibrillation is needed.

Monophasic and biphasic defibrillators

Two types of defibrillators are available: monophasic and biphasic.

Monophasic defibrillators

Monophasic defibrillators deliver a single current of electricity that travels in one direction between the two pads or paddles on the patient's chest. To be effective, a large amount of electrical current (360 joules) is frequently required.

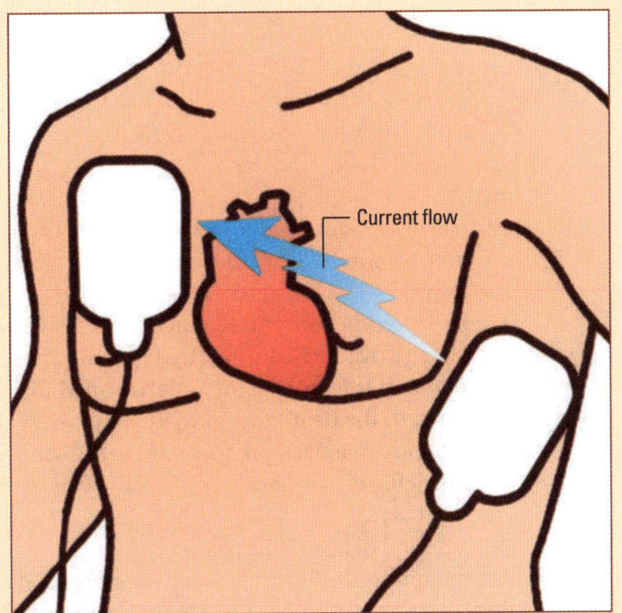

(*continued*)

Monophasic and biphasic defibrillators *(continued)*

Biphasic defibrillators

With a biphasic defibrillator, the discharged electrical current travels in a positive direction for a specified duration. The charge then reverses and flows in a negative direction for the remaining time of the electrical discharge, delivering two currents of electricity. Using two currents lowers the defibrillation threshold of the heart muscle, increasing the likelihood for successful defibrillation of ventricular fibrillation with smaller amounts of energy (120 to 200 joules). Biphasic defibrillators also adjust for differences in impedance or resistance, which reduces the number of shocks needed. Most newer defibrillators are biphasic.

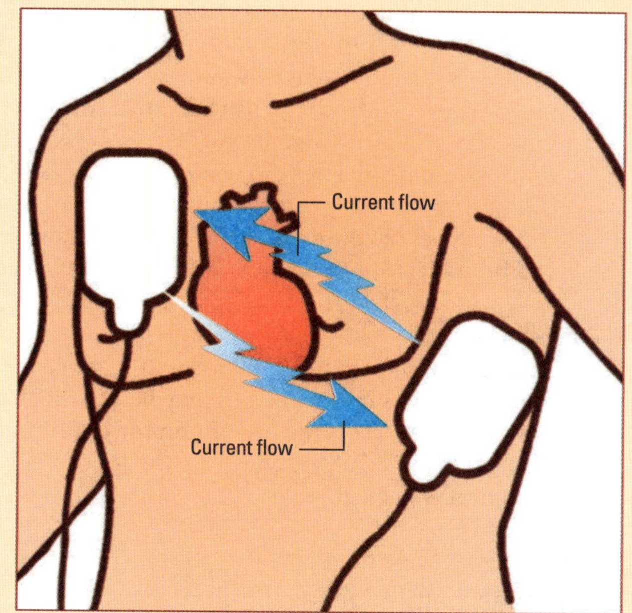

Conventional wisdom

To perform defibrillation with a conventional defibrillator:

- Expose the patient's chest.
- Apply "hands-off" pads, and connect to the defibrillator.
  - For anterolateral pad placement: Place one pad to the right of the upper sternum, just below the right clavicle, and the other over the fifth or sixth intercostal space at the left anterior axillary line.
  - For anteroposterior pad placement: Place the anterior pad directly over the heart at the precordium to the left of the lower sternal border; place the posterior pad under the patient's body beneath the heart and immediately below the scapula.
  - If hands-free pads are not available, place conductive gel to the defibrillator paddles or conduction pads to the patient's chest wall.
- Turn on the defibrillator.
- Set the monophonic defibrillator energy level to 360 joules, or set the biphasic energy level to 120 to 200 joules for an adult patient. Follow manufacturer and ACLS recommendations for biphasic dosing. If you don't know which type of defibrillator you're using, set the energy level to 200 joules.

- If using paddles, place over the conduction pads and press firmly against the patient's chest using a minimum of at least 25 lbs of pressure. If using gel, ensure adequate paddle coverage and then place the paddles in the appropriate positions.
- If using hands-free patches, place the patches in the appropriate positions.
- Charge the defibrillator by pressing the CHARGE button located on the machine. If using paddles, the defibrillator may also be charged by pressing the CHARGE button located on the paddle handle.
- When the machine is fully charged, instruct everyone to STAND CLEAR of the patient and the bed. Turn off any oxygen flow.
- When everyone is clear of the patient and bed and the oxygen is off, press the DISCHARGE or SHOCK button on the machine or paddles.

After the shock is delivered, immediately resume CPR, beginning with chest compressions. Perform five cycles (about 2 minutes). Reassess the patient's cardiac rhythm on the monitor, and defibrillate again if indicated.

Restoration station

If defibrillation successfully restores cardiac rhythm:

- Check the patient for a palpable pulse.
- Obtain a blood pressure reading, treat hypotension, and monitor the patient's heart rhythm, respiratory rate, and pulse oximetry.
- Assess the patient's level of consciousness (LOC), breath sounds, skin color, and urine output.
- Obtain blood for laboratory tests, such as cardiac markers, electrolytes, and blood gas analysis. Obtain a chest X-ray and 12-lead ECG.
- Treat hypoxemia and provide supplemental oxygen, ventilation, fluids, and medications, as needed.
- Be prepared to provide therapeutic hypothermia for comatose patients, if appropriate.

What to consider

- Familiarize yourself with your facility's equipment and policies for a quick and accurate response to cardiac arrest situations.
- A defibrillator can be a dangerous piece of equipment because it delivers electricity to whatever it's in contact with. To avoid injury to others, be diligent in checking that no one is in contact with the patient or bed before discharging a shock, and that there is no free-flowing oxygen that may ignite on contact with an electrical shock.

- Check defibrillator equipment regularly to make sure that it's in working condition. Keep the defibrillator's battery charged by connecting it to alternating current.
- When delivering a shock using paddles, use firm pressure to maintain full contact with the patient's skin. If the paddles are lifted off the patient's chest while delivering a shock, a dangerous "arc" of electricity may occur, causing electrical injury. Ensure that oxygen is off and that care providers are clear before delivering the shock.
- When performing synchronized cardioversion, it is important to synchronize the electrical charge with the R wave by pressing the SYNC button.

Synchronized cardioversion

Synchronized cardioversion (synchronized countershock) is used to treat tachyarrhythmias (such as atrial tachycardia, atrial flutter, atrial fibrillation, and unstable VT (with a pulse)). It is performed as either an elective or an emergent procedure and may be performed when the arrhythmia does not respond to drug therapy or vagal maneuvers such as carotid sinus massage. (See *Carotid sinus massage*.)

Peak technique

Carotid sinus massage

Carotid sinus massage is used to interrupt paroxysmal atrial tachycardia. Only expert practitioners trained and experienced (and within their scope of practice) in this procedure should perform carotid sinus massage. Massaging the carotid sinus stimulates the vagus nerve, which inhibits firing of the sinoatrial (SA) node and slows atrioventricular (AV) node conduction. As a result, the SA node can resume its function as primary pacemaker.

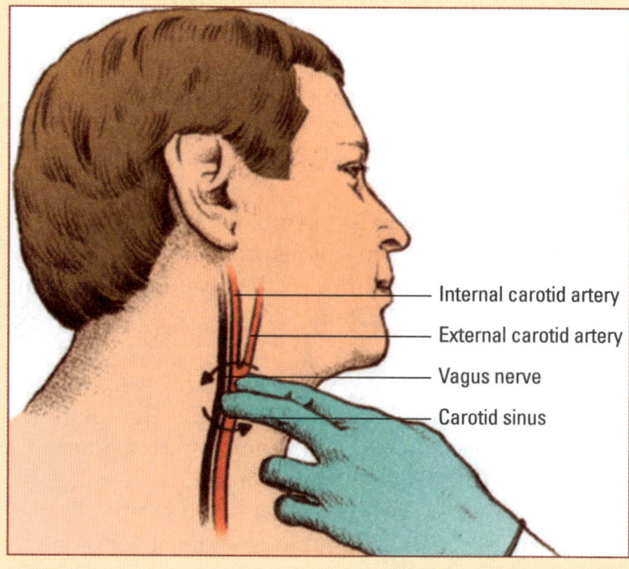

To perform carotid massage, place the patient in a supine position and turn their head to the left to massage the right carotid sinus (as shown). Firmly massage the patient's carotid sinus for no longer than 5 to 10 seconds. Don't perform carotid massage on both sides simultaneously because it may cause cardiac arrest.

Carotid sinus massage is contraindicated in patients with severe carotid stenosis. Risks of the procedure include decreased heart rate, syncope, sinus arrest, increased degree of AV block, cerebral emboli, stroke, and asystole.

It's electric

Synchronized cardioversion delivers electrical charge to the myocardium at the peak of the R wave. This causes immediate depolarization, interrupting reentry circuits, and allowing the sinoatrial node to resume control. Synchronizing the electrical charge with the R wave ensures that the current won't be delivered on the vulnerable T wave and disrupt repolarization. This reduces the risk that the current will strike during the relative refractory period of the cardiac cycle and induce VF.

Elective synchronized cardioversion

Elective synchronized cardioversion is a scheduled procedure that delivers an electric shock in the attempt to restore normal cardiac rhythm. It is the treatment of choice for arrhythmias that do not respond to drug therapy or vagal maneuvers.

How it's done

Before beginning elective cardioversion:

- Perform hand hygiene.
- Done appropriate PPE including gloves, gown, eye shield, and facial coverings including an N95 respirator if appropriate.
- Identify the patient using two patient identifiers.
- Explain the procedure to the patient and answer all questions.
- Verify that the patient has a signed informed consent.
- Ensure that the patient withheld food and fluids for 6 to 12 hours before the procedure.
- Perform hand hygiene.
- Obtain a 12-lead ECG to serve as a baseline.
- Connect the patient to a pulse oximeter and blood pressure cuff.
- Obtain IV access or check existing IV access for patency.
- Administer a sedative, as ordered.
- Place the leads on the patient's chest and assess cardiac rhythm to determine if cardioversion is still appropriate.
- Apply pads to the chest wall, positioning the pads so that one pad is to the right of the sternum just below the clavicle, and the other at the fifth or sixth intercostal space at the left anterior axillary line. Alternatively, pads may be placed anteriorly at the precordium to the left of the lower sternal border and posteriorly under the patient's body beneath the heart and immediately below the scapula.

  To perform elective synchronized cardioversion:
- Turn on the defibrillator.
- Select the appropriate energy level (joules) based on the patient's cardiac rhythm. The monophasic energy level is usually between 100 and 200 joules. Biphasic machines may achieve effective

Correct joules for synchronized cardioversion using a biphasic defibrillator

Use these joule levels for synchronized cardioversion with a biphasic defibrillator:

- narrow, regular tachycardia—50 to100 joules
- narrow irregular tachycardia—100 to 200 joules
- wide, regular tachycardia—100 joules

cardioversion at a lower energy setting, usually 50 to 200 joules. (See *Correct joules for synchronized cardioversion using a biphasic defibrillator.*)

- Activate the synchronize mode by depressing the SYNCHRONIZE button.
- Check to verify that the machine is sensing the R wave correctly by noting a marker (appears as a "dot") on the R wave.
- Charge the machine to the appropriate joules.
- Instruct other personnel to STAND CLEAR of the patient and the bed to avoid the risk of an electric shock. Ensure that there is no free-flowing oxygen.
- Discharge the current by pressing the SHOCK button on the machine. Unlike defibrillation, the discharge won't occur immediately; you'll notice a slight delay while the defibrillator synchronizes with the R wave before delivering the shock.

If at first you don't succeed...

If initial synchronized cardioversion is unsuccessful, repeat the procedure up to three more times, as ordered, gradually increasing the energy level with each additional countershock. If normal rhythm is restored, check for a pulse and continue to monitor the patient. Obtain an ECG to document successful cardioversion. If the patient's cardiac rhythm changes to VF, switch from a synchronized mode to defibrillation and immediately charge the machine to the appropriate joules and deliver a shock. Perform CPR as needed.

What to consider

- Perform synchronized cardioversion with a practitioner present.
- Be sure to warn the patient when a shock will be delivered. Explain to them that you may need to deliver additional shocks to achieve successful cardioversion.
- If the patient's cardiac rhythm converts to pulseless VT or VF, defibrillate them with an unsynchronized shock. Make sure that the SYNCHRONIZE button is off or a shock won't be delivered.

Emergency synchronized cardioversion

Emergency synchronized cardioversion is used to rapidly convert an abnormal cardiac rhythm when the patient is displaying a deteriorating hemodynamic state (chest pain, shortness of breath, systolic blood pressure less than 90, altered LOC).

How it's done

Before beginning emergency synchronized cardioversion:

- Place defibrillator cardiac monitor leads on the patient, if they aren't already in place.
- Explain the procedure to the patient, if possible.
- Connect the patient to a pulse oximeter and blood pressure cuff.
- Obtain IV access or check existing IV access for patency.
- Administer a sedative if possible.
- Apply pads so that one pad is to the right of the sternum, just below the clavicle, and the other is at the fifth or sixth intercostal space in the left anterior axillary line. Alternatively, pads may be placed anteriorly at the precordium to the left of the lower sternal border and posteriorly under the patient's body beneath the heart and immediately below the scapula.

To perform emergency synchronized cardioversion:

- Turn on the defibrillator.
- Select the appropriate energy level (joules) based on the patient's cardiac rhythm. The monophasic energy level is usually between 100 and 200 joules. Biphasic machines may achieve effective cardioversion at a lower energy setting, usually 50 to 200 joules.
- Activate the synchronize mode by depressing the SYNCHRONIZE button.
- Check to verify that the machine is sensing the R wave correctly, by noting a marker (appears as a "dot") on the R wave.
- Charge the machine to the appropriate joules.
- Instruct health care providers to STAND CLEAR of the patient and the bed to avoid the risk of an electric shock. Ensure that there is no free-flowing oxygen.
- Discharge the current by pressing the SHOCK button on the machine. Unlike defibrillation, the discharge will not occur immediately. A slight delay will be noted while the defibrillator synchronizes with the R wave before delivering the shock.

What to consider

- Perform synchronized cardioversion with a practitioner present.
- Be sure to warn the patient when a shock will be delivered. Explain to them that you may need to deliver additional shocks to achieve successful cardioversion.
- If the patient's cardiac rhythm converts to pulseless VT or VF, defibrillate them using an unsynchronized shock. Make sure that the SYNCHRONIZE button is off or a shock won't be delivered.

Temporary pacemakers

A temporary pacemaker is a non-surgically implanted device that is used in an emergency situation. These situations include when the patient shows signs of decreased cardiac output such as chest pain, hypotension, altered mental status, or syncope. It is often required for patients with symptomatic bradycardia that is unresponsive to drug therapy. A temporary pacemaker can also serve as a bridge until a permanent pacemaker is inserted.

If a patient's condition requires a temporary pacemaker and if his condition doesn't improve, a permanent pacemaker may be inserted. Pacemakers should be used without delay for an unstable patient with second-degree atrioventricular (AV) block (type II) or third-degree AV block. They also may be used for the following conditions:

- hemodynamically unstable patient with symptomatic bradycardia, especially if the patient doesn't respond to drug therapy
- significant bradycardia associated with poisoning or drug overdose
- paroxysmal supraventricular tachycardia.

Pacemakers are contraindicated in patients with:

- severe hypothermia with a bradycardic rhythm. (Ventricles are more prone to fibrillation and more resistant to defibrillation as core temperature drops.)
- asystole or pulseless electrical activity.

Types of temporary pacemakers include transcutaneous and transvenous pacemakers.

Transcutaneous pacemaker

The transcutaneous pacemaker, also known as an *external pacemaker*, is the best choice in life-threatening situations when time is critical. It is a temporary noninvasive pacing method that uses the defibrillator to send electrical impulses to the patient's chest. One pad is placed to the right of the sternum just below the clavicle, and the other is placed at the fifth or sixth intercostal space in the left anterior axillary line. Alternatively pads may be placed anteriorly at the precordium to the left of the lower sternal border, and posteriorly under the patient's body beneath the heart and immediately below the scapula.

Setting the pace

A transcutaneous pacemaker is used to stabilize the patient's heart rhythm until a practitioner can insert a transvenous or permanent pacemaker.

Peak technique

Pad placement for transcutaneous pacing

One option for pad placement for transcutaneous pacing is the anterior and posterior placement. Place the two pacing pads at heart level on the patient's chest and back, as shown. This placement ensures that the electrical stimulus need only travel a short distance to the heart. Alternatively, pads may be placed as described for defibrillation.

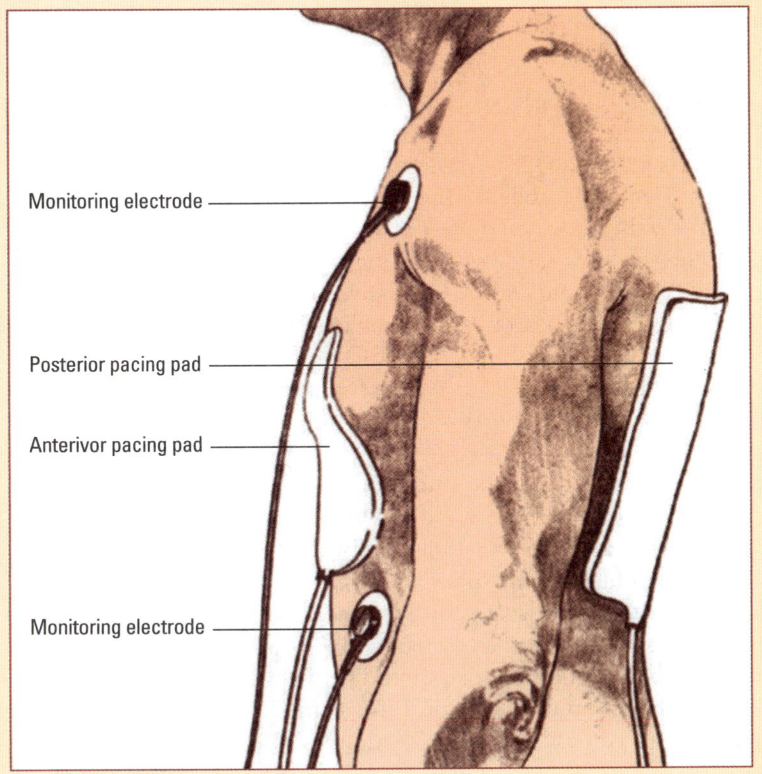

How it's done

Before initiating transcutaneous pacing:

- If necessary, clip the patient's hair over the areas of electrode and pad placement. In addition to defibrillator pads, ECG electrodes must also be placed in order for the defibrillator to read the patient's underlying cardiac rhythm. Defibrillator pads deliver the energy needed to pace the heart. Make sure the patient's skin is clean and dry to ensure good skin contact. (See *Pad placement for transcutaneous pacing*.)
- Set the selector switch to the "Monitor On" position.

Attach monitoring cable from the defibrillator to the electrodes, and program the machine to read in the lead I, II, or III position.

- An ECG waveform should be visible on the monitor.
- Adjust the R-wave beeper volume to a suitable level.
- Activate the ALARM ON button; set the alarm for 10 to 20 beats lower and 20 to 30 beats higher than the patient's target pacing rate.
- Obtain a printout of the baseline waveform, and place in the patient's medical record.

To begin transcutaneous pacing:

- If the patient is awake, them that they may feel a twitching sensation and that you can administer a sedative to help tolerate the discomfort, if needed.

Turn the pacer function on by either turning a switch or pressing the *PACER* button.

- Check the waveform, looking for a tall QRS complex in lead II.
- Choose either a "Fixed" or "Demand" mode for the pacemaker, if the option is presented. A "fixed" mode will deliver an electrical stimulus continuously at the rate set, regardless of the patient's own underlying heart rate. The "demand" mode will deliver an electrical stimulus if the patient's own heart rate drops below the demand rate set on the defibrillator.
- Set the dial to a target pacing heart rate of 60 to 70 beats/minute.
- Press the *START* button to begin pacing, if needed, based on the machine.
- Look for pacer artifact spikes. Slowly increase the amount of energy (mA) delivered to the heart by adjusting the OUTPUT dial. Do this until capture is achieved—you'll see a pacer spike followed by a widened QRS complex that resembles a premature ventricular contraction. This is the pacing threshold (the usual pacing threshold is between 40 and 80 mA). To ensure capture, increase output by 10%.
- When full capture is achieved, the patient's pulse should be the same as the pacemaker rate shown on the machine. Print a strip that documents the patient's paced rhythm and place in his medical record.

What to consider

- Pacing can cause discomfort. Provide sedation and analgesia as needed.
- The practitioner may order a transcutaneous pacemaker to be on "stand-by" when the patient has a bradycardic rhythm but doesn't have symptoms of hemodynamic instability. If instability develops, the pacemaker can be quickly turned on.
- Work to correct underlying causes of the bradycardia. If the patient is waiting for a transvenous or permanent pacemaker, provide emotional support until the procedure is completed.

Transvenous pacemaker

A transvenous pacemaker is an inserted pacemaker that is more comfortable and typically less painful for the patient than a transcutaneous pacemaker. Inserting it is an invasive procedure, which carries a risk for complications.

Pulse power

With a transvenous pacemaker, an electrode catheter is threaded through a large vein into the patient's right atrium or right ventricle. The electrode is then attached to a pulse generator, which can provide an electrical stimulus directly to the endocardium. (See *Pulse generator features*.)

How it's done

- Done appropriate PPE including gloves, eye protection, and facial coverings including an N95 respirator if appropriate.
- Identify the patient using two patient identifiers.
- If possible, explain the procedure to the patient and answer all questions.

Pulse generator features

This illustration describes the features of a temporary pulse generator.

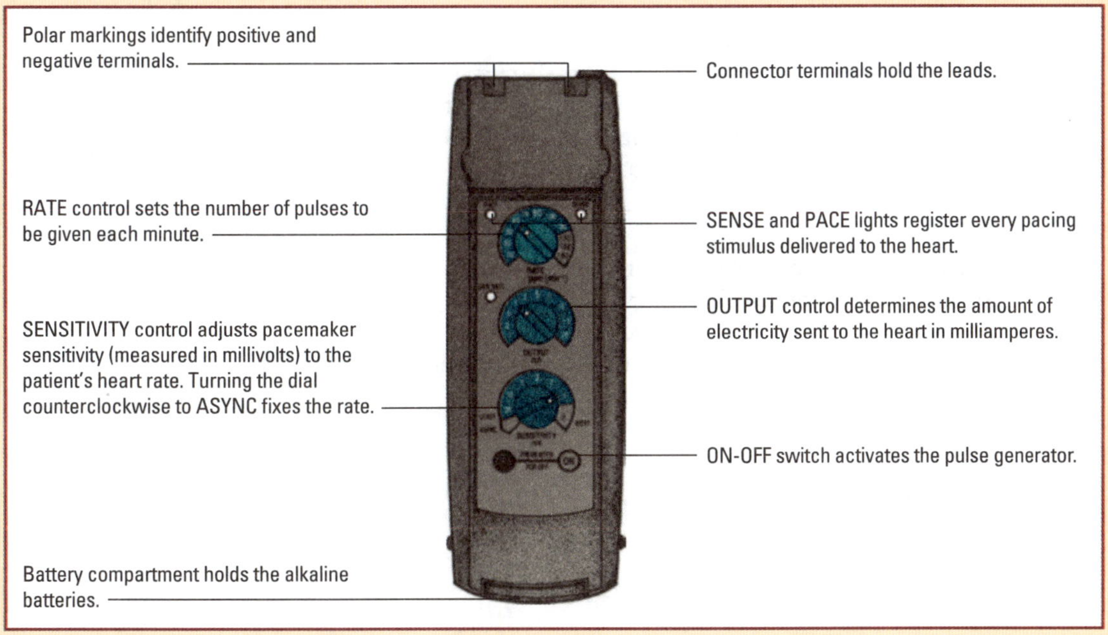

Polar markings identify positive and negative terminals.

Connector terminals hold the leads.

RATE control sets the number of pulses to be given each minute.

SENSE and PACE lights register every pacing stimulus delivered to the heart.

OUTPUT control determines the amount of electricity sent to the heart in milliamperes.

SENSITIVITY control adjusts pacemaker sensitivity (measured in millivolts) to the patient's heart rate. Turning the dial counterclockwise to ASYNC fixes the rate.

ON-OFF switch activates the pulse generator.

Battery compartment holds the alkaline batteries.

- If the procedure is not being done emergently, obtain informed consent.
- Attach the patient to a cardiac monitor and obtain a baseline cardiac rhythm. Print a rhythm strip, and place in the patient's medical record.
- Perform a baseline assessment including the patient's vital signs, oxygen saturation, skin color, and LOC.
- Ensure that the patient has a patent peripheral IV line.
- Put a new battery into the external pacemaker generator, and test it to make sure it has a strong charge.
- Connect the bridging cable to the generator, and align the positive and negative poles.
- Place the patient in a supine position and perform hand hygiene.
- Put on sterile gown and gloves and then open the supply tray (maintain a sterile field).
- Using an antibacterial solution, clean the insertion site and cover it with a sterile drape.
- The practitioner will puncture the brachial, femoral, subclavian, or jugular vein and insert the guide wire or introducer, advancing the electrode catheter.
- Watch the cardiac monitor as the catheter is advanced into the heart and identify and treat arrhythmias appropriately.
- When the electrode catheter is in place, attach the catheter leads to the bridging cable, lining up the positive and negative poles.
- Check the battery's charge again by pressing the BATTERY TEST button.
- Set the pacemaker adjusting the output and sensitivity until it fires at the preset rate and 100% capture occurs. Each pacemaker spike should be followed by a wide QRS complex on the cardiac monitor. Print a strip showing the patient's paced rhythm and place in the patient's medical record.

What to consider

- Inserting a transvenous pacemaker is an invasive procedure. Monitor for complications, such as bleeding or pneumothorax. Be sure to obtain a chest X-ray after the procedure.
- Monitor the patient's movement and positioning carefully, so the pacemaker wires do not dislodge.
- Monitor cardiac rhythm continuously for appropriate pacemaker function.
- Prepare the patient for permanent pacemaker insertion, if appropriate.

Evaluating pacemaker function

As part of performing ACLS, you may need to evaluate a patient's temporary pacemaker. Follow these steps:

- Review the patient's 12-lead ECG.
- Select a monitoring lead that clearly shows the pacemaker spikes.
- When you evaluate the ECG tracing, consider the pacemaker settings and be sure to answer these questions:
  - Is there capture?
  - Is there a P wave or QRS complex after each pacer spike?
  - Do P waves and QRS complexes stem from intrinsic activity?
  - If intrinsic activity is present, what's the pacemaker's response? (See *Pacemaker spikes*)
- Determine the rate by quickly counting the number of complexes in a 6-second ECG strip or, more accurately, by counting the number of small boxes between complexes and dividing by 1,500.

After you have evaluated the pacemaker, you can then determine if any of the four common pacemaker problems that can occur with a temporary pacemaker are present: failure to capture, failure to pace, failure to sense, or oversensing.

Pacemaker spikes

Pacemaker impulses (stimuli that travel from the pacemaker to the heart) are visible on the patient's electrocardiogram tracing as spikes. Whether large or small, the spikes appear above or below the isoelectric line. This example shows an atrial and a ventricular pacemaker spike.

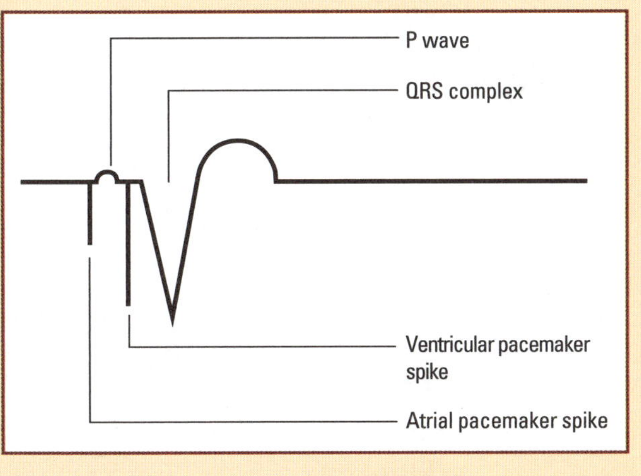

Failure to capture

Failure to capture appears on an ECG as a pacemaker spike without the appropriate atrial or ventricular response (a spike without a complex). Failure to capture indicates the pacemaker's inability to stimulate the heart chamber. (See *Failure to capture.*)

Causes of failure to capture include:

- battery depletion
- incorrect lead position or connection
- low mA setting
- myocardial infarction
- acidosis or electrolyte imbalance
- fibrosis
- broken or cracked leadwire
- perforation of the leadwire through the myocardium

To treat failure to capture:

- change the battery.
- check all connections and gradually increase mA setting to see if capture occurs, according to your facility's protocol.
- obtain a chest X-ray to determine lead placement.
- treat metabolic or electrolyte disturbances.
- prepare to initiate transcutaneous pacing if a transvenous or permanent pacemaker continues being unable to capture, especially if the patient becomes symptomatic.

Failure to capture

This illustration shows failure to capture, in which the pacemaker spike is seen, but there's no response from the heart.

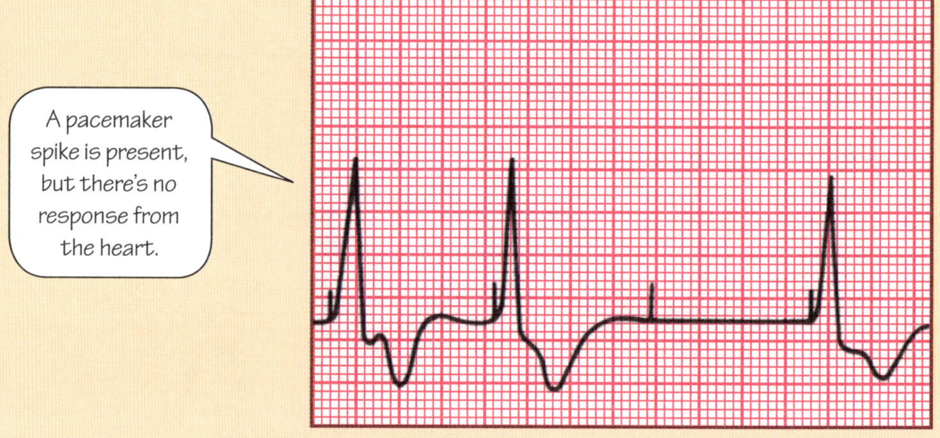

Failure to pace

Failure to pace is seen as no pacemaker activity on an ECG. It can lead to asystole. (See *Failure to pace*.)

Causes of failure to pace include the following:
- Battery or circuit failure
- Cracked or broken leads

Failure to pace can lead to asystole. To treat failure to pace:
- Change the battery if the pulse generator is turned on but the indicators aren't flashing.
- If the pacing or indicator light of the pulse generator flashes, check the connections to the cable; obtain a chest X-ray to check the position of the pacing electrode with a transvenous pacer.
- Make sure transcutaneous pacing pads are adhering adequately to the skin and are in the correct position.
- Initiate CPR if the patient becomes unresponsive and does not have a palpable pulse.

Uh oh! If a temporary pacemaker fails to pace, it could result in asystole.

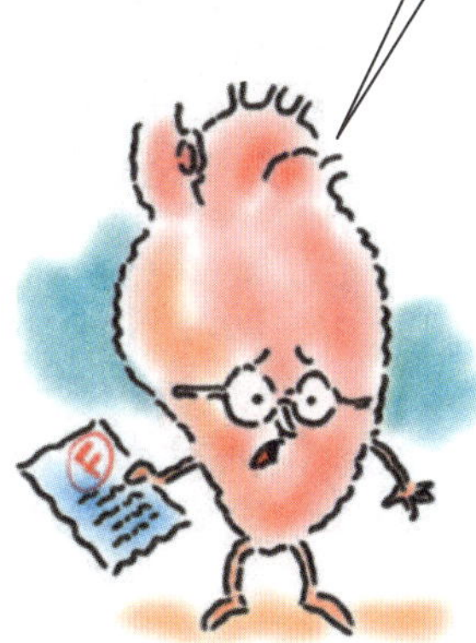

Failure to pace

This illustration shows failure to pace, in which the pacemaker spike isn't seen and no electrocardiogram complex occurs.

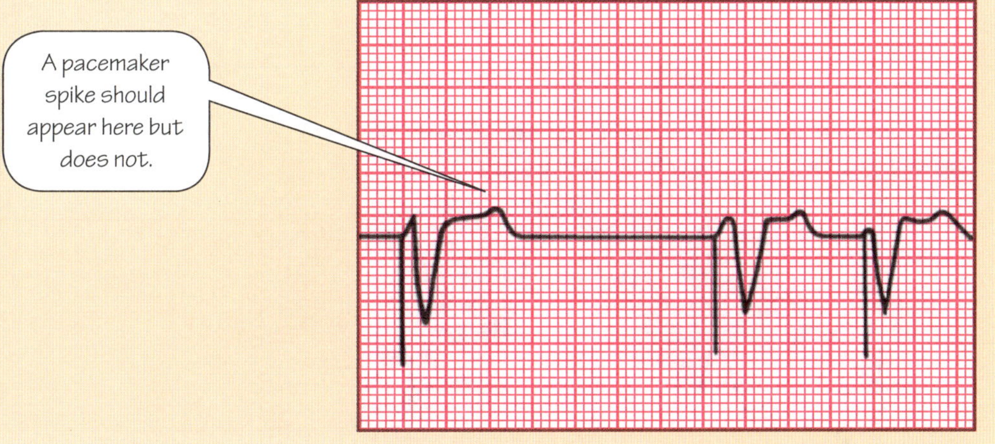

Failure to sense

Failure to sense, or *undersensing*, is indicated by a pacemaker spike that occurs abnormally when intrinsic cardiac activity is already present. If a spike falls on the T wave, it can result in VT or VF. (See *Failure to sense*.)

Causes of failure to sense include:

- Electrolyte imbalances
- Disconnection of a lead
- Improper lead placement
- Increased sensing threshold from edema or fibrosis at the electrode tip
- Drug interactions
- Ineffective pacemaker battery

To treat failure to sense:

- If the pacemaker is undersensing (it fires but at the wrong times or for the wrong reasons), adjust the SENSITIVITY setting, according to your facility's protocol.
- Change the battery or pulse generator.
- Remove items in the room that may be causing electromechanical interference.
- Check to ensure that the equipment is grounded.
- If the pacemaker is firing on the T wave and all corrective actions have failed, turn it off. Be prepared to initiate ACLS protocol, depending on the resulting rhythm.

Failure to sense

This illustration shows failure to sense intrinsic beats, in which the pacemaker spike is seen firing at the wrong time or for the wrong reason.

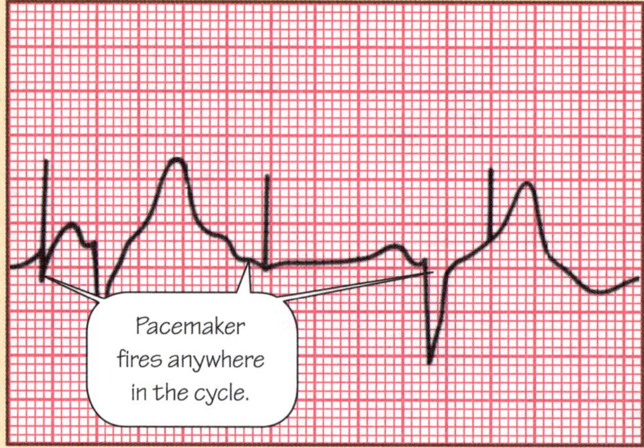

Oversensing

If the pacemaker is too sensitive, it can misinterpret muscle movement or other events in the cardiac cycle as depolarization. It won't pace the patient when needed, and their heart rate and AV synchrony will not be maintained.

Causes of oversensing include the following:

- Pacemaker not programmed accurately
- Improper lead placement
- Disconnection of a lead

To treat oversensing, adjust the sensitivity setting, according to your facility's protocol.

Quick quiz

1. A hospitalized 68-year-old patient is found unresponsive during hourly rounding. They have no pulse and are not breathing. CPR is initiated, and help is called. Defibrillator pads are placed, and the rhythm on the cardiac monitor is identified as VF. What is the appropriate biphasic energy level (joules) for defibrillation of this patient?
   - A. 100 joules
   - B. 200 joules
   - C. 300 joules
   - D. 360 joules

Answer: B. The appropriate biphasic energy level for defibrillation is 120 to 200 joules.

2. A 70-year-old patient collapses on the golf course. CPR is initiated by bystanders, and an AED is brought to the scene. The next appropriate action is:
   - A. Turn the AED on.
   - B. Apply the AED pads.
   - C. Stop CPR so the AED may be utilized.
   - D. Charge the AED to shock the patient as soon as possible.

Answer: A. Turn the AED on and follow instructions provided by the machine.

3. A patient presents to the emergency room with the complaint of weakness and chest tightness. The patient is connected to the cardiac monitor and found to be in third degree ventricular block with a rate of 32 beats/minute. The patient then becomes unresponsive with a blood pressure of 70/40. Which intervention would be most appropriate for immediate treatment?

A. Initiate CPR.
B. Obtain a stat electrocardiogram.
C. Initiate transcutaneous pacing.
D. Obtain laboratory specimens to help identify the cause of the arrhythmia.

Answer: C. The patient has an unstable bradycardic rhythm. Initiation of a transcutaneous pacemaker is an appropriate emergent intervention.

4. A patient is in the intensive care unit with a transvenous pacemaker in place. Their nurse notes several pacemaker spikes on the cardiac monitor without a following QRS complex. This occurrence may be interpreted as:

A. failure to sense
B. failure to capture
C. failure to pace
D. overpacing.

Answer: B. A spike occurring without a complex following it indicates that the pacemaker isn't capturing or stimulating the heart chamber.

5. A 50-year-old patient is experiencing supraventricular tachycardia (SVT) at a rate of 215 that has not responded to vagal maneuvers of drug therapy. The patient's blood pressure is dropping and they are becoming more lethargic. The next treatment to be considered is:

A. pacemaker insertion
B. defibrillation
C. CPR
D. synchronized cardioversion.

Answer: D. Synchronized cardioversion is an appropriate treatment for the deteriorating patient with SVT.

Scoring

☆☆☆ If you answered all five questions correctly, super! Your knowledge is electrifying.

☆☆ If you answered four questions correctly, good for you! You're pacing yourself very well.

☆ If you answered fewer than four questions correctly, don't worry! With just a little stimulus, you'll generate a perfect score next time.

Suggested references

American Heart Association (2020). *Advanced cardiovascular life support provider manual,* E-book edition.

American Heart Association. (2020). *Highlights of the 2020 American Heart Association guidelines update for CPR and ECC.* Dallas, TX: American Heart Association.

Rea, T. D., & Eisenberg, M. S. (2015). Automated external defibrillators. In R. L. Page (Ed.), *UpToDate.* Retrieved from www.uptodate.com

Chapter 6

Cardiovascular pharmacology

Just the facts

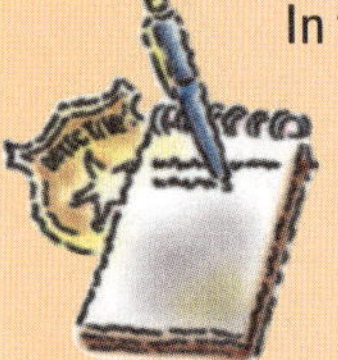

In this chapter, you'll learn:

- guidelines for administering emergency medications
- medications commonly used when following advanced cardiovascular life support (ACLS) algorithms
- medication indications and dosages
- antidotes for the most common medication overdoses

Emergency medication administration

Emergency medications used during ACLS situations are given most frequently by IV push or IV infusion. If you can't obtain peripheral or central IV access, then you may give medications via the intraosseous (IO) route (bone marrow cavity is accessed) and some medications via an endotracheal (ET) tube during cardiac arrest. Depending on the specific situation, you may also give medications subcutaneously, orally, or sublingually.

Here are some general pointers to remember when administering medication:

- Keep in mind that elderly patients usually require smaller dosages than do other adult patients.
- You may need to reduce the dosage for an adult patient with organ impairment (especially kidney or liver) because medication metabolism and excretion may be altered significantly.
- Remember that a patient may be taking over-the-counter (OTC) medications, illegal drugs, or herbal remedies or may be consuming food or beverages that interact with the medication.
- Be aware that a patient may have known or unknown medication allergies; any medication has the potential to cause an anaphylactic or hypersensitivity reaction.
- After you administer a medication, continually monitor the patient for the medication's effects, including adverse reactions. This includes continuous cardiac monitoring; assessing vital signs before, during, and after giving the medication; and additional assessment indicated by the medication use.

ACE inhibitors

Angiotensin-converting enzyme (ACE) inhibitors are used to reduce mortality and improve left ventricular function in patients with postacute myocardial infarction (MI). They prevent adverse left ventricular remodeling, delay the progression of heart failure, and decrease sudden death and recurrent MI. They also reduce mortality and alleviate symptoms in patients with symptomatic heart failure and heart failure with reduced ejection fraction.

Usually given within the first 24 hours after the onset of acute MI symptoms and after blood pressure has stabilized, ACE inhibitors are indicated for suspected MI and ST-segment elevation in two or more precordial leads, hypertension, and heart failure (without hypotension). ACE inhibitors should also be used when clinical signs of acute MI with left ventricular dysfunction are present and left ventricular ejection fraction is less than 40%. (See *General precautions for ACE inhibitors*.)

ACE-ing hypertension

ACE inhibitors reduce blood pressure by interrupting the renin-angiotensin-aldosterone cycle. They specifically prevent the conversion of angiotensin I to angiotensin II, a potent vasoconstrictor. Reduced formation of angiotensin II decreases peripheral arterial resistance, thus decreasing aldosterone secretion, sodium and water retention, and blood pressure. ACE inhibitors also decrease sys-

General precautions for ACE inhibitors

Observe these general precautions when you administer angiotensin-converting enzyme (ACE) inhibitors:

- Use with caution in patients with renal impairment.
- Excessive hypotension may occur when given with diuretics or other antihypertensives.
- The risk of hypoglycemia and hyperkalemia is increased in patients with diabetes.
- The risk of hyperkalemia is increased in patients also taking potassium-sparing diuretics.
- Hyperkalemia may occur in patients also taking potassium-containing salt substitutes.
- Don't give to patients taking lithium because ACE inhibitors may increase lithium levels and cause toxicity.
- Don't give to pregnant women because fetal injury or death may occur.

temic vascular resistance (afterload) and pulmonary artery wedge pressure (PAWP; preload), thus increasing cardiac output in patients with heart failure. (See *How ACE inhibitors work.*)

Commonly prescribed ACE inhibitors include captopril, enalapril, lisinopril, and ramipril.

Enalapril

Enalapril (Vasotec) is used to treat hypertension and heart failure. Like captopril, it prevents the conversion of angiotensin I to angiotensin II, thus reducing blood pressure. You may also give the IV form of enalapril—enalaprilat (Vasotec IV).

How to give it

Here's how to administer enalapril:

- Orally—Give 2.5 mg as a single dose initially and then increase to 20 mg two times per day.
- IV—Give an initial 1.25 mg IV dose slowly over 5 minutes and then 1.25 to 5 mg IV every 6 hours. Alternatively, you can dilute the medication in 50 mL of a compatible solution (such as dextrose 5% in water [D_5W], normal saline solution for injection, dextrose 5% in lactated Ringer's solution, dextrose 5% in normal saline solution for injection, or Isolyte E) and infuse it over 15 minutes.

What can happen

Adverse reactions to enalapril include hypotension; tachycardia; angina; angioedema; persistent, dry nonproductive cough; hyperkalemia; leukopenia; and agranulocytosis.

What to consider

- Closely monitor blood pressure response to the medication.
- Monitor the patient's potassium intake and potassium level. Patients with diabetes, those with impaired renal function, and those receiving medications that may increase the potassium level may develop hyperkalemia.
- Assess renal function before and throughout therapy; monitor the patient for increased blood urea nitrogen (BUN) and creatinine levels.
- Aspirin and other NSAIDs may decrease the antihypertensive effect of enalapril.
- Enalapril is contraindicated during pregnancy and in patients with angioedema or bilateral renal artery stenosis.

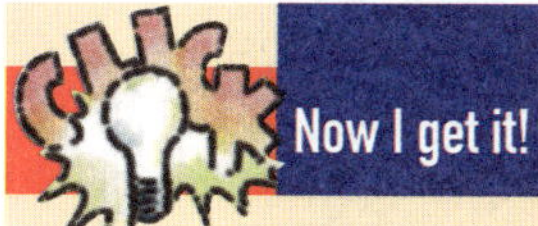

Now I get it!

How ACE inhibitors work

Angiotensin-converting enzyme (ACE) inhibitors reduce blood pressure by interrupting the renin-angiotensin-aldosterone system, which prevents the conversion of angiotensin I to angiotensin II.

The renin-angiotensin-aldosterone system pathway

Sodium depletion, reduced blood pressure, dehydration

↓

Juxtaglomerular cells of the kidney release renin.

↓

Renin

↓

Renin reacts with angiotensinogen and angiotensinogen converted to angiotensin I.

↓

Angiotensin I

↓

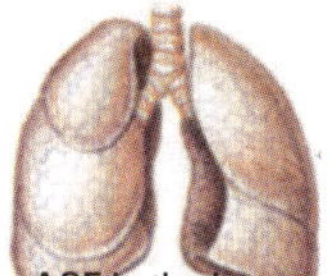

ACE in the lungs ← * ← *ACE inhibitor—inhibits angiotensin-converting enzyme and prevents conversion of angiotensin I to angiotensin II.

ACE in the lungs → Angiotensin II → Aldosterone production

- Angiotensin II → Vasoconstriction of arterioles → Increased blood pressure
- Aldosterone production → Sodium and water retained by kidneys → Increased blood volume and increased blood pressure

*ACE inhibitor:

- Arterioles dilate and peripheral vascular resistance is reduced. → Reduced blood pressure
- Reduced aldosterone secretion → Increased sodium and water secretion → Reduced blood pressure

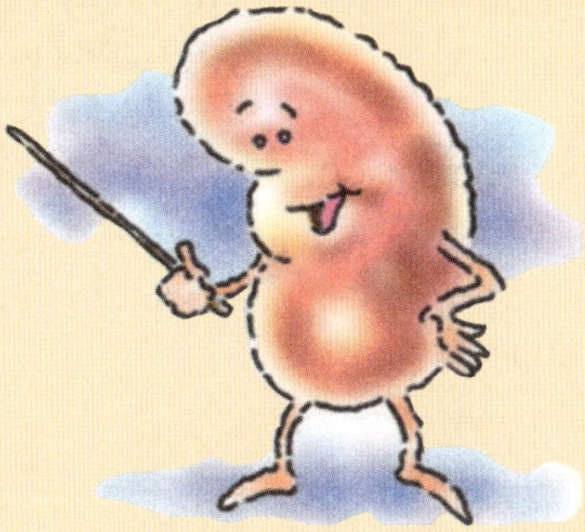

Key: * = Treatment with ACE inhibitor blocks rest of renin-angiotensin-aldosterone system pathway.

Lisinopril

Lisinopril (Prinivil, Zestril) is used to treat hypertension and heart failure as well as to improve patient survival after acute MI. Like the other ACE inhibitors, it lowers blood pressure by preventing the conversion of angiotensin I to angiotensin II.

When administering lisinopril, carefully monitor your patient's blood pressure response.

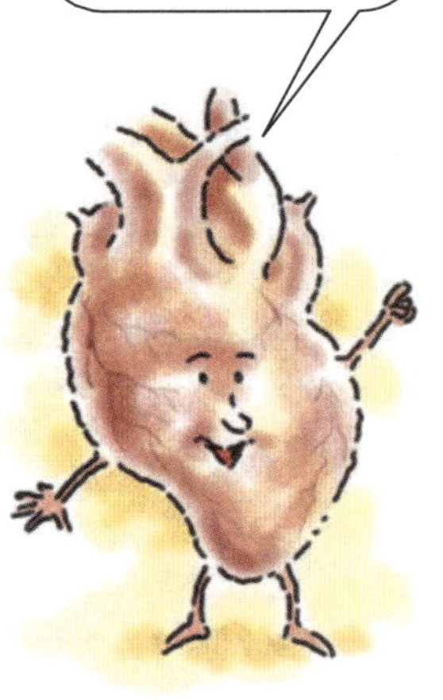

How to give it

Here's how to administer lisinopril:

- For heart failure—Give 5 mg orally once per day, increase as tolerated to 40 mg once per day.
- For acute MI—Give 5 mg orally within the first 24 hours of symptom onset, 5 mg after 24 hours, and 10 mg once per day.

What can happen

Adverse reactions to lisinopril include hypotension; tachycardia; angina; angioedema; persistent, dry nonproductive cough; hyperkalemia; and leukopenia.

What to consider

- Closely monitor blood pressure response to the medication.
- Monitor the patient's potassium intake and potassium level. Patients with diabetes, those with impaired renal function, and those receiving medications that may increase the potassium level may develop hyperkalemia.
- Use lisinopril cautiously in patients with impaired renal function because hyperkalemia may occur. BUN and creatinine levels may increase.
- Aspirin and other NSAIDs may decrease the antihypertensive effect of lisinopril.
- Lisinopril is contraindicated during pregnancy and for patients with a history of angioedema.
- Take caution administering lisinopril with concomitant IV dye in cardiac Cath lab as this can worsen renal function.

Adrenergics

Adrenergic medications are also called *sympathomimetic medications* because they produce effects similar to those produced by the sympathetic nervous system (SNS). These medications are typically used for ACLS as cardiac stimulants to restore heart rate, rhythm, and blood pressure while resuscitating the patient. Adrenergic medications include epinephrine, dopamine hydrochloride, dobutamine hydrochloride, norepinephrine, and isoproterenol. Vasopressin, or antidiuretic hormone, is a posterior pituitary hormone that has adrenergic properties and is used to treat adult shock.

Epinephrine

Epinephrine is a naturally occurring catecholamine used for its bronchodilator, vasopressor, and cardiac stimulant effects. It's used to treat cardiac arrest (VF, pulseless ventricular tachycardia [VT], asystole, and pulseless electrical activity [PEA]), symptomatic bradycardia (after atropine), severe hypotension, and severe allergic reactions (when combined with large fluid volumes, corticosteroids, or antihistamines).

Epinephrine acts directly by stimulating alpha- and beta-adrenergic receptors in the SNS. Its main therapeutic effects include relaxation of bronchial smooth muscle, cardiac stimulation, and the dilation of skeletal muscle vasculature.

Relax...

At lower doses, epinephrine relaxes bronchial smooth muscle by stimulating $beta_2$-adrenergic receptors and constricts bronchial arterioles by stimulating alpha-adrenergic receptors, resulting in relief of bronchospasm, reduced congestion and edema, and increased tidal volume and vital capacity. By inhibiting histamine release, it may reverse bronchiolar constriction, vasodilation, and edema. This action is beneficial in asthma exacerbation and anaphylaxis.

...Stimulate

As a cardiac stimulant, higher doses of epinephrine produces positive chronotropic and inotropic effects by acting on $beta_1$ receptors in the heart and increasing cardiac output, myocardial oxygen consumption, and the force of contraction. At higher doses it becomes a nearly pure alpha agent resulting in vasoconstriction.

How to give it

Here's how to administer epinephrine:

- During resuscitation—Give 1 mg (10 mL of 1:10,000 solution) IV or IO push every 3 to 5 minutes; follow each dose with a 20-mL IV flush and elevate the arm for 10 to 20 seconds if administering via a peripheral IV line in the arm. Dosages of up to 0.2 mg/kg may be considered and used with caution.
- For continuous infusion—Add a 1-mg dose (1 mL of 1:1,000 solution) to 500 mL of normal saline solution or D_5W; use an

initial IV infusion rate of 1 mcg/minute; increase to 2 to 10 mcg/minute.

- For profound bradycardia or hypotension—Add 1 mg of 1:1,000 solution to 500 mL of normal saline solution and infuse at a titrated dosage of 2 to 10 mcg/minute.

You can also give epinephrine via an ET tube with confirmed placement by administering 2 to 2.5 mg; diluted in 10 mL of normal saline solution or sterile water every 3 to 5 minutes until IV/IO access is established or spontaneous circulation occurs. Follow each administration with several positive pressure ventilations.

What can happen

Adverse reactions to epinephrine include anxiety, excitability, angina, cardiac arrhythmias, palpitations, hyperglycemia, hypertension, hypertensive crisis, and cerebral hemorrhage.

When epinephrine is given with antihistamines or tricyclic antidepressants, adverse cardiac effects may be potentiated; avoid concomitant use. When used with beta-adrenergic blockers, the cardiac and bronchodilating effects of epinephrine may be antagonized. Additionally, cardiac glycosides may sensitize the myocardium to the effects of epinephrine, causing arrhythmias.

What to consider

- Monitor the patient's heart rate and rhythm and blood pressure response to the medication. Increased heart rate and blood pressure may cause myocardial ischemia.
- Use with caution in patients with myocardial ischemia and hypoxia because epinephrine increases myocardial oxygen demand.
- Don't administer epinephrine with alpha-adrenergic blockers because its vasoconstrictive and hypertensive effects may be counteracted.
- Dosage adjustments may be necessary if the patient is taking antidiabetics because the effect of epinephrine may be decreased.
- Monitor the patient's serum glucose levels because epinephrine may cause hyperglycemia.
- Higher doses of epinephrine (up to 0.2 mg/kg) may result in postresuscitation myocardial dysfunction.
- Epinephrine is incompatible with alkaline solutions (sodium bicarbonate).
- Tissue necrosis and sloughing may occur if IV epinephrine leaks into surrounding tissue.
- Although highly recommended in ACLS, studies have shown that epinephrine does not decrease overall mortality or morbidity despite an increase in ROSC.

Epinephrine

- Produces positive chronotropic and inotropic effects by action on beta1 receptors in the heart
- Indications: cardiac arrest, symptomatic bradycardia, severe hypotension, severe allergic reaction
- Administer 1 mg (10 mL of 1:10,000 solution) IV every 3 to 5 minutes during resuscitation
- May be given via endotracheal tube: 2 to 2.5 mg in 10 mL normal saline solution

Dopamine hydrochloride

Although it's an adrenergic, dopamine is also classified as a vasopressor. Dopamine is used as a secondary medication (after atropine) for symptomatic bradycardia. It's also used to treat hypotension accompanied by signs and symptoms of shock.

Dopamine stimulates the dopaminergic, beta-adrenergic, and alpha-adrenergic receptors of the SNS. It has a direct stimulating effect on beta-1 receptors and little or no effect on beta-2 receptors.

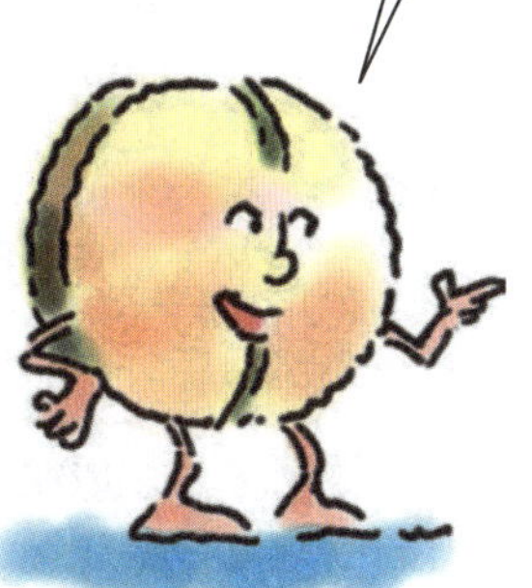

Dose dependence

The effects of dopamine are dose dependent. With IV doses of 0.5 to 5 mcg/kg/minute, it acts on dopaminergic receptors (dopaminergic response), causing vasodilation in the renal, mesenteric, coronary, and intracerebral vascular beds. Low to moderate doses (5 to 10 mcg/kg/minute) produce a beta effect, which results in cardiac stimulation. With IV doses greater than 10 mcg/kg/minute, it stimulates alpha receptors, which results in increased peripheral resistance and renal vasoconstriction. At higher doses (greater than 15mcg/kg/min), it is a pure alpha agent resulting in vasoconstriction.

How to give it

Here's how to administer dopamine:

- Give an IV infusion of 5 to 20 mcg/kg/minute and titrate to the patient's response; taper the infusion slowly.
- Adjust the dosage to meet individual patient needs and to achieve the desired response. Reduce the dosage as soon as the patient's hemodynamic condition is stabilized.

Livin' large

It is best practice to administer dopamine on an infusion pump into a large vein (central venous access is recommended) to prevent the possibility of extravasation. Phentolamine (Regitine) is recommended for all vasoactive agent infiltration, epineprhine, norepinephrine, dopamine, dobutamine, and neosyneprhine.

What can happen

Adverse reactions to dopamine include bradycardia, tachycardia, ventricular arrhythmias, conduction disturbances, hypertension, anxiety, and dyspnea. Severe hypotension may result with abrupt withdrawal of dopamine; remember to taper the dosage gradually.

What to consider

- Before giving dopamine, use the appropriate plasma volume expanders to correct hypovolemia.

- Monitor the patient's heart rate and rhythm and blood pressure response to medication.
- Don't give dopamine to patients with uncorrected tachyarrhythmias, pheochromocytoma, or VF.
- Use caution when giving beta-adrenergic blockers with dopamine because these medications may antagonize cardiac effects.
- Use caution when giving phenytoin (Dilantin) with dopamine because it may cause hypotension and bradycardia.
- Dopamine is incompatible with alkaline solutions (sodium bicarbonate).
- Tissue necrosis medication may occur if the IV medication leaks into surrounding tissue.
- Central line access should be initiated within 12 hours.

Key points

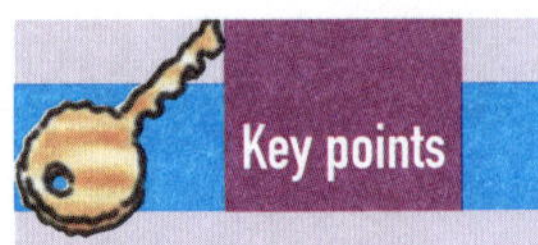

Dopamine hydrochloride
- Vasopressor and adrenergic
- Indications: symptomatic bradycardia, hypotension with signs and symptoms of shock
- Continuous IV infusion: low dose, 0.5 to 5 mcg/kg/minute; cardiac dose, 5 to 10 mcg/kg/minute; vasopressor dose, 10 to 20 mcg/kg/minute

Dobutamine hydrochloride

Dobutamine is used to increase cardiac output in patients experiencing cardiac decompensation with a systolic blood pressure of 70 to 100 mm Hg and no accompanying signs of shock.

Selective stimulator

Dobutamine selectively stimulates beta-1 adrenergic receptors to increase myocardial contractility and stroke volume. This results in increased cardiac output (a positive inotropic effect). Systolic blood pressure and pulse pressure may remain unchanged or may increase as a result of increased cardiac output.

At therapeutic doses, dobutamine decreases peripheral resistance (afterload), reduces ventricular filling pressure (preload), and may facilitate atrioventricular (AV) node conduction.

Dobutamine really helps me get a steady beat going!

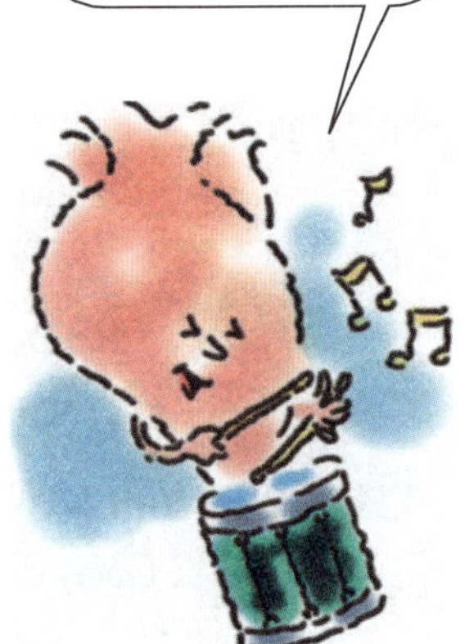

How to give it

Here's how to administer dobutamine:
- Give an IV infusion of 2.5 to 20 mcg/kg/minute; titrate so that the patient's heart rate isn't greater than 10% of baseline.
- Use an infusion pump or other device to control the flow rate.

What can happen

Adverse reactions to dobutamine include tachycardia, fluctuations in blood pressure (hypertension, hypotension), bronchospasm, headache, and nausea.

What to consider

- Before giving dobutamine, use the appropriate plasma volume expanders to correct hypovolemia.

- Monitor the patient's heart rate and rhythm and blood pressure response to the medication; hemodynamic monitoring is recommended to monitor the medication effect.
- Avoid administering dobutamine when systolic blood pressure is less than 100 mm Hg and signs of shock exist.
- Don't give dobutamine if poisoning or medication-induced shock is suspected.
- Don't give beta-adrenergic blockers with dobutamine because these medications may antagonize cardiac effects.
- Don't give tricyclic antidepressants with dobutamine because these medications may potentiate pressor response and cause arrhythmias.
- Don't give in the same IV line with other medications.
- Tissue necrosis and sloughing may occur if the IV medication leaks into surrounding tissue.

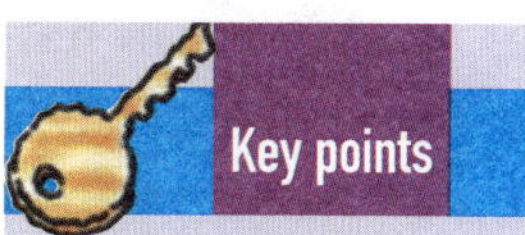

Dobutamine hydrochloride
- Increases cardiac output
- Indications: cardiac decompensation situation with systolic blood pressure of 70 to 100 mm Hg and no signs of shock
- Continuous IV infusion: 2.5 to 20 mcg/kg/minute, titrated so that cardiac rate isn't greater than 10% of baseline

Norepinephrine

Norepinephrine (Levophed) is used to treat hypotension and shock. It's the initial vasopressor of choice in septic, cardiogenic, and hypovolemic shock.

Norepinephrine stimulates alpha- and beta-1 receptors within the SNS. It primarily produces vasoconstriction and cardiac stimulation. At higher doses, it is a pure alpha agent resulting in vasoconstriction.

How to give it

Here's how to administer norepinephrine:

For continuous infusion, add a 4-mg or 8-mg dose to 250 mL of D_5W or dextrose 5% in normal saline solution titrated to the desired effect.

- **Hypotension/shock:** Initially, 0.05 to 0.1 mcg/kg/minute; titrate to desired effect; maximum dose, 2 mcg/kg/minute
- **Post–cardiac arrest care:** Initial, 0.1 to 0.5 mcg/kg/minute (7 to 35 mcg/minute in a 70 kg patient); titrate to desired response.
- **Sepsis and septic shock:** Range from clinical trials, 0.01 to 3 mcg/kg/minute

You may need to give a higher dosage to achieve adequate perfusion in patients with poison-induced hypotension.

Centrally speaking

Remember to administer norepinephrine via a central venous catheter using an infusion pump to minimize the risk of extravasation. Phentolamine 5 to 10 mg in 10 to 15 mL of normal saline solution is used to infiltrate the area to minimize tissue necrosis if extravasation occurs in a peripheral site; must be done within 12 hours of extravasation.

Phentolamine (Regitine) is recommended for all vasoactive agent infiltration. This includes: epinephrine, norepinephrine, dopamine, dobutamine, and neosynephrine.

What can happen

Adverse reactions to norepinephrine include anxiety, excitability, angina, cardiac arrhythmias, palpitations, hypertension, hypertensive crisis, and cerebral hemorrhage.

What to consider

- Administering norepinephrine isn't a substitute for blood or fluid replacement therapy. If the patient has a volume deficit, replace fluid before administering vasopressors.
- Monitor the patient's heart rate and rhythm and blood pressure response to the medication.
- Monitor the patient's extremities for color and temperature.
- Don't give alpha-adrenergic blockers with norepinephrine because these medications may antagonize its effects.
- Severe hypotension may occur when norepinephrine is used with monoamine oxidase inhibitors, methyldopa, or tricyclic antidepressants.
- Norepinephrine is incompatible with alkaline solutions (sodium bicarbonate).
- Tissue necrosis and sloughing may occur if the IV medication leaks into surrounding tissue. Consider phentolamine.

Key points

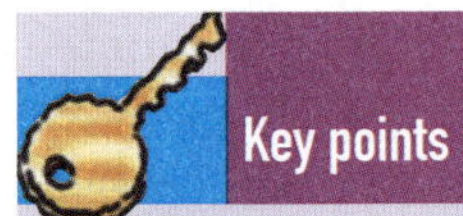

Norepinephrine
- Primarily produces vasoconstriction and cardiac stimulation
- Indications: severe cardiogenic shock, significant hypotension, ischemic heart disease, and shock
- Continuous infusion: 0.5 to 1 mcg/kg/minute titrated to desired blood pressure.

Isoproterenol

Isoproterenol (Isuprel) is a temporary measure for treating symptomatic bradycardia if atropine is ineffective and an external pacemaker isn't available. Due to the availability of alternative agents and its higher cost relative to them, isoproterenol is rarely used; it is primarily reserved for post-heart transplant patients. Dopamine and epinephrine drips are considered for use before administering isoproterenol. It's also used to treat torsades de pointes that doesn't respond to magnesium sulfate, for temporary control of bradycardia in heart transplant patients, and for counteracting beta-adrenergic blocker poisoning. Isoproterenol is contraindicated in cardiac arrest.

Quite an actor

Isoproterenol acts on B1 and B2 adrenergic receptors in a nonselective manner, in the heart, producing a positive chronotropic and inotropic effect. It usually increases cardiac output. In patients with AV block, isoproterenol shortens conduction time and the refractory period of the AV node and increases the rate and strength of ventricular contraction.

I hear isoproterenol shortens the heart's conduction time. Good thing! I could really use an intermission about now.

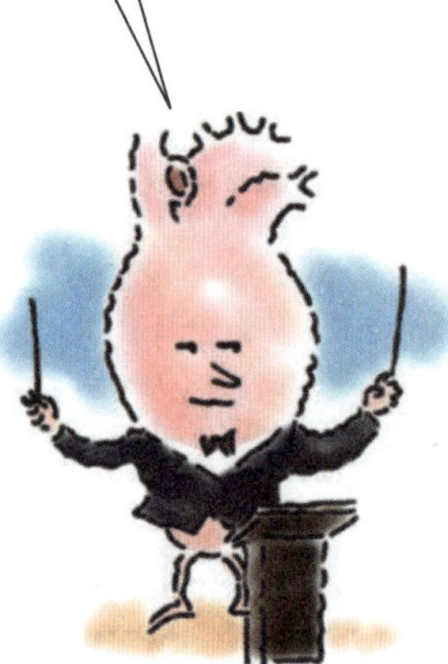

How to give it

Here's how to administer isoproterenol:

- For continuous infusion, add a 1- to 2-mg dose to 500 mL of D_5W and give an IV infusion rate of 2 to 10 mcg/minute; titrate to an adequate heart rate.
- For torsades de pointes, titrate until the rhythm is suppressed.
- Always use an infusion pump for administration.

Because of the danger of arrhythmias, the infusion rate is usually decreased or temporarily stopped if the patient's heart rate exceeds 110 beats/minute. The order for the IV infusion rate should include specific guidelines for regulating the flow or terminating the infusion in relation to heart rate, premature beats, electrocardiogram (ECG) changes, myocardial ischemia, blood pressure, and urine output.

What can happen

Adverse reactions to isoproterenol include anxiety, excitability, angina, cardiac arrhythmias, palpitations, and hypertension.

What to consider

- Remember that isoproterenol doesn't replace the administration of blood, plasma, fluids, or electrolytes in patients with blood volume depletion.
- Monitor the patient's heart rate and rhythm and blood pressure response to the medication. Increased heart rate and blood pressure may cause myocardial ischemia.
- Don't give isoproterenol to patients with tachycardia caused by digoxin toxicity, preexisting arrhythmias (other than those that may respond to treatment with isoproterenol), and angina pectoris.
- Giving isoproterenol with epinephrine or another adrenergic may cause additive reactions and result in VT and VF; allow for at least 4 hours to elapse between administrating the two medications.
- The patient is at increased risk for arrhythmias when isoproterenol is used with cardiac glycosides, potassium-depleting medications, and other medications that affect cardiac rhythm. Additionally, beta-adrenergic blockers antagonize the effects of isoproterenol.

Vasopressin

Vasopressin (antidiuretic hormone) is a nonadrenergic peripheral vasoconstrictor that also causes coronary and renal vasoconstriction. Vasopressin provides hemodynamic support in vasodilatory shock by maintaining coronary perfusion pressure. When given at high doses, vasopressin is a powerful vasoconstrictor of capillaries and small arterioles. One of the benefits of vasopressin is its ability to work in academic environments as compared to other vasopressors.

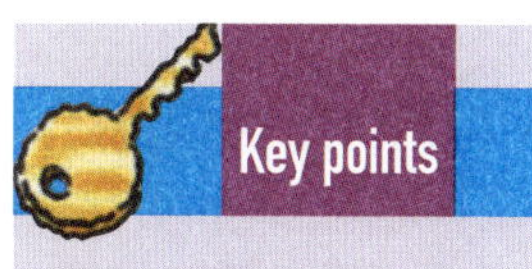

Key points

Vasopressin

- Indications: adult shock: Give 0.03 units per minute (along with norepinephrine) to raise MAP to target.

Totally tubular

Vasopressin acts at the renal tubular level to increase cyclic adenosine monophosphate (cAMP), which, in turn, increases water permeability at the renal tubule and collecting duct. This results in increased urine osmolality and a decreased urine flow rate.

How to give it

Here's how to administer vasopressin:

- For septic shock: Give 0.01 to 0.07 units/min (0.04 units/min is considered a starting dose) along with norepinephrine to raise mean arterial pressure (MAP) to target.
- For hypovolemic shock, GI bleeding dose is: 0.2-0.4 units/min. It may be increased to 0.8 units/min IV.

What can happen

Adverse reactions to vasopressin include cardiac ischemia, angina, bronchoconstriction, and water intoxication.

What to consider

- Monitor the patient's heart rate and rhythm and blood pressure response to the medication. Potent vasoconstrictor medication effects may cause myocardial ischemia.
- Assess for hypersensitivity reactions, including urticaria, angioedema, bronchoconstriction, and anaphylaxis.

Analgesics

Morphine sulfate is the analgesic used most often in patients with ST elevation myocardial infarction (STEMI) to help alleviate chest pain unrelieved by nitrates. It should be used with caution in patients with unstable angina and non-ST elevation myocardial infarction (NSTEMI). It's also used to promote relaxation.

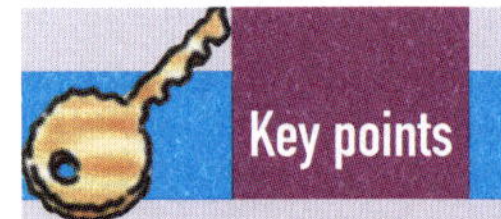

Morphine sulfate

- Opioid agonist that alters the perception of pain
- Indications: pain, acute pulmonary edema
- 2 to 4 mg IV over 1 to 5 minutes; repeat every 5 to 30 minutes and titrate to effect

Morphine sulfate

The most commonly used analgesic in ACLS, morphine is an opioid agonist. It's a schedule II controlled substance indicated for chest pain that doesn't respond to nitrates. Morphine is also given to patients with acute pulmonary edema (if blood pressure is adequate) because it dilates peripheral blood vessels and decreases preload, thus reducing pulmonary congestion and relieving shortness of breath.

The doors of perception

As an opium alkaloid, morphine is thought to work through opiate receptors, altering the patient's perception of pain. It also has a central depressant effect on respiration and the cough reflex center.

How to give it

Here's how to administer morphine:

- Give 2 to 4 mg IV over 1 to 5 minutes; repeat every 5 to 30 minutes based on patient response and condition.
- Rapid IV administration of morphine may result in overdose because of the delay in maximum central nervous system (CNS) effect (30 minutes).

What can happen

Adverse reactions to morphine include respiratory depression, hypotension, bradycardia, shock, cardiac arrest, tachycardia, and hypertension. Apnea and respiratory arrest may also occur. Additionally, morphine may cause hypotension in volume-depleted patients. Correct hypovolemia before giving morphine.

What to consider

- Use morphine with caution in patients with a compromised respiratory state because it may compromise respirations.
- Don't give CNS depressants with morphine because these medications may potentiate its respiratory, sedative, and hypotensive effects.
- If needed, reverse the effects of morphine with naloxone.

Antiarrhythmics

In general, antiarrhythmics are used to treat, suppress, or prevent three major mechanisms of arrhythmias: increased automaticity, decreased conductivity, and reentry. (See *Antiarrhythmic medications and the action potential.*)

Class is in session

Four classes of antiarrhythmic medications exist: I, II, III, and IV. Class I is further subdivided into class IA, IB, and IC. Class IA alters the myocardial cell membrane; class IB blocks the rapid influx of sodium ions; and class IC slows conduction. (See *Guide to common antiarrhythmic medications.*) Several antiarrhythmic medications aren't included in the four classes. These medications include adenosine and atropine. Epinephrine is also considered an antiarrhythmic medication. For class II antiarrhythmics, see *Beta-adrenergic blockers.* For class IV antiarrhythmics, see *Calcium channel blockers.*

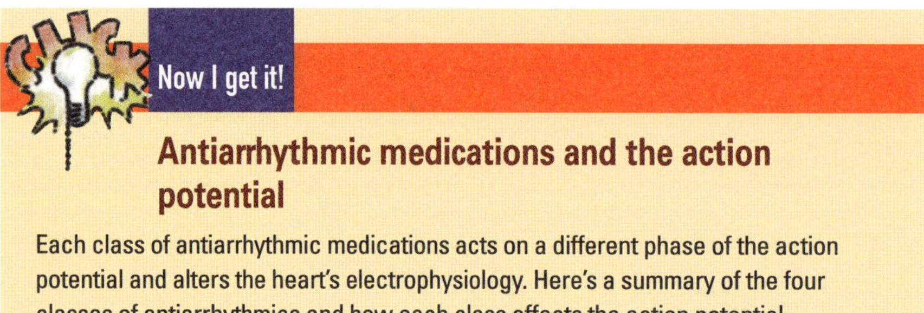

Antiarrhythmic medications and the action potential

Each class of antiarrhythmic medications acts on a different phase of the action potential and alters the heart's electrophysiology. Here's a summary of the four classes of antiarrhythmics and how each class affects the action potential.

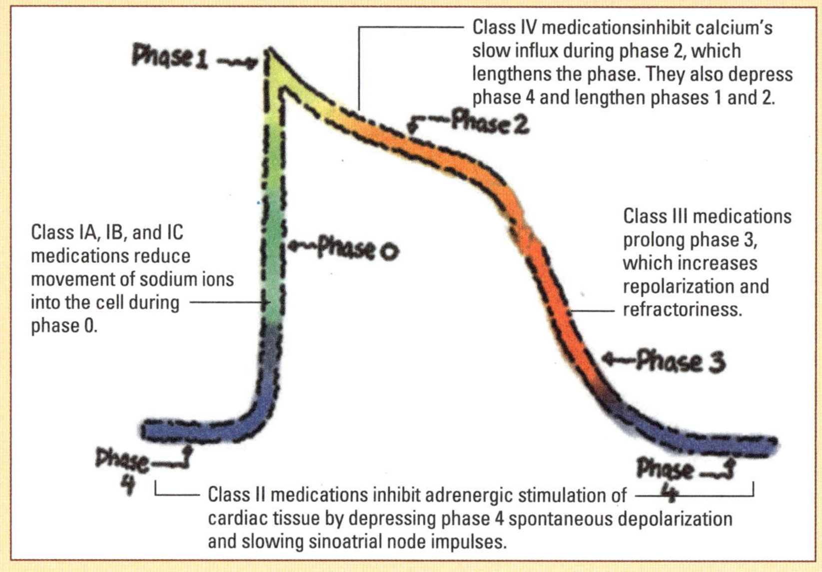

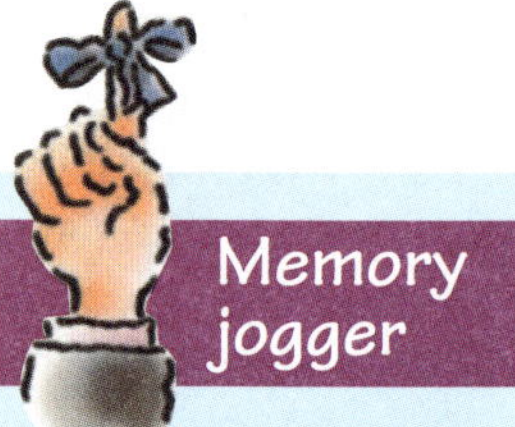

To remember the main differences among class IA, class IB, and class IC antiarrhythmics, just think of their names:

Class I**A**: **A**lters the myocardial cell membrane

Class I**B**: **B**locks the rapid influx of sodium ions

Class I**C**: Slows **C**onduction.

IV antiarrhythmics used during ACLS situations include adenosine, amiodarone hydrochloride, atropine sulfate, lidocaine, ibutilide fumarate, procainamide hydrochloride, and sotalol. Keep in mind that antiarrhythmics may have a more powerful effect when used in combination.

Adenosine

Adenosine (Adenocard) is classified as a miscellaneous antiarrhythmic. A naturally occurring nucleoside, it's used to diagnose and treat paroxysmal supraventricular tachyarrhythmia (PSVT). Adenosine may also be considered for use with regular, monomorphic wide-complex tachycardia (with a pulse) as a diagnostic maneuver. It acts on the AV node to slow conduction and inhibit reentry pathways.

How to give it

Here's how to administer adenosine:

- Give 6 mg IV by rapid bolus injection (due to its short half-life), followed by a rapid flush with 20 mL of normal saline solution.
- If the arrhythmia isn't disrupted in 1 to 2 minutes, give 12 mg IV
- If necessary, you may give a third dose of 12 mg IV Remember, transient arrhythmias or asystole may occur after a rapid IV push.

What can happen

Adverse reactions to adenosine include hypotension, transient bradycardia, ventricular arrhythmias, flushing, chest pain, light-headedness, nausea, and a metallic taste. However, because the half-life of adenosine is less than 10 seconds, adverse effects usually dissipate rapidly and are self-limiting.

What to consider

- Monitor the patient's heart rate and rhythm and blood pressure response to the medication.
- Don't give adenosine to patients with second- or third-degree heart block unless the patient has a pacemaker.
- Don't give to patients with asthma.
- Use adenosine cautiously with other medications:
  - With carbamazepine (Tegretol)—Higher degrees of heart block may occur with concurrent use.
  - With dipyridamole—A smaller dosage may be needed because the medication may potentiate the effects of adenosine.
  - With methylxanthines—These medications antagonize the effects of adenosine.
- Caffeine may antagonize the effects of adenosine; a higher dosage may be needed or the patient may not respond at all.

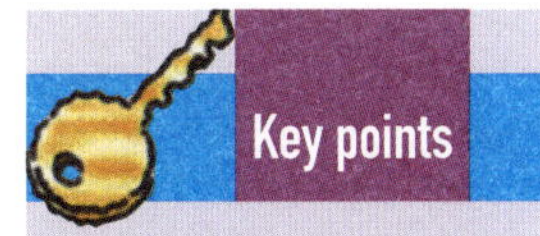

Adenosine

- Acts on the atrioventricular node to slow conduction and inhibit reentry pathways
- Indications: first-line medication for paroxysmal supraventricular tachyarrhythmia
- 6 mg IV by rapid bolus injection
- 12 mg IV if arrhythmia isn't eliminated in 1 to 2 minutes (a third dose of 12 mg IV may be given if necessary)
- Has a short half-life: Must be given as a very rapid IV push

Amiodarone hydrochloride

Amiodarone (Cordarone, Nexterone, Pacerone) is a ventricular and supraventricular antiarrhythmic used to treat recurrent VF, unstable VT, supraventricular arrhythmias, or rapid atrial fibrillation.

Take a load off

Amiodarone has mixed class IC and III antiarrhythmic effects, but it's considered a class III medication. It increases the action potential duration (repolarization inhibition) and has alpha- and beta-adrenergic blocking properties. With prolonged therapy, amiodarone slows conduction through the AV node and prolongs the refractory period. Its vasodilating effect decreases cardiac workload and myocardial oxygen consumption. It also affects sodium, potassium, and calcium channels.

How to give it

Here's how to administer amiodarone:

- For cardiac arrest—Give 300 mg by IV or IO push ; repeat with 150 mg IV push or IO in 3 to 5 minutes; dilute in 20 to 30 mL D_5W.
- For wide-complex tachycardia (life-threatening ventricular arrhythmias)—Give a IV infusion of 150 mg over the first 10 minutes (15 mg/minute) and repeat every 10 minutes as needed; follow with a slow infusion of 360 mg IV over 6 hours (1 mg/minute).
- Maintenance infusion—Give 540 mg IV over 18 hours (0.5 mg/minute).
- Maximum cumulative dose—Give 2.2 g IV over 24 hours.

Remember that amiodarone IV infusions exceeding 2 hours must be administered in glass or polyolefin bottles containing D_5W.

What can happen

Adverse reactions to amiodarone include bradycardia, hypotension, heart failure, arrhythmias, heart block, or sinus arrest. Such adverse reactions are more prevalent with high doses but usually resolve within about 4 months after medication therapy stops. Additional adverse reactions include pulmonary fibrosis, hepatotoxicity, hyperthyroidism, photosensitivity and skin discoloration, and corneal microdeposits.

What to consider

- Watch the patient for hypersensitivity reactions to amiodarone.
- Monitor the patient's heart rate and rhythm and blood pressure response to the medication and monitor the ECG for QT prolongation.
- Don't give amiodarone to patients with severe sinoatrial (SA) node disease resulting in preexisting bradycardia, syncope caused by bradycardia, or, unless a pacemaker is present, second- or third-degree AV block.
- When used with beta-adrenergic blockers or calcium channel blockers, amiodarone may cause sinus bradycardia, sinus arrest, and AV block; use together cautiously.
- Remember that amiodarone can't be removed by dialysis.
- The half-life of amiodarone is up to 40 days.

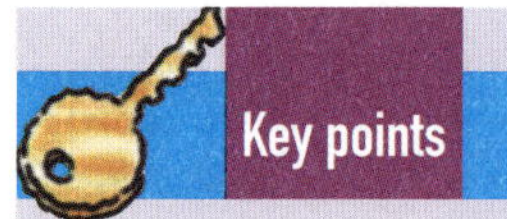

Amiodarone hydrochloride

- Antiarrhythmic that increases the action potential duration
- Indications: recurrent VF, unstable VT, supraventricular arrhythmias, atrial fibrillation, angina, and hypertrophic cardiomyopathy
- For cardiac arrest: give 300 mg IV or IO push; repeat with 150 mg IV or IO push in 3 to 5 minutes.
- For wide-complex tachycardia (stable): Give bolus infusion of 150 mg IV over first 10 minutes (15 mg/minute) and repeat every 10 minutes as needed; slow infusion of 360 mg IV over 6 hours (1 mg/minute) may be given.
- Maintenance infusion is 540 mg IV over 18 hours (0.5 mg/minute).
- Maximum cumulative dose is 2.2 g IV per 24 hours.
- Medication half-life is up to 40 days.

Atropine sulfate

Atropine is classified as a miscellaneous antiarrhythmic. It's used to treat symptomatic bradycardia and bradyarrhythmia (junctional or escape rhythm).

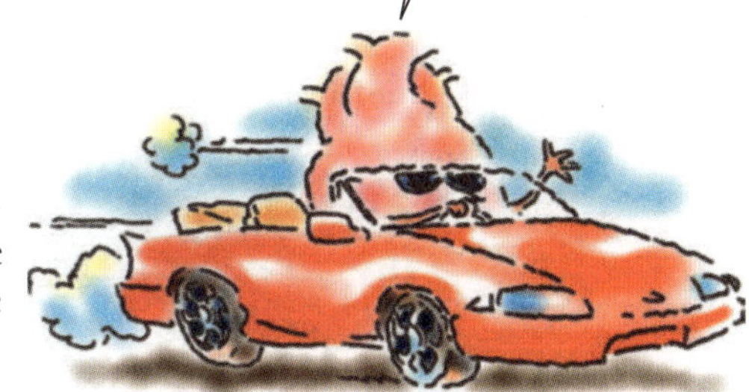

Rate increase

Atropine is an anticholinergic (parasympatholytic) that blocks the effects of acetylcholine on the SA and AV nodes, thereby increasing SA and AV node conduction velocity. It also increases the sinus node discharge rate and decreases the effective refractory period of the AV node. The result is increased heart rate. (See *How atropine speeds the heart rate.*)

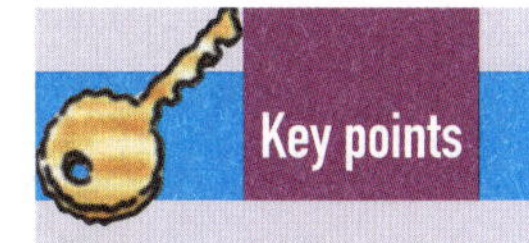

Atropine sulfate

- Blocks the effects of acetylcholine on the sinoatrial (SA) and atrioventricular (AV) nodes, thereby increasing SA and AV node conduction velocity
- Indications: symptomatic bradycardia, bradyarrhythmia (junctional or escape rhythm)
- For bradycardia: 0.5 mg IV every 3 to 5 minutes as needed, not to exceed total dose of 3 mg; shorter dosing interval of 3 minutes and a higher dose may be used with severe clinical condition.

How to give it

Here's how to administer atropine:

- To treat bradycardia—Give 0.5 mg IV every 3 to 5 minutes as needed, not to exceed a total dose of 3 mg. Shorter dosing interval of 3 minutes and a higher dose may be used in severe clinical condition.

Remember that effects on the patient's heart rate peak within 2 to 4 minutes after IV administration.

What can happen

Tachycardia may occur after higher doses of atropine. Signs of atropine overdose reflect excessive cardiovascular and CNS stimulation; treat with physostigmine (Antilirium).

What to consider

- Transplanted hearts lack vagal nerve innervation so atropine won't be effective.
- Monitor the patient's heart rate and rhythm with medication administration.
- Avoid using atropine for hypothermic bradycardia.
- IV administration of less than 0.5 mg may cause paradoxical slowing of the heart rate.
- Use atropine with caution in patients with myocardial ischemia and hypoxia because it increases myocardial oxygen demand.
- Don't give atropine with other anticholinergics or with medications that have anticholinergic effects.
- Atropine is ineffective for infranodal (type II) AV block and new third-degree AV block with wide QRS complexes because paradoxical slowing may occur.

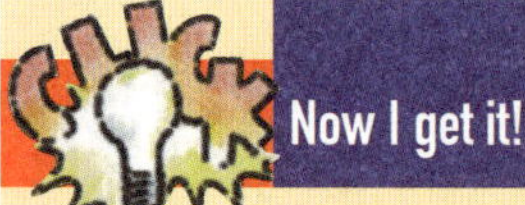

How atropine speeds the heart rate

When acetylcholine is released, the vagus nerve stimulates the sinoatrial (SA) and atrioventricular (AV) nodes, which inhibits electrical conduction. This slows the heart rate. The cholinergic blocker atropine competes with acetylcholine for binding with cholinergic receptors on SA and AV nodal cells. By blocking the effects of acetylcholine, atropine speeds the heart rate.

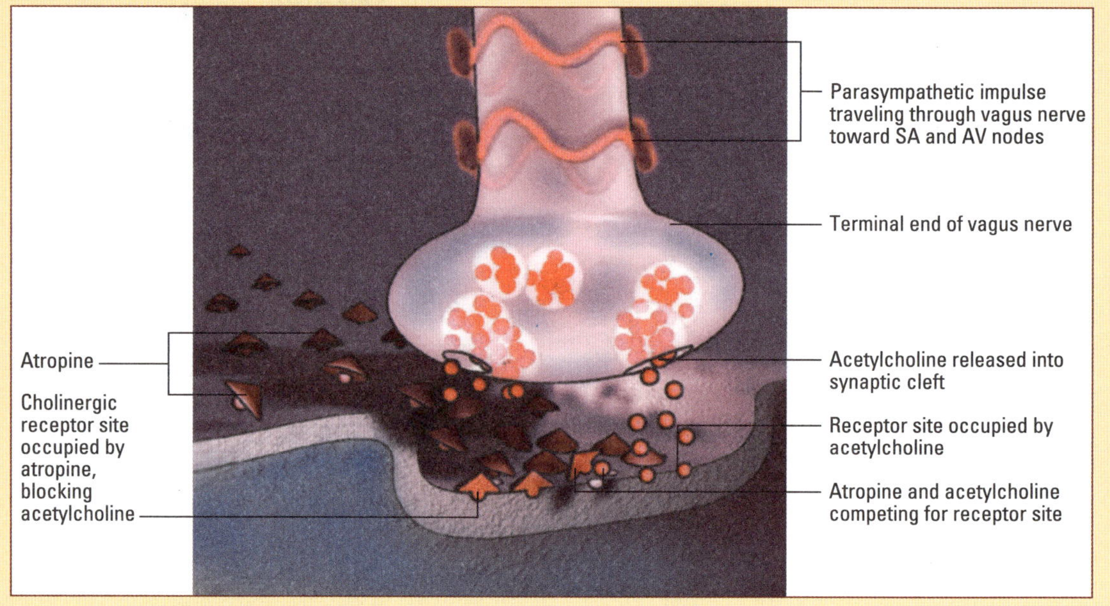

Lidocaine

Lidocaine is a ventricular antiarrhythmic used for cardiac arrest caused by VF or VT, stable VT, wide-complex tachycardia of an uncertain type, or wide-complex PSVT if amiodarone is unavailable. It seems to act preferentially on diseased or ischemic myocardial tissue.

Super suppressant

As a class IB antiarrhythmic, lidocaine suppresses automaticity and shortens the effective refractory period and action potential duration of the His-Purkinje fibers. It also suppresses spontaneous ventricular depolarization during diastole. By exerting its effects on the conduction system, it inhibits reentry mechanisms and halts ventricular arrhythmias.

How to give it

Here's how to administer lidocaine:

- For cardiac arrest—Give a 1 to 1.5 mg/kg IV push or IO dose initially; in refractory VF, you may give an additional 0.5 to 0.75 mg/kg by IV push or IO and repeat in 5 to 10 minutes. The maximum total dosage is 3 mg/kg. A single dose of 1.5 mg/kg by IV push may suffice as treatment in cardiac arrest.
- For endotracheal administration—Give 2 to 3.75 mg/kg diluted in 5 to 10 mL of normal saline solution of sterile water. Follow with several ventilated breaths.
- For perfusing arrhythmia with stable VT, wide-complex tachycardia of uncertain type, or significant ectopy—Give 0.5 to 0.75 mg/kg up to 1.5 mg/kg by IV push; repeat 0.5 to 0.75 mg/kg every 5 to 10 minutes. The maximum total dosage is 3 mg/kg.
- Maintenance infusion—Give 1 to 4 mg/minute IV (20 to 50 mcg/kg/minute).

Remember to use an infusion pump to precisely monitor the lidocaine infusion. Never exceed the infusion rate of 4 mg/minute. A faster rate greatly increases the risk of toxicity.

What can happen

Adverse reactions to lidocaine include hypotension, bradycardia, AV block, confusion, dizziness, restlessness, paresthesia, tinnitus, and agitation. Effects of lidocaine overdose include signs and symptoms of CNS toxicity, such as seizures or respiratory depression, and cardiovascular toxicity resulting in cardiovascular collapse and cardiac arrest.

If you notice signs of excessive cardiac conductivity depression when administering lidocaine, reduce the dosage or stop giving the medication altogether.

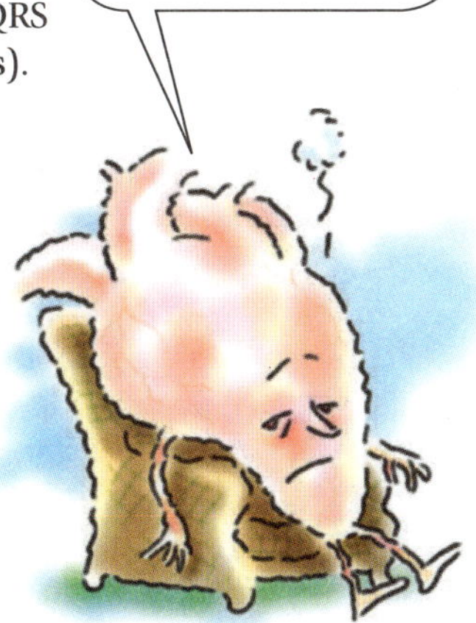

What to consider

- Monitor the patient's heart rate and rhythm.
- Watch the patient for signs of excessive cardiac conductivity depression (such as sinus node dysfunction, PR interval prolongation, QRS interval widening, and appearance or exacerbation of arrhythmias). If they occur, reduce the dosage or stop the medication.
- Don't give lidocaine to patients with hypersensitivity to amide-type local anesthetics, Stokes-Adams syndrome, Wolff-Parkinson-White (WPW) syndrome, and severe degrees of SA, AV, or intraventricular block in the absence of a pacemaker.
- Use caution when giving lidocaine with beta-adrenergic blockers or cimetidine because these medications may cause lidocaine toxicity from reduced hepatic clearance. Other antiarrhythmics (such as phenytoin, procainamide, propranolol, and quinidine) may also cause additive or antagonist effects and additive toxicity when given with lidocaine.

Ibutilide fumarate

Ibutilide (Corvert) is used for supraventricular arrhythmias. It's most effective for the conversion of new-onset atrial fibrillation or atrial flutter. Ibutilide prolongs the action potential in isolated cardiac myocytes and increases atrial and ventricular refractoriness, namely, class III electrophysiologic effects.

How to give it

Here's how to administer ibutilide:

- For adults weighing 132 lb (60 kg) or more—Give a 1 mg IV infusion over 10 minutes, diluted or undiluted; a second dose may be repeated after 10 minutes.
- For adults weighing less than 132 lb—Give a 0.01-mg/kg IV infusion over 10 minutes; a second dose may be given after 10 minutes.

What can happen

Adverse reactions to ibutilide include AV block, bradycardia, bundle-branch block, hypotension, monomorphic and polymorphic VT, palpitations, prolonged QT interval, and ventricular extrasystoles. Polymorphic VT, including torsades de pointes, develops in 2% to 5% of patients after ibutilide is administered. Additionally, ibutilide may worsen ventricular arrhythmias.

What to consider

- Monitor the patient's ECG continuously during medication administration and for at least 4 hours afterward or until QT interval returns to baseline.
- Make sure that a cardiac monitor, defibrillator, and emergency medication to treat sustained VT or VF are available.
- Don't give class IA and class III antiarrhythmics within 4 hours of administering the ibutilide infusion because they can cause prolonged refractoriness.
- Don't give medications that prolong the QT interval, phenothiazines, tricyclic and tetracyclic antidepressants, or certain antihistamines, such as H1 receptor antagonists, with ibutilide because they may cause arrhythmias.
- Patients with atrial fibrillation that lasts more than 2 to 3 days must be adequately anticoagulated, generally for at least 2 weeks, before ibutilide is administered.

Procainamide hydrochloride

Procainamide is a ventricular and supraventricular antiarrhythmic. It's used for several arrhythmias, including PSVT, stable wide-complex tachycardias, and atrial fibrillation with a rapid ventricular rate in WPW syndrome. Procainamide is also recommended for VF or pulseless VT that recurs after periods of non-VF rhythms during cardiac arrest. In all instances, procainamide must be given as a slow IV infusion; therefore, it is not always the optimal treatment.

Procainamide hydrochloride

- The need for slow IV infusion minimizes the medication usefulness in ACLS situations.
- Depresses phase 0 of the action potential: decreases myocardial excitability and conduction velocity and may depress myocardial contractility; also possesses anticholinergic activity that may modify direct myocardial effects
- Indications: wide variety of arrhythmias
- For cardiac arrest and arrhythmia suppression: 20 mg/minute IV infusion with a maximum total dose of 17 mg/kg; doses of up to 50 mg/minute IV may be used.
- Maintenance infusion: 1 to 4 mg/minute

Depress...

As a class IA antiarrhythmic, procainamide depresses the upstroke velocity of the action potential (phase 0 of the depolarization cycle). It's considered a myocardial depressant because it decreases myocardial excitability and conduction velocity and may depress myocardial contractility. Procainamide also acts as an anticholinergic, which may modify direct myocardial effects. In therapeutic doses, the medication reduces conduction velocity in the atria, ventricles, and His-Purkinje system.

...Prolong...

Procainamide also prolongs the PR and QT intervals. It controls atrial tachyarrhythmias by prolonging the effective refractory period and increasing the action potential duration in the atria, ventricles, and His-Purkinje system; the tissue remains refractory even after returning to resting membrane potential.

...Shorten

Procainamide shortens the effective refractory period of the AV node. The medication anticholinergic action may also increase AV node conductivity. Suppression of automaticity in the His-Purkinje system and ectopic pacemakers accounts for the effectiveness of procainamide in treating ventricular premature beats.

How to give it

Here's how to administer procainamide:

- For hemodynamically stable monomorphic VT or pre-excited atrial fibrillation—Give a loading dose by infusing 20 to 50 mg/minute **or** 100 mg every 5 minutes until arrhythmia is controlled, hypotension occurs, QRS complex widens by 50% of its original width, or total of 17 mg/kg is given.
- Follow with a continuous infusion of 1 to 4 mg/minute.

What can happen

Adverse reactions to procainamide include dizziness, heart block, hypotension, liver failure, agranulocytosis, and lupus erythematosus-like syndrome. Medication toxicity may cause severe hypotension, widening QRS complex, junctional tachycardia, intraventricular conduction delay, VF, oliguria, and confusion.

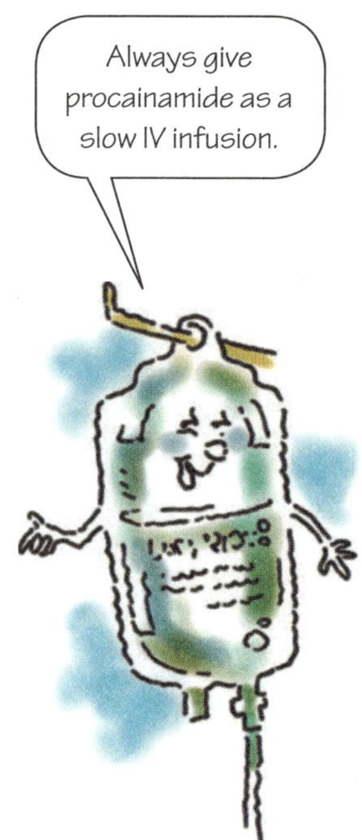

What to consider

- Monitor the patient's heart rate and rhythm and blood pressure response to the medication.
- Watch the patient for prolonged QT and QRS intervals (50% or greater widening), heart block, or increased arrhythmias. If these appear, stop the medication and monitor the patient closely.
- Don't give procainamide to patients with hypersensitivity to procaine and related medication, second- or third-degree AV block in the absence of a pacemaker, myasthenia gravis, systemic lupus erythematosus, or torsades de pointes.
- Use caution when giving procainamide with antihypertensives because these medications may cause additive hypotensive effects. Other antiarrhythmics may cause additive or antagonistic cardiac effects and possible additive toxic effects.
- Procainamide is not recommended for use in ongoing VF or pulseless VT due to the need for slow IV infusion and uncertain efficacy.

Anticoagulants

Unfractionated heparin (UFH) and its derivatives (low-molecular-weight heparin [LMWH], fondaparinux, and bivalirudin) are anticoagulant medications used in cardiac patients to prevent clot formation. These medications are used as adjuvant therapy with fibrinolytic agents and in combination with aspirin to treat patients with acute coronary syndrome (ACS).

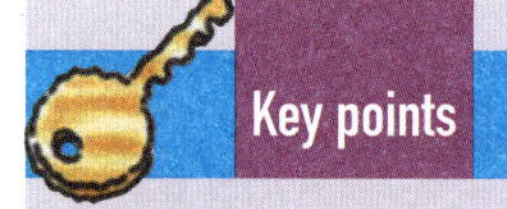

Sotalol

- Depresses sinus heart rate, slows atrioventricular (AV) conduction, increases AV nodal refractoriness, and prolongs the refractory period of atrial and ventricular muscle and AV accessory pathways in anterograde and retrograde directions

Heparin and heparin derivatives

UFH is prepared commercially from animal tissue. Because heparin doesn't affect clotting factor synthesis, it can't dissolve clots that have already formed. LMWH, such as enoxaparin (Lovenox), is derived by decomposing UFH into simpler compounds.

Clots need not apply

Heparin potentiates the effects of antithrombin, which inhibits the conversion of fibrinogen to fibrin. It also inhibits the action of factors IX, X, XI, and XII. Heparin inactivates the fibrin-stabilizing factor, preventing the formation of a stable fibrin clot.

How to give it

Here's how to administer UFH:

- For ST-segment elevation MI—Give an initial IV bolus of 60 units/kg and then 12 units/kg/hour by IV infusion.
- For non–ST-segment elevation MI—Give an initial IV bolus of 60 to 70 units/kg and then 12 units/kg/hour by IV infusion.

Remember to follow your facility's policy for heparin protocol. Adjust the dosage to maintain the partial thromboplastin time (PTT) 1½ to 2 times the control values for 48 hours or until angiography; for activated coagulation time, use 2 to 3 times the control. (The target range for PTT after the first 24 hours is between 50 and 70 seconds but may vary by laboratory.) Anti-Xa monitoring is considered more reliable than aPTT and may be utilized at some facilities. Check your local laboratory for therapeutic value.

To reverse heparin, give 1% solution of protamine sulfate by slow infusion. Remember, hemodialysis doesn't remove heparin.

Here's how to administer LMWH:

- For ST-segment elevation MI as an adjuvant therapy with fibrinolytics—Give enoxaparin 30 mg by IV bolus and then 1 mg/kg subcutaneously every 12 hours.
- For non–ST-segment elevation MI—Give enoxaparin 1 mg/kg subcutaneously every 12 hours; the first dose may be preceded by a 30-mg IV bolus.

Remember to adjust the dosage for patients with a creatinine clearance of less than 30 mL/minute. Follow the prescriber's orders and use cautiously in patients with renal insufficiency.

What can happen

Adverse reactions to UFH and LMWH include bleeding, bruising, hematoma formation, skin irritation, and thrombocytopenia. When used with antihistamines and cardiac glycosides, the anticoagulant effects of heparin may be diminished.

What to consider

- Monitor platelet count and coagulation tests frequently, such as PTT, prothrombin time, and activated coagulation time.
- Monitor the patient for signs of bleeding, which may be difficult to detect. Monitor hematocrit (HCT) frequently and check stools for occult blood to detect asymptomatic bleeding. Inspect venipuncture and wound sites and the skin regularly for bleeding.
- Use heparin cautiously in patients with hemorrhaging (or who are at risk for it) or GI conditions, such as ulcerative colitis, because severe hemorrhage, acute thrombocytopenia, and new thrombus formation (white clot syndrome) may occur.

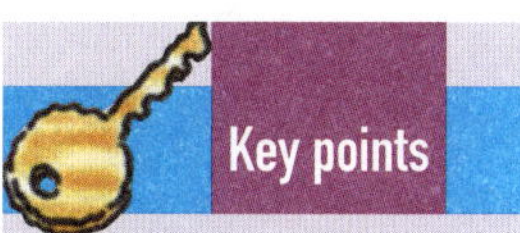

Key points

Heparin

- Potentiates the effects of antithrombin, which inhibits conversion of fibrinogen to fibrin
- Also inhibits the action of factors IX, X, XI, and XII; inactivates fibrin-stabilizing factor and prevents formation of a stable fibrin clot
- Indications: adjuvant therapy in acute myocardial infarction and fibrinolytic therapy
- For ST-segment elevation MI: initial bolus of 60 units/kg and then 12 units/kg/hour IV infusion
- Adjust dosage to maintain partial thromboplastin time 1½ to 2 times the control values for 48 hours or until angiography
- For non–ST-segment elevation MI: initial bolus dose of 60 units/kg and then 12 units/kg/hour IV infusion

- These medications are contraindicated in patients with a platelet count of less than 100,000/mm^3 (SI, 100 × 10^9 /L) or in patients with heparin-induced thrombocytopenia.
- When these medications are used with aspirin, dipyridamole (Persantine), other NSAIDs, or indomethacin (Indocin), impaired platelet aggregation and a possible increased risk of bleeding may occur.
- Heparin is incompatible with alteplase, amiodarone, diazepam, diltiazem, dobutamine, furosemide, morphine sulfate, phenytoin sodium, quinidine gluconate, solutions with a phosphate buffer, sodium carbonate, or sodium oxalate.

Factor Xa inhibitor: Fondaparinux (Arixtra)

Fondaparinux is a synthetic factor Xa inhibitor anticoagulant used to prevent clot formation in patients undergoing surgical procedures. It is also used to treat deep vein thrombus (DVT) and pulmonary emboli (PE) when administered in conjunction with warfarin and as an adjunctive anticoagulant in patients with STEMI who are not undergoing percutaneous coronary intervention (PCI).

How to give it

Here's how to administer fondaparinux:

- Give 2.5 mg IV followed by 2.5 mg subcutaneously once daily (for patients with STEMI being managed medically) (not approved by the US Food and Drug Administration for this use).
- Give 2.5 mg IV as a bolus followed by a subcutaneous dose of 2.5 mg once daily to patients receiving fibrinolytic therapy.
- Give 2.5 mg subcutaneously once daily to patients with NSTEMI managed with a not undergoing PCI.
- For patients who undergo PCI after initial medical therapy with fondaparinux, subsequent dosing depends upon which anticoagulant was given initially.

What can happen

Adverse reactions that can occur with the use of fondaparinux include bleeding and mild local irritation (injection site bleeding, rash, and pruritus). Additionally, anemia, insomnia, increased wound drainage, hypokalemia, dizziness, hypotension, confusion, hematoma, postoperative hemorrhage, and purpura may occur.

What to consider

- Avoid use in patients with estimated creatinine clearance less than 30 mL/minute.
- Not recommended for use in patients undergoing primary PCI

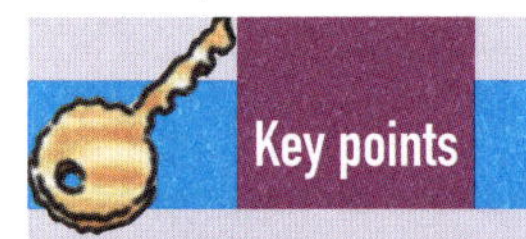

Fondaparinux:

- FDA approved as an anticoagulant in STEMI or NSTEMI
- Not recommended for use in patients undergoing primary PCI
- Contraindicated in patients with a CrCl less than 30 mL/minute and concomitant use of indwelling epidural catheters and other medications that affect hemostasis, such as nonsteroidal anti-inflammatory medications (NSAIDs), platelet inhibitors, or other anticoagulants
- Contraindicated in patients with a history of traumatic or repeated epidural or spinal puncture or a history of spinal deformity or spinal surgery

- Increased bleeding risk in patients with renal impairment or body weight less than 50 kg
- Patient should be monitored for signs of bleeding and thrombocytopenia, such as bruising, hypotension, and decreased hematocrit.
- Should not be used for patients with latex sensitivity because the packaging (needle guard) contains dry natural rubber, which may cause an allergic reaction

Direct thrombin inhibitor—Bivalirudin (Angiomax)

Bivalirudin is a synthetic congener of hirudin and works as an anticoagulant by directly inhibiting thrombin in the clotting cascade thereby preventing the formation of clots. It is used as an anticoagulant in patients with unstable angina undergoing percutaneous transluminal coronary angioplasty (PTCA) and in patients with STEMI/NSTEMI undergoing PCI and is especially useful in patients with heparin-induced thrombocytopenia (HIT) or heparin-induced thrombocytopenia and thrombosis syndrome (HITTS). It is not approved for use in patients with acute coronary syndromes who are not undergoing PTCA or PCI.

How to give it

Here's how to administer bivalirudin:

- PCI/PTCS (without HIT/HITTS): 0.75 mg/kg IV bolus followed by an infusion of 1.75 mg/kg/hour for the duration of the procedure. Five minutes after the bolus dose has been administered, ACT should be performed and an additional 0.3 mg/kg should be given if needed. The infusion may be continued for up to 4 hours for up to 20 more hours at a rate of 0.2 mg/kg/hour.
- PCI (with HIT): 0.75 mg/kg IV bolus followed by an infusion of 1.75 mg/kg/hour for the duration of the procedure. The infusion may be continued for up to 4 hours for up to 20 more hours at a rate of 0.2 mg/kg/hour.
- For patients with CrCl less than 30: 1 mg/kg/hour, for patients undergoing dialysis, the infusion rate should be reduced to 0.25 mg/kg/hour.

What can happen

Common adverse reactions associated with the use of bivalirudin include bleeding, hemorrhage, headache, thrombocytopenia, and fever.

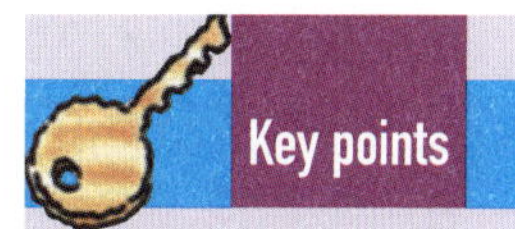

Bivalirudin:

- Intended for use with aspirin 300 to 325 mg/day
- Should be dose adjusted in patients with significant renal impairment, that is, CrCl less than 30 or patients who are undergoing dialysis
- Not indicated for patients with acute coronary syndromes who are not undergoing PTCA or PCI
- Certain patients undergoing PCI may require the additional use of a glycoprotein IIb/IIIa inhibitor.

What to consider

- Monitor the patient for signs of bleeding and thrombocytopenia, such as bruising, hypotension, and decreased hematocrit.
- Monitor complete blood counts (including platelet counts), serum, creatinine level, and stool occult blood tests.

Antiplatelet medications

Antiplatelet medications block the final common pathway of platelet aggregation, improving the prognosis of patients with ST-segment depression and ischemia. They're also used as adjuncts to PCI. The antiplatelet medications used during ACLS and in the immediate postresuscitative period to treat patients with ACS include aspirin, the glycoprotein (GP) IIb/IIIa inhibitors (abciximab, eptifibatide, and tirofiban), and the thienopyridines (clopidogrel, prasugrel, ticlopidine, ticagrelor, and cangrelor).

Awesome analgesic

Aspirin is a nonopioid analgesic with antipyretic, anti-inflammatory, and antiplatelet effects. It's used for all patients with ACS, especially reperfusion candidates, and for anyone with signs of ischemic pain (chest pain described as pressure, heavy weight, squeezing, or crushing). Early administration of aspirin, either in the out-of-hospital setting or emergency department, has decreased mortality in patients with suspected ACS.

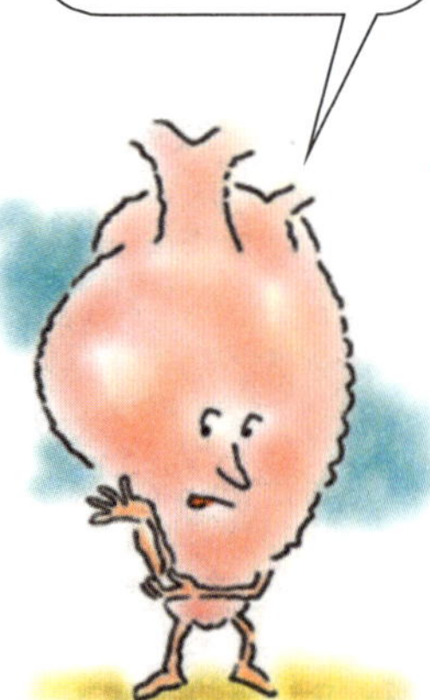

Uninhibited inhibitors

GP IIb/IIIa inhibitors are used to treat ACS without ST-segment elevation. These agents may also be used in a select group of STEMI patients who have no coronary reflow or have a large thrombus burden at the time of PCI. These medications inhibit the integrin GP IIb/IIIa receptor in the membrane of platelets, preventing platelet aggregation and thrombus growth. Be aware of bleeding precautions and other general precautions when using glycoproteins. (See *Bleeding precautions for glycoproteins*.)

Thienopyridines reduce platelet aggregation through a different mechanism than aspirin. They are used in ACS and have been shown to reduce mortality and morbidity in non-STEMI and STEMI.

Aspirin

Aspirin works as an analgesic by affecting the hypothalamus (central action) and blocking the generation of pain impulses (peripheral action). As an anti-inflammatory, aspirin is believed to inhibit prostaglandin synthesis.

Bleeding precautions for glycoproteins

The patient given glycoprotein IIb/IIIa inhibitors may experience bleeding at the arterial access site for cardiac catheterization or internal bleeding involving the GI, genitourinary, or retroperitoneal areas. Follow these precautions when administering glycoproteins:

- Before infusion, measure platelet count, prothrombin time, activated clotting time, and partial thromboplastin time to identify preexisting hemostatic abnormalities.
- Monitor the platelet count before treatment, 2 to 4 hours after treatment, and 24 hours after treatment or before discharge.
- Administer the medication in a separate IV line. (Don't add other medications to infusion solution.)
- Keep emergency medications available in case of anaphylaxis.
- Monitor the patient closely for bleeding.
- Discontinue heparin at least 4 hours before sheath removal.
- Minimize or avoid (if possible) arterial and venous punctures and intramuscular (IM) injections.
- Avoid invasive procedures (if possible), such as nasotracheal intubation or the insertion of urinary catheters and nasogastric tubes.
- Avoid the use of constrictive devices, such as automatic blood pressure cuffs and tourniquets.
- Remember that antiplatelet medications, heparin, nonsteroidal anti-inflammatory medications, thrombolytics, and other anticoagulants may increase the risk of bleeding.

Aspirin

- At low doses, impedes clotting by blocking prostaglandin synthetase action, preventing formation of platelet-aggregating substance thromboxane A2
- Indications: acute coronary syndrome and ischemic pain
- 162 to 325 mg PO and ask the patient to chew it if possible; give rectally if patient can't take PO.
- Give as soon as possible when chest pain occurs.

At low doses, aspirin appears to impede clotting by blocking prostaglandin synthetase action, preventing formation of the platelet-aggregating substance thromboxane A_2. This interference with platelet activity is irreversible and can prolong bleeding time. *At high doses (1,000 mg), aspirin interferes with prostacyclin production, a potent vasoconstrictor and inhibitor of platelet aggregation, possibly negating its anticlotting properties.*

How to give it

Here's how to administer aspirin:

- Give 162 to 325 mg orally, and ask the patient to chew it if possible.
- Give 300 mg rectally if the patient can't take it orally or has a GI problem.
- Give aspirin as soon as possible when chest pain occurs.
- Avoid enteric-coated aspirin.

What can happen

Adverse reactions to aspirin include heartburn, GI distress, GI bleeding, occult bleeding, bruising, and tinnitus.

What to consider

- Don't give aspirin to patients with bleeding disorders or NSAID-induced sensitivity reactions.
- Use aspirin cautiously in patients with GI lesions, impaired renal function, hypoprothrombinemia, vitamin K deficiency, thrombotic thrombocytopenic purpura, or hepatic impairment.
- Use caution when giving aspirin with other GI irritants, such as antibiotics, corticosteroids, and other NSAIDs, because they may potentiate the adverse GI effects of aspirin.
- Anticoagulants and thrombolytics may potentiate the platelet-inhibiting effects of aspirin.
- Enteric-coated products are absorbed slowly and aren't suitable for acute therapy.

Abciximab

Abciximab (ReoPro) binds to the GP IIb/IIIa receptor of human platelets and inhibits platelet aggregation. Abciximab is used to treat patients with medically managed unstable angina or non-STEMI. They are occasionally used in STEMI patients with no reflow or a large thrombus burden at the time of PCI. It's also used for planned PCI within 24 hours.

How to give it

Here's how to administer abciximab:

- For ACS with PCI—Give an IV bolus of 0.25 mg/kg 10 to 60 minutes before the start of the procedure and then give a continuous IV infusion of 0.125 mcg/kg/minute; the maximum dosage is 10 mcg/minute for 12 hours.
- For ACS with planned PCI within 24 hours—Give an IV bolus of 0.25 mg/kg and then give an IV infusion of 10 mcg/minute for 18 to 24 hours, concluding 1 hour after PCI.

Remember to withdraw the necessary amount of abciximab for the bolus injection through a sterile, nonpyrogenic, low-protein-binding 0.2- or 0.22-millipore filter into a syringe. If opaque particles are present, discard the solution and obtain a new vial.

For a continuous IV infusion, inject abciximab into sterile normal saline solution or D_5W, as ordered, and infuse through a continuous infusion pump equipped with an in-line filter. Discard the unused portion at the end of the 12-hour infusion.

What can happen

Adverse reactions to abciximab include bleeding, thrombocytopenia, bradycardia, and hypotension.

What to consider

- Abciximab is intended for use with aspirin and heparin.
- Monitor the patient closely for bleeding at the arterial access sites and for internal bleeding involving the GI or genitourinary (GU) tract or retroperitoneal sites.
- Platelet function recovers in about 48 hours but abciximab remains in the patient's circulation for up to 10 days in a platelet-bound state.

Clopidogrel

Clopidogrel (Plavix) is a thienopyridine that inhibits platelet function by binding to the adenosine diphosphate (ADP) P2Y12 receptors on platelets. It's used for patients up to age 75 with non-STEMI or STEMI (in addition to standard treatment, including fibrinolysis), for patients with suspected ACS who can't take aspirin, and for patients with recent stroke.

How to give it

Here's how to administer clopidogrel:

For patients younger than age 75 with suspected ACS, non-STEMI, or STEMI, give a loading dose of 600 mg PO followed by 75 mg. PO daily. For patients with stroke, give 75 mg PO daily.

What can happen

Major adverse reactions to clopidogrel include bleeding (which may be life threatening), thrombotic thrombocytopenic purpura, anemia, bradycardia, atrial fibrillation, hypertension, and hypotension.

What to consider

- Clopidogrel should be withheld for 5 days before coronary artery bypass graft (CABG) or other major surgery because its effects last the life of the platelet cells.
- Carefully monitor patients for bleeding.
- Monitor patients for signs and symptoms of thrombotic thrombocytopenic purpura (thrombocytopenia, hemolytic anemia, neurologic changes, renal impairment, and fever).
- Patients who are genetically poor metabolizers of clopidogrel may have higher rates of cardiovascular events. Genetic tests can identify these patients and can be used to plan alternative treatment.

Eptifibatide

Eptifibatide (Integrilin) functions as a platelet aggregation inhibitor. It's used to treat patients with medically managed unstable angina or non-STEMI. It's also used during PCI.

How to give it

- Here's how to administer eptifibatide:
- For ACS—Give an IV bolus of 180 mcg/kg and then give an IV infusion of 2 mcg/kg/minute for up to 72 hours.
- For PCI—Give an IV bolus of 180 mcg/kg over 1 to 2 minutes and then begin an IV infusion of 2 mcg/kg/minute for 18 to 24 hours. The bolus may be repeated 10 minutes after the initial bolus is given.
- In patients with creatinine clearance less than 50 mL/minute, reduce the infusion to 1 mcg/kg/minute.

Eptifibatide may be administered in the same IV line as alteplase, atropine, dobutamine, heparin, lidocaine, meperidine (Demerol), metoprolol (Lopressor), midazolam, morphine, nitroglycerin, verapamil (Calan), normal saline solution, or dextrose 5% in normal saline solution. The main infusion may also contain up to 60 mEq/L of potassium chloride. **However, don't administer eptifibatide in an IV line with furosemide**.

What can happen

Adverse reactions to eptifibatide include bleeding, thrombocytopenia, and hypotension.

What to consider

- Eptifibatide is intended for use with heparin and aspirin.
- Monitor the patient closely for bleeding.
- Platelet function recovers within 4 to 8 hours after discontinuing eptifibatide.
- If the patient is undergoing coronary artery bypass graft surgery, stop the infusion before surgery.

Prasugrel

Prasugrel (Effient) is a thienopyridine that inhibits platelet function by binding to the ADP P2Y12 receptors on platelets. It's used in place of clopidogrel after angiography in patients with non-STEMI or STEMI who aren't at high risk for bleeding. It shouldn't be given to STEMI patients treated with fibrinolytics, to non-STEMI patients before angiography, to patients age 75 and older, or to patients with a history of transient ischemic attack or stroke.

How to give it

Here's how to administer prasugrel:

For patients who weigh 132 lb (60 kg) or more and are managed with PCI, give a loading dose of 60 mg PO followed by a maintenance dose of 10 mg PO daily. For patients weighing less than 132 lb, consider reducing dosage to 5 mg PO daily.

What can happen

Adverse reactions include bleeding (which may be life threatening), anemia, bradycardia, atrial fibrillation, hypertension, and hypotension.

What to consider

- Prasugrel should be withheld for 7 days before CABG or other major surgery because its effects last the life of the platelet cells.
- Don't use prasugrel in patients with active bleeding. Carefully monitor patients for signs of bleeding. Suspect bleeding in patients with hypotension.
- If possible, manage bleeding without discontinuing prasugrel. Discontinuing the medication, particularly in the first few weeks after ACS, increases the risk of more cardiovascular events.

Ticagrelor

Ticagrelor (Brilinta) is a thienopyridine that inhibits platelet function by binding to the ADP P2Y12 receptors on platelets. It's used in place of clopidogrel to reduce the rate of cardiovascular death, MI, and stroke in patients with ACS or history of MI. It also prevents stent thrombosis in patients who have been stented for treatment of ACS.

How to give it

Here's how to administer ticagrelor:

- For the management of ACS, give a loading dose of 180 mg PO followed by a maintenance dose of 90 mg PO bid for 1 year following the ACS event.
- After 1 year, reduce the dose to 60 mg PO bid.

What can happen

Adverse reactions include bleeding (which may be life threatening) and difficulty breathing.

Use cautiously in patients with a history of asthma.

What to consider

- Ticagrelor should be withheld for 5 days before CABG or other major surgery because its effects last the life of the platelet cells.

- Don't use prasugrel in patients with active bleeding. Carefully monitor patients for signs of bleeding. Suspect bleeding in patients with hypotension.
- If possible, manage bleeding without discontinuing ticagrelor. Discontinuing the medication, particularly in the first few weeks after ACS, increases the risk of more cardiovascular events.

Cangrelor

Cangrelor (Kengreal) is a thienopyridine that inhibits platelet function by binding to the ADP receptors on platelets. It is used as an adjunct to PCI in patients who have not been treated with a P2Y12 platelet inhibitor and who are not being given a GP IIb/IIIa inhibitor.

How to give it

Here's how to administer cangrelor:

- Prior to PCI, give 30 mcg/kg IV bolus followed immediately by a 4 mcg/kg/minute IV infusion.
- Continue a maintenance infusion for at least 2 hours or for the duration of PCI, whichever is longer.
- To maintain platelet inhibition after discontinuation of the cangrelor infusion, an oral P2Y12 platelet inhibitor should be administered, such as ticagrelor, prasugrel, or clopidogrel.

What can happen

The most common adverse reaction is bleeding (which may be life threatening).

What to consider

- Cangrelor must be administered through a dedicated IV line.
- To maintain platelet inhibition after the infusion is discontinued, an oral thienopyridine must be administered.
- Don't use cangrelor in patients with active bleeding. Carefully monitor patients for signs of bleeding. Suspect bleeding in patients with hypotension.

Tirofiban

Tirofiban (Aggrastat) functions as a platelet aggregation inhibitor. It's used to treat patients with medically managed unstable angina or non–ST-segment elevation MI. It's also used during PCI.

How to give it

Here's how to administer tirofiban:

- For ACS or PCI: Give a high-dose bolus of 25 mcg/kg over 5 minutes followed by a maintenance infusion of 0.15 mcg/kg/minute for 18 hours.
- Decrease infusion dose by 50% to 0.075 mcg/kg/minute for CrCl less than or equal to 60 mL/minute.

What can happen

Adverse reactions to tirofiban include bradycardia, coronary artery dissection, bleeding, and thrombocytopenia.

What to consider

- Monitor the patient's hemoglobin level, HCT, and platelet count before starting tirofiban, 6 hours following the loading dose, and at least daily during therapy.
- Tirofiban is intended for use with aspirin and heparin.
- Monitor the patient closely for bleeding.
- Platelet function recovers within 4 to 8 hours after discontinuing tirofiban.

Beta-adrenergic blockers

Used for patients with ACS, including acute MI, suspected MI, and unstable angina in the absence of complications, beta-adrenergic blockers are effective antianginal agents that can reduce morbidity and mortality, nonfatal reinfarction, and recurrent ischemia. Beta-adrenergic blockers are also used as second-line agents (after adenosine, diltiazem, and digoxin) for conversion to normal sinus rhythm or to slow ventricular response (or both) in SVTs, such as PSVT, atrial fibrillation, or atrial flutter.

Beta-adrenergic blockers

- Used in patients with acute coronary syndromes to:
- reduce morbidity and mortality
- treat and manage angina
- reduce the incidence of nonfatal reinfarction
- slow ventricular response and convert to sinus rhythm.

Angina busters

These medications help treat chronic stable angina by decreasing myocardial contractility and heart rate (negative inotropic and chronotropic effect), thus reducing myocardial oxygen consumption. The mechanism of action in patients with MI is unknown. However, beta-adrenergic blockers do reduce the frequency of PVCs, chest pain, and enzyme level elevation. (For precautions that apply to all beta-adrenergic blockers, see *General precautions for beta-adrenergic blockers*.)

General precautions for beta-adrenergic blockers

Observe these general precautions when you administer beta-adrenergic blockers:

- Severe hypotension can occur if given IV with IV calcium channel blocking agents, such as verapamil or diltiazem.
- Avoid use in patients with severe bronchospastic diseases, severe heart failure, or severe abnormalities in conduction.
- Myocardial depression may occur.
- Beta-adrenergic blockers are contraindicated in the presence of severe bradycardia, systolic blood pressure less than 100 mm Hg, severe left-sided heart failure, hypoperfusion, or second- or third-degree atrioventricular block.
- Beta-adrenergic blockers may require altered dosage requirements in stable patients with diabetes.
- Signs and symptoms of overdose include severe hypotension, bradycardia, heart failure, and bronchospasm.

Pressure reducer

Beta-adrenergic blockers may reduce blood pressure by adrenergic receptor blockade. This decreases cardiac output by decreasing sympathetic outflow from the CNS and suppressing renin release. (See *Major effects of beta-adrenergic blockers*.)

ACLS guidelines point the way

ACLS guidelines and best practice recommend that all patients with ischemic chest pain and ST-segment elevation receive a beta-adrenergic blocker within 12 hours of infarction, unless contraindications exist. Beta-adrenergic blockers are also used for emergency antihypertensive therapy for hemorrhagic and acute ischemic stroke. The beta-adrenergic blockers used during ACLS include atenolol, esmolol, labetalol, metoprolol, and propranolol.

Esmolol hydrochloride

Esmolol (Brevibloc) is a class II antiarrhythmic and ultrashort-acting selective beta-adrenergic blocker used to decrease heart rate, contractility, and blood pressure. It's recommended for the acute treatment of PSVT and rate control in non–pre-excited atrial fibrillation or atrial flutter, ectopic atrial tachycardia, and polymorphic VT due to torsades de pointes.

Major effects of beta-adrenergic blockers

Beta-adrenergic blockers block the action of endogenous catecholamines and other sympathomimetic agents at beta-receptor sites, thus counteracting the stimulating effects of those agents. Pulmonary effects produce constriction of bronchial smooth muscle and peripheral vascular effects produce constriction of peripheral vessels (beta-2 receptor). This illustration depicts the effects of beta-adrenergic blockers on the heart.

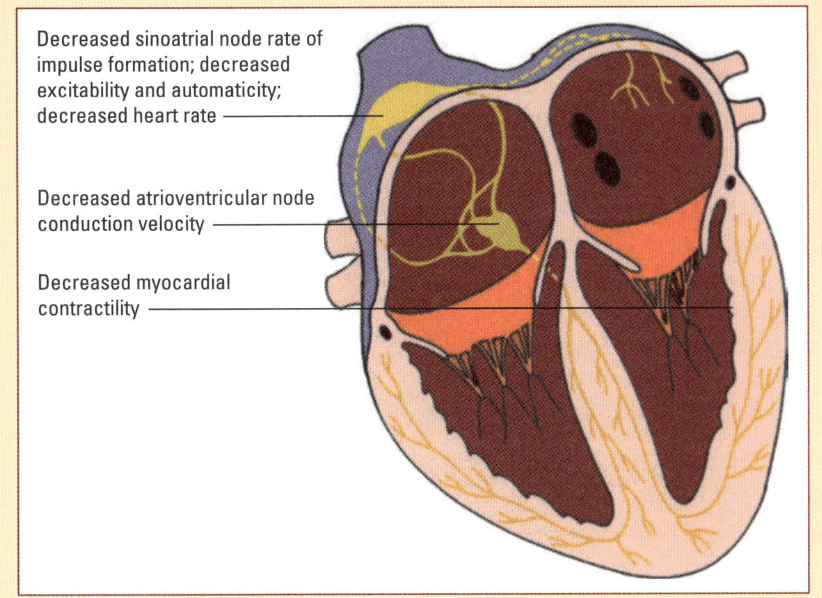

How to give it

Here's how to administer esmolol hydrochloride:

- Give 0.5 mg/kg as an IV infusion over 1 minute, followed by a continuous 4-minute IV infusion of 50 mcg/kg/minute with a maximum infusion of 300 mcg/kg/minute. Titrate the dosage to maintain effect.
- Esmolol is recommended only for short-term use; discontinue after 48 hours.
- Don't mix esmolol with other IV medication.

What can happen

Adverse reactions to esmolol include bradycardia, AV block, hypotension, heart failure, bronchospasm, and light-headedness.

What to consider

- Monitor the patient's heart rate and rhythm and blood pressure response to the medication.

- Check the patient's apical pulse before giving esmolol. If extremes in the pulse rate occur, withhold the medication and notify the prescriber immediately.
- Report significant lengthening of the PR interval and monitor for AV block.
- Esmolol may mask common signs of shock and hypoglycemia in diabetic patients.
- Use cautiously in patients with reactive airway disease.
- Remember that the half-life of esmolol is 2 to 9 minutes.
- Morphine may increase esmolol blood levels.
- If the patient's heart rate becomes stable, replace esmolol with alternative (longer-acting) antiarrhythmics such as propranolol.
- Esmolol may increase serum digoxin levels by 10% to 20% with patients taking digoxin.
- Up to 50% of patients treated with esmolol develop hypotension, which can be reversed within 30 minutes by decreasing the dosage or, if needed, by stopping the infusion.
- When used with catecholamine-depleting medications, esmolol may cause additive bradycardia and hypotension.

Labetalol hydrochloride

Labetalol is used to treat hypertension. labetalol is a combined alpha1 and beta-adrenergic blocking agent. Blood pressure is lowered by reducing heart rate, and vasodilation from inhibition of alpha 1. It's recommended as emergency antihypertensive therapy for hemorrhagic and acute ischemic stroke.

How to give it

Here's how to administer labetalol:

- Give a 10-mg IV push over 1 to 2 minutes; repeat injections of 10 to 20 mg every 10 minutes to a maximum dosage of 150 mg IV
- As an alternative, give an initial IV bolus dose and then start an IV infusion of 2 to 8 mg/minute until you obtain a satisfactory response.
- maximum dose is considered 300 mg per day

What can happen

Adverse reactions to labetalol include bradycardia, AV block, ventricular arrhythmias, hypotension, heart failure, bronchospasm, and lightheadedness.

What to consider

- Monitor the patient's heart rate and rhythm and blood pressure response to the medication.

- Check the patient's apical pulse before giving labetalol. If extremes in the pulse rate occur, withhold the medication and notify the prescriber immediately.
- Report significant lengthening of the PR interval and monitor for AV block.
- Labetalol may mask common signs of shock and hypoglycemia in diabetic patients.
- Use cautiously in patients with reactive airway disease.

Metoprolol tartrate

Metoprolol (Lopressor) is used to treat hypertension and as an adjunctive treatment for acute MI to reduce the incidence of VF. The exact mechanism of how metoprolol decreases blood pressure isn't known; however, it may decrease blood pressure by blocking adrenergic receptors and decreasing cardiac output.

How to give it

Here's how to administer metoprolol tartrate:

- Give a slow IV dose of 5 mg at 5-minute intervals for a total dosage of 15 mg.
- Fifteen minutes following the last IV dose, give 50 mg orally every 6 hours.

What can happen

Adverse reactions to metoprolol include bradycardia, AV block, hypotension, heart failure, bronchospasm, and light-headedness.

What to consider

- Monitor the patient's heart rate and rhythm and blood pressure response to the medication.
- Check the patient's apical pulse before giving metoprolol. If extremes in the pulse rate occur, withhold the medication and notify the prescriber immediately.
- Report significant lengthening of the PR interval and monitor for AV block.
- Metoprolol may mask signs of hypoglycemia in diabetic patients.
- Use cautiously in patients with reactive airway disease.
- Use metoprolol cautiously with adrenergic agonists.
- Don't give metoprolol to patients with sinus bradycardia, second- or third-degree AV block, cardiogenic shock, or overt cardiac failure when treating hypertension or angina.

Calcium channel blockers

In oral forms, calcium channel blockers are used to prevent angina that doesn't respond to other antianginal agents. They are additionally utilized in chronic hypertension management and chronic rate control for patients with chronic atrial fibrillation. IV calcium channel blockers are used to control the ventricular rate in atrial fibrillation and atrial flutter. They reduce electrical impulse formation in cardiac pacemaker cells and can convert reentry arrhythmias. (For precautions that apply to all calcium channel blockers, see *General precautions for calcium channel blockers*.)

You look like you could use some diltiazem. Try it! You'll be dilated and feeling less pain in no time.

Demand decrease

Calcium channel blockers work by decreasing myocardial oxygen demand, the force of myocardial contractility, and afterload. They also increase the oxygen supply to the myocardium by dilating the coronary arteries. (See *How calcium channel blockers work.*) The calcium channel blockers used during ACLS include diltiazem and verapamil.

Diltiazem hydrochloride

Diltiazem (Cardizem) is used to treat angina, to control the ventricular rate in atrial fibrillation and atrial flutter, and, after adenosine, to treat refractory reentry SVT in patients with narrow QRS complex and adequate blood pressure. By impeding the slow inward influx of calcium at the AV node, it decreases conduction velocity and increases the refractory period, thereby decreasing the impulses transmitted to the ventricles in atrial fibrillation or atrial flutter. Ventricular rate then decreases.

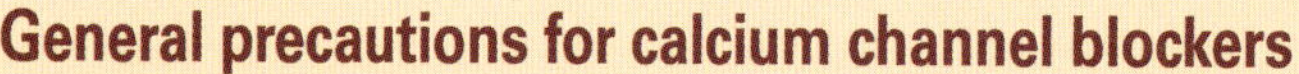

General precautions for calcium channel blockers

Adverse reactions to calcium channel blockers include hypotension, arrhythmias, and heart failure. Follow these general precautions when you administer calcium channel blockers:

- Don't use for wide-complex tachycardias of uncertain origin or for poison- or medication-induced tachycardia.
- Avoid use in patients with WPW syndrome plus rapid atrial fibrillation or flutter, sick sinus syndrome, or atrioventricular block without a pacemaker.
- Avoid use in patients receiving oral beta-adrenergic blockers.
- Don't give IV with IV beta-adrenergic blockers because severe hypotension may result.

In patients with Prinzmetal's angina, it inhibits coronary artery spasm, increasing myocardial oxygen delivery.

Dilation = decrease

Diltiazem works by dilating systemic arteries. This dilation decreases total peripheral resistance and afterload, slightly reduces blood pressure, and increases the cardiac index when given in high doses. Afterload reduction and the resulting decrease in myocardial oxygen consumption account for its effectiveness in controlling chronic stable angina.

Diltiazem also decreases myocardial oxygen demand and cardiac workload by reducing heart rate, relieving coronary artery spasm (through coronary artery vasodilation), and dilating peripheral vessels. These effects serve to relieve ischemia and pain.

How to give it

Here's how to administer diltiazem hydrochloride:

- Give 0.25 mg/kg IV over 2 minutes. After 15 minutes, you may give another 0.35 mg/kg IV over 2 minutes.
- Give 5 to 15 mg/hour IV, titrated to the patient's heart rate, as a maintenance infusion.
- Sublingual nitroglycerin may be administered with diltiazem, as needed, if the patient has acute angina symptoms.

What can happen

Adverse reactions to diltiazem include bradycardia, AV block, hypotension, dizziness, edema, heart failure, and acute hepatic injury.

What to consider

- Monitor the patient's heart rate and rhythm and blood pressure response to the medication.
- Don't give diltiazem to patients with severe left ventricular dysfunction, cardiogenic shock, second- or third-degree AV block (except in the presence of a functioning pacemaker), atrial fibrillation, atrial flutter, or sick sinus syndrome in the presence of WPW syndrome.
- Don't give IV diltiazem to patients receiving IV beta-adrenergic blockers or to patients with VT or other wide-complex tachycardia.
- Use reduced doses for patients with severely compromised cardiac function or for those receiving beta-adrenergic blockers.
- Diltiazem may increase serum levels of digoxin.

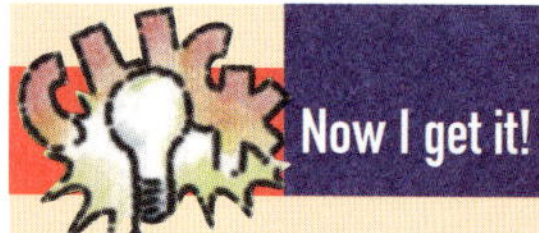

How calcium channel blockers work

Calcium channel blockers increase the myocardial oxygen supply and slow the heart rate. By blocking the slow calcium channel, they inhibit the influx of extracellular calcium ions across both myocardial and smooth muscle membranes. Calcium channel blockers achieve this blockade without changing serum calcium concentrations.

Who are you calling normal?
Under normal conditions, a protein complex prevents muscle contraction by keeping actin and myosin (the contractile proteins) apart. Actin and myosin must interact for a muscle to contract. When the muscle cell is stimulated, calcium ions enter the cell. This influx of calcium releases more calcium from the sarcoplasmic reticulum inside the muscle cell.

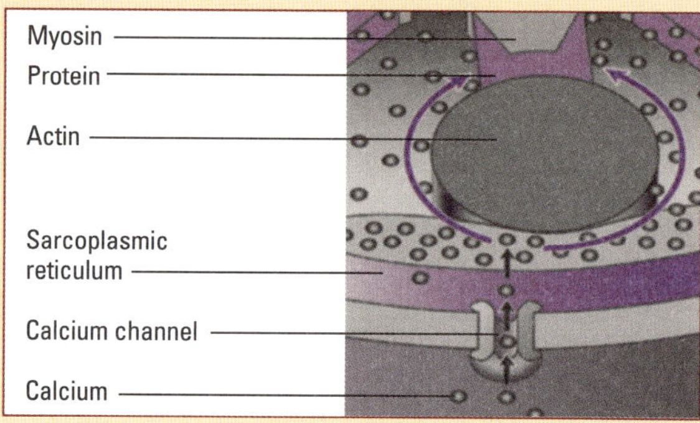

A binding proposition
When enough calcium is released, it binds with the protein complex. The actin and myosin can then interact and the muscle contracts.

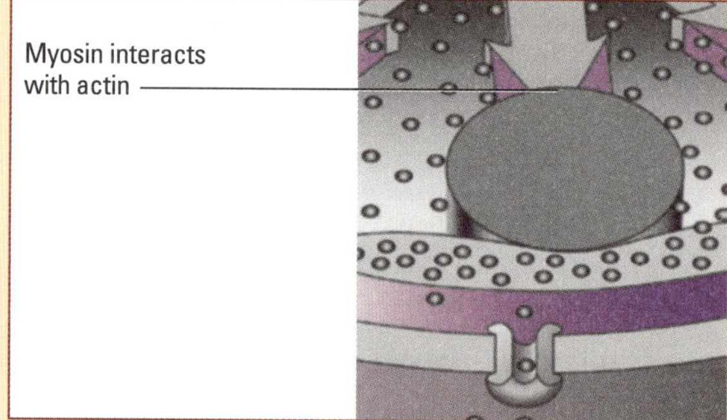

An ounce of prevention
Calcium channel blockers prevent calcium transport across the cell membrane, thereby preventing calcium release from the sarcoplasmic reticulum. This causes the cardiac muscle and the smooth muscle of the coronary arteries to dilate.

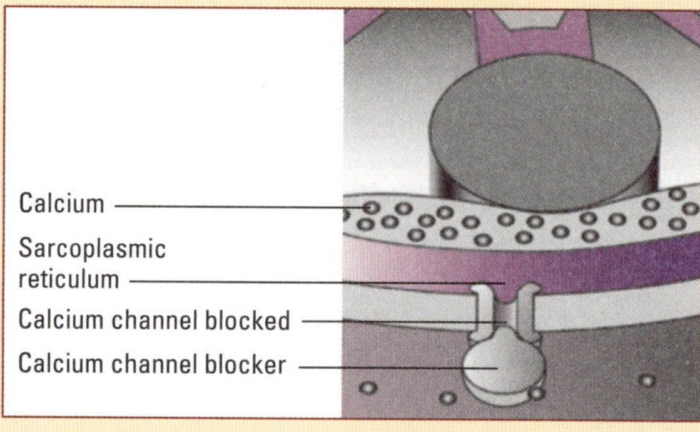

Verapamil hydrochloride

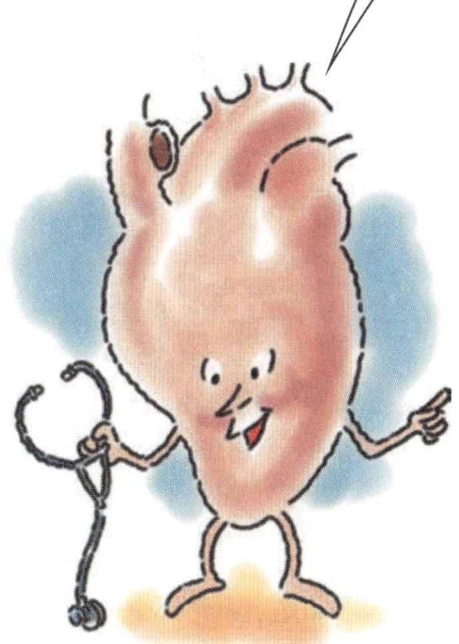

Verapamil (Calan) is used to treat angina, hypertension, and arrhythmias. It's indicated as an alternative medication (after adenosine) to terminate PSVT with narrow QRS complex, adequate blood pressure, and preserved left ventricular function. Verapamil controls ventricular response with atrial fibrillation, atrial flutter, or multifocal atrial tachycardia. Its primary effect is on the AV node; slowed conduction reduces the ventricular rate in atrial tachyarrhythmias and blocks re-entry paths in paroxysmal supraventricular arrhythmias.

This medication got it under control

Verapamil manages unstable and chronic stable angina by reducing afterload, thereby decreasing oxygen consumption. It also decreases myocardial oxygen demand and cardiac workload by exerting a negative inotropic effect: reducing heart rate, relieving coronary artery spasm (via coronary artery vasodilation), and dilating peripheral vessels. Verapamil reduces blood pressure mainly by dilating peripheral vessels. Its negative inotropic effect blocks reflex mechanisms that lead to increased blood pressure. Verapamil is utilized as a secondary agent or in the event of a shortage of diltiazem.

How to give it

Here's how to administer verapamil hydrochloride:

- Give an IV bolus of 2.5 to 5 mg over 2 minutes with a second dose of 5 to 10 mg, if needed, in 15 to 30 minutes. The maximum dosage is 20 mg.
- For elderly patients, remember to administer IV doses over at least 3 minutes to minimize the risk of adverse reactions.

What can happen

Adverse reactions to verapamil include bradycardia, AV block, ventricular arrhythmias, hypotension, dizziness, edema, and heart failure.

What to consider

- Monitor the patient's heart rate and rhythm and blood pressure response to the medication.
- Don't give verapamil to patients with severe left ventricular dysfunction, cardiogenic shock, second- or third-degree AV block (except in the presence of a functioning pacemaker), atrial fibrilla-

tion, atrial flutter, or sick sinus syndrome in the presence of WPW syndrome.
- Don't give IV verapamil to patients receiving IV beta-adrenergic blockers or to patients with VT or other wide-complex tachycardia.
- Use reduced doses for patients with severely compromised cardiac function or for those receiving beta-adrenergic blockers.
- Verapamil has an increased risk of hypotension when compared to diltiazem.

Statins

Statins are used to treat hypercholesterolemia and hyperlipidemia. They work by inhibiting HMG-CoA reductase, the rate-limiting step in cholesterol biosynthesis. Cardiovascular morbidity and mortality vary directly with the level of total cholesterol and LDL cholesterol and inversely with the level of HDL cholesterol. Statins decrease total cholesterol and LDL cholesterol and increase HDL cholesterol. Statin therapy should be instituted prior to hospital discharge, with some data supporting initiation at the time of diagnosis of STEMI or NSTEMI. Initial intensive statin therapy, rather than gradual dose titration upward, is recommended. It is also recommended for acute ischemic stroke prior to discharge as secondary stroke prophylaxis.

Atorvastatin

Atorvastatin (Lipitor) lowers plasma cholesterol and lipoprotein levels by inhibiting HMG-CoA reductase and cholesterol synthesis in the liver and by increasing the number of hepatic LDL receptors on the cell surface to enhance uptake and catabolism of LDL. It also reduces LDL production and the number of LDL particles.

How to give it

Here's how to administer atorvastatin:

- High-intensity statin therapy is recommended in patients with ACS at a dose of 80 mg PO daily.

What can happen

Adverse reactions to atorvastatin include nasopharyngitis, arthralgia, diarrhea, pain in extremity, and urinary tract infection.

What to consider

- Do not administer statins to patients with contraindications such as liver disease or unexplained persistent elevations in liver enzymes and women who are pregnant or may become pregnant or nursing mothers.

- Monitor patients for skeletal muscle effects (for example, myopathy and rhabdomyolysis) especially in patients who may be predisposed such as patients greater than 65 years old, uncontrolled hypothyroidism, and renal impairment.
- Advise patients to promptly report to their physician unexplained and/or persistent muscle pain, tenderness, or weakness.
- Discontinue therapy if myopathy is diagnosed or suspected.
- Check liver enzyme tests before initiating therapy and as clinically indicated thereafter.
- Atorvastatin is metabolized by cytochrome P450 3A4. Concomitant administration with strong inhibitors of CYP 3A4 can lead to increased plasma concentrations of atorvastatin.

Diuretics

Diuretics are used to promote the excretion of water and electrolytes by the kidneys. These medications are used to treat hypertension as well as other cardiovascular conditions, such as edema, heart failure, and pulmonary edema. Frequently used diuretics include furosemide and mannitol.

Furosemide

A highly potent loop diuretic, furosemide (Lasix) is also an antihypertensive. It's used as adjunctive therapy for acute pulmonary edema in patients with systolic blood pressure greater than 90 to 100 mm Hg without signs and symptoms of shock. Furosemide is also used in hypertensive emergencies and in cases of increased intracranial pressure (ICP).

In the loop

Furosemide inhibits sodium and chloride reabsorption in the proximal part of the ascending loop of Henle, promoting sodium, water, chloride, and potassium excretion. Its antihypertensive effect may result from renal and peripheral vasodilation, a temporary increase in the glomerular filtration rate, and a decrease in peripheral vascular resistance.

How to give it

Here's how to administer furosemide:

- Give a slow IV infusion of 0.5 to 1 mg/kg over 1 to 2 minutes; if there's no response, increase to 2 mg/kg IV and give slowly over 1 to 2 minutes.
- If high-dose furosemide therapy is needed, administer the medication as a controlled infusion not exceeding 4 mg/minute. Remember to dilute furosemide in D_5W, normal saline solution, protect from light and use the infusion within 24 hours.
- Furosemide dose orally is 20 to 80 mg per dose, with a maximum daily dose of 600 mg.

What can happen

Adverse reactions to furosemide include dizziness, ototoxicity, hypotension, volume depletion and dehydration, hypokalemia, agranulocytosis, and leukopenia. Signs and symptoms of furosemide overdose include profound electrolyte and volume depletion, which may precipitate circulatory collapse. When given with antihypertensives, furosemide may increase the risk of hypotension.

What to consider

- Monitor the patient's weight, heart rate and rhythm, and blood pressure response to the medication.
- Closely monitor electrolyte levels and accurately assess fluid balance.
- Furosemide may decrease hypoglycemic effects in patients with diabetes.
- Use caution when giving NSAIDs with furosemide because they may inhibit the diuretic response.
- Cardiac glycosides and lithium may increase the risk of toxicity when given with furosemide because of furosemide-induced hypokalemia.

Mannitol

Mannitol (Osmitrol) is an osmotic diuretic used to reduce increased ICP during neurologic emergencies. It may also be used to prevent acute renal failure.

Mannitol increases the osmotic pressure of glomerular filtrate. This inhibits tubular reabsorption of water and electrolytes, promoting diuresis and the urinary elimination of certain medications. Reduced ICP occurs because the medication elevates plasma osmolality, enhancing the flow of water into extracellular fluid.

Stop right there! Never use solutions with undissolved crystals.

How to give it

Here's how to administer mannitol:

- Give 0.5 to 1 g/kg IV over 5 to 10 minutes for increased ICP; additional doses of 0.25 to 2 g/kg IV may be given every 4 to 6 hours.

- Remember to always administer mannitol by IV line with an in-line filter. If the mannitol solution crystallizes (a common occurrence at low temperatures), place the crystallized solution in a hot water bath, shake vigorously to dissolve the crystals, and cool to body temperature before use. Don't use solutions with undissolved crystals.

What can happen

Adverse reactions to mannitol include dizziness, seizures, tachycardia, angina-like chest pain, dehydration, hypotension, hypertension, and thrombophlebitis.

What to consider

- Monitor the patient's serum and urine sodium and potassium levels daily.
- Don't give mannitol to patients with severe pulmonary congestion, pulmonary edema, severe heart failure, severe dehydration, metabolic edema, progressive renal disease or dysfunction, or active intracranial bleeding except during craniotomy.
- Use mannitol with extreme caution in patients with compromised renal function because fluid overload may result; monitor vital signs (including central venous pressure) hourly as well as intake and output, weight, renal function, and fluid balance.
- Mannitol may enhance the possibility of digoxin toxicity.

Electrolytes and buffers

Electrolytes and buffering agents are used for electrolyte replacement therapy. Calcium chloride, magnesium sulfate, and sodium bicarbonate are the medications most frequently used in ACLS.

Calcium chloride

Calcium chloride is a calcium supplement used for patients experiencing electrolyte imbalances. It's indicated for known or suspected hyperkalemia (as in renal failure) and in hypocalcemia. It serves as an antidote for calcium channel blocker or beta-adrenergic blocker overdose. It may also be given prophylactically before IV calcium channel blockers to prevent hypotension but isn't used routinely in cardiac arrest.

Calcium chloride is essential for maintaining the functional integrity of the nervous, muscular, and skeletal systems as well as for maintaining cell membrane and capillary permeability.

How to give it

Here's how to administer calcium chloride:

- Prophylaxis for IV calcium channel blockers—Give 500 to 1,000 mg/kg (5 to 10 mL of a 10% solution) by slow IV push and repeat, as needed.
- For hyperkalemia and calcium channel blocker overdose—Give 500 to 1,000 mg/kg (5 to 10 mL of a 10% solution) by slow IV push.

Only give calcium chloride by IV line, slowly through a small-bore needle into a large vein. Severe necrosis and sloughing of tissue may occur after extravasation.

Calcium gluconate is less irritating to veins and tissue than calcium chloride. Crash carts usually contain gluconate and chloride; be sure to double-check which form is ordered. Bioavailable calcium concentrations differ between calcium chloride and calcium gluconate; roughly 1 g of calcium chloride is equal to 3 g of calcium gluconate.

What can happen

Adverse reactions to calcium chloride include hypercalcemia when large doses of calcium chloride are given to patients with chronic kidney disease. Acute hypercalcemia syndrome is characterized by a markedly elevated plasma calcium level, lethargy, weakness, nausea and vomiting, and coma; it may lead to sudden death.

What to consider

- Initially, assess the patient with hypocalcemia for Trousseau's and Chvostek's signs periodically to check for tetany. (See *Checking for Trousseau's and Chvostek's signs.*)
- Monitor the patient for symptoms of hypercalcemia (nausea, vomiting, lethargy, headache, mental confusion, anorexia). Remember to report symptoms immediately.
- Don't use calcium chloride routinely for cardiac arrhythmias.
- Administer calcium chloride very cautiously, if at all, to patients receiving digoxin because of the increased risk of digoxin toxicity.
- Don't mix calcium chloride with sodium bicarbonate.
- Use caution when giving calcium chloride and magnesium together because calcium decreases the amount of bioavailable magnesium.
- Calcium chloride may antagonize the therapeutic effects of calcium channel blockers such as verapamil.

Peak technique

Checking for Trousseau's and Chvostek's signs

Here's how to check for Trousseau's and Chvostek's signs, which aid in the diagnosis of tetany associated with hypocalcemia.

Trousseau's sign

To check for Trousseau's sign, apply a blood pressure cuff to the patient's upper arm and inflate it to a pressure 20 mm Hg above the systolic pressure. Trousseau's sign (carpal spasm) may appear after 1 to 4 minutes. The patient will experience an adducted thumb, flexed wrist and metacarpophalangeal joints, and extended interphalangeal joints (with fingers together) indicating tetany, a major sign of hypocalcemia.

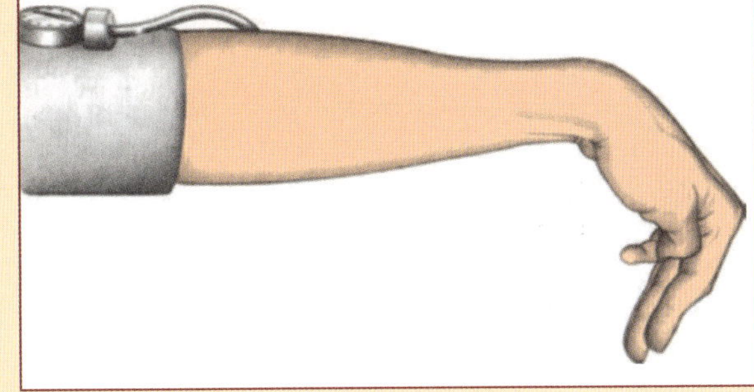

Chvostek's sign

You can induce Chvostek's sign by tapping the patient's facial nerve adjacent to the ear. A brief contraction of the upper lip, nose, or side of the face indicates Chvostek's sign.

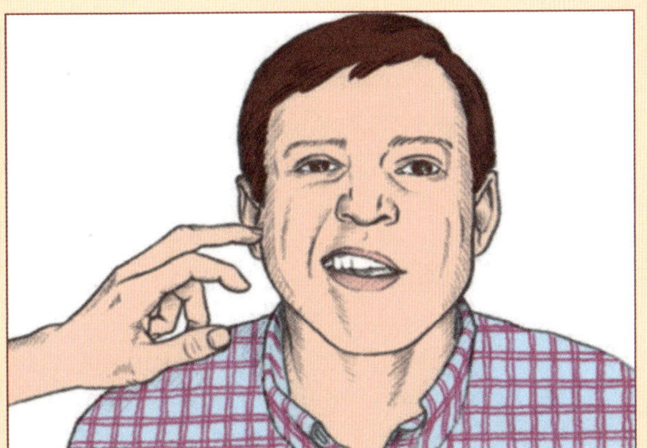

Magnesium sulfate

Magnesium sulfate is a mineral and electrolyte used in cardiac arrest only when torsades de pointes is suspected or hypomagnesemia is present. It isn't likely to be effective in terminating irregular polymorphic VT in patients with a normal QT interval. It may also be used for life-threatening ventricular arrhythmias due to digoxin toxicity.

Magnesium sulfate depresses the CNS and respiratory system. It acts peripherally, causing vasodilation. Moderate doses result in flushing and sweating, while high doses may lead to hypotension.

How to give it

Here's how to administer magnesium sulfate:

- For cardiac arrest (hypomagnesia or torsades de pointes)—Give 1 to 2 g (2 to 4 mL of 50% solution) diluted in 10 mL of D_5W by IV or IO over 5 to 20 minutes.
- For torsades de pointes without cardiac arrest or acute MI with hypomagnesemia—Give a loading dose of 1 to 2 g IV in 50 to 100 mL of D_5W over 5 to 60 minutes; follow with 0.5 to 1 g/hour IV If indicated, titrate to control torsades de pointes.

Remember, in IV bolus form, magnesium sulfate must be injected slowly to avoid hypotension.

What can happen

Adverse reactions to magnesium sulfate include hypotension, circulatory collapse, depressed cardiac function, and respiratory paralysis.

What to consider

- Use caution when giving magnesium sulfate with cardiac glycosides because it may exacerbate arrhythmias.
- Magnesium sulfate coadministered with IV calcium can cause changes in cardiac conduction in patients taking digoxin and may lead to heart block; avoid concomitant use.

Sodium bicarbonate

Sodium bicarbonate is an alkalinizing agent used as a systemic hydrogen ion buffer to treat metabolic acidosis. It restores the buffering capacity of the body and neutralizes excess acid. (See *When to use sodium bicarbonate*.) Sodium bicarbonate may be given to treat certain medication intoxications, such as a salicylate overdose, or for hemolytic reaction to a blood transfusion to alkalinize the urine.

Dissociative property

Sodium bicarbonate dissociates to provide bicarbonate ions. Excess bicarbonate (bicarbonate not needed to buffer hydrogen ions) causes systemic alkalinization and, when excreted, urinary alkalinization as well.

How to give it

Here's how to administer sodium bicarbonate:

- Give an IV bolus of 1 mEq/kg (depending on arterial blood gas [ABG] values, if rapidly available).
- Calculate the dosage based on bicarbonate concentration.
- For persistent metabolic acidosis, sodium bicarbonate may be given in a continuous infusion until the cause of the metabolic acidosis is identified and treated.

What can happen

Adverse reactions to sodium bicarbonate include clinical signs of sodium overdose: depressed consciousness and obtundation from hypernatremia, tetany from hypocalcemia, arrhythmias from hypokalemia, and seizures from alkalosis.

What to consider

- Monitor the patient's vital signs and fluid and electrolyte levels closely.
- Remember that adequate ventilation and cardiopulmonary resuscitation are the first-line buffering agents in cardiac arrest.
- Sodium bicarbonate isn't recommended for routine use during cardiac arrest.
- Don't give calcium salts with sodium bicarbonate because they may cause precipitate.
- Sodium bicarbonate is incompatible with dobutamine, dopamine, epinephrine, and norepinephrine.
- Monitor serum sodium levels with increased dosage or prolonged usage of sodium bicarbonate.

When to use sodium bicarbonate

Use sodium bicarbonate to treat:

- hyperkalemia
- known preexisting bicarbonate-responsive acidosis (diabetic ketoacidosis)
- overdose from medications, such as tricyclic antidepressants, cocaine, and diphenhydramine (Benadryl)
- aspirin or other overdose (alkalizes urine)

It's also used for prolonged resuscitation with effective ventilation. However, sodium bicarbonate isn't useful or effective for treating hypercarbic acidosis (a condition that can result from cardiac arrest and cardiopulmonary resuscitation without intubation). It isn't recommended for routine use for patients in cardiac arrest.

Fibrinolytics

Fibrinolytics are thrombolytic enzymes that promote the enzyme plasmin, which in turn dissolves fibrin and fibrous strands that bind clots. They're used for acute MI in adults with:

- ST-segment elevation (greater than or equal to 1 mm in two or more leads)
- evidence of new left bundle-branch block on the ECG and a history and symptoms strongly suspicious of myocardial injury
- onset of acute MI symptoms of less than 12 hours and PCI isn't available within 90 minutes of first medical contact

Note that certain conditions contraindicate the use of fibrinolytics. (See *Contraindications and precautions for fibrinolytics used in ST-segment elevation MI.*) The fibrinolytics used during ACLS include alteplase, reteplase, and tenecteplase.

Alteplase

Alteplase (recombinant alteplase [Activase] tissue plasminogen activator) is a thrombolytic enzyme used to treat acute MI. In addition, alteplase is the only thrombolytic agent approved for the treatment of acute ischemic stroke. Although alteplase can be given within 12 hours of acute MI symptoms, it can only be given within 3 hours of known onset of acute stroke.

Conversion catalyst

Alteplase exerts thrombolytic action because of an enzyme that catalyzes the conversion of tissue plasminogen to plasmin in the presence of fibrin. This fibrin specificity produces local fibrinolysis in the area of recent clot formation, with limited systemic proteolysis. In patients with acute MI, this allows for reperfusion of ischemic cardiac muscle and improved left ventricular function with a decreased risk of heart failure.

How to give it

Here's how to administer alteplase:

- For acute MI with ST-segment elevation—Give an accelerated infusion over 1½ hours. For patients greater than 67 kg, give an initial IV bolus of 15 mg IV and then administer 50 mg over the next 30 minutes and 35 mg/kg over the next 30 minutes. The total dosage shouldn't exceed 100 mg.
- For patients less than or equal to 67 kg, give an initial IV bolus of 15 mg and then 0.75 mg/kg over the next 30 minutes, followed by 0.5 mg/kg over the following 30 minutes.
- For acute ischemic stroke—Infuse 0.9 mg/kg (maximum dose of 90 mg) IV over 60 minutes; give 10% of the total dosage as an ini-

Contraindications and precautions for fibrinolytics used in ST-segment elevation MI

The American Heart Association has provided criteria that must be met before a patient with ST-segment elevation myocardial infarction (MI) may be considered for fibrinolytic therapy.

Criteria that must *not* be present

- Active bleeding
- Known structural cerebral vascular lesion (arteriovenous malformation) or malignancy
- Ischemic stroke within 3 months except for acute ischemic stroke within 3 to 4.5 hours of symptom onset
- Significant closed head trauma or facial trauma within 3 months
- History of intracranial hemorrhage or any prior hemorrhagic stroke
- Suspected aortic dissection
- Intracranial neoplasm or arteriovenous malformation
- Intracranial or intraspinal surgery within 2 months
- Severe uncontrolled hypertension
- For streptokinase treatment within 6 months

Criteria that shouldn't be present

- Active peptic ulcer
- Major surgery or serious trauma within 21 days, or more than 10 minutes of CPR
- Pregnancy
- Lumbar puncture performed within 7 days
- Recent noncompressible arterial puncture
- Internal bleeding within past 2 to 4 weeks
- Current medications include anticoagulants
- BP greater than 180/110 mm Hg on presentation or history of poorly controlled hypertension
- History of ischemic stroke greater than 3 months prior
- Recent internal bleeding within 2 to 4 weeks

Special precautions

- Monitor the patient for adverse reactions, including cerebral hemorrhage; hypotension; arrhythmias; severe, spontaneous bleeding (cerebral, retroperitoneal, genitourinary, GI); and bleeding at puncture sites.
- Avoid IM injections, venipuncture, and arterial puncture during therapy; use pressure dressings or ice packs on recent puncture sites to prevent bleeding. If arterial puncture is needed, select a site on the arm and apply pressure for 30 minutes afterward.

Source: 2015 American Heart Association Guidelines for Cardiopulmonary Resuscitation and Emergency Cardiovascular Care.

tial IV bolus over 1 minute and give the remaining dose over the next 60 minutes.

Remember to prepare the alteplase solution for injection using sterile water, not bacteriostatic water. Alteplase may be further diluted with an injection of normal saline solution or D_5W to yield a concentration of 0.5 mg/mL. When preparing a dose from a 50-mg vial, use an 18-G needle for preparing the solution—aim the water stream at the lyophilized cake. Expect a slight foaming to occur and don't use if a vacuum isn't present. When preparing a dose from a 100-mg vial, use a transfer device for reconstitution and remember that the 100-mg vial doesn't have a vacuum. Reconstituted or diluted solutions are stable for up to 8 hours at room temperature.

ASAP is the key

Expect to begin alteplase infusions as soon as possible after the onset of MI symptoms. Administer alteplase within 3 hours after the onset of stroke symptoms but only after excluding intracranial hemorrhage by computed tomography scan or another diagnostic imaging method.

Eligibility requirements for alteplase in acute ischemic stroke

Inclusion criteria:

- Clinical diagnosis of ischemic stroke causing measurable neurologic deficit
- Onset of symptoms less than 4.5 hours before beginning treatment; if the exact time of stroke onset is not known, it is defined as the last time the patient was known to be normal.
- Age greater than or equal to 18 years

Exclusion criteria:

- Significant stroke or head trauma in the previous 3 months
- Previous intracranial hemorrhage
- Intracranial neoplasm, arteriovenous malformation, or aneurysm
- Recent intracranial or intraspinal surgery
- Arterial puncture at a noncompressible site in the previous 7 days
- Symptoms suggestive of subarachnoid hemorrhage
- Persistent blood pressure elevation (systolic greater than or equal to 185 mm Hg or diastolic greater than or equal to 110 mm Hg)
- Serum glucose less than 50 mg/dL (less than 2.8 mmol/L)
- Active internal bleeding
- Platelet count less than 100,000/mm^3
- Current anticoagulant use with an INR greater than 1.7 or PT greater than 15 seconds
- Heparin use within 48 hours and an abnormally elevated aPTT
- Current use of a direct thrombin inhibitor or direct factor Xa inhibitor with evidence of anticoagulant effect by laboratory tests such as aPTT, INR, ECT, TT, or appropriate factor Xa activity assays
- Evidence of hemorrhage

Relative contraindications:

- Only minor and isolated neurologic signs
- Major surgery or serious trauma in the previous 14 days
- Gastrointestinal or urinary tract bleeding in the previous 21 days
- Myocardial infarction in the previous 3 months
- Seizure at the onset of stroke with postictal neurologic impairments
- Pregnancy

Additional relative exclusion criteria for treatment from 3 to 4.5 hours from symptom onset

- Age greater than 80 years
- Oral anticoagulant use regardless of INR
- Severe stroke (National Institutes of Health Stroke Scale score greater than 25)
- Combination of both previous ischemic stroke and diabetes mellitus

What can happen

Adverse reactions to alteplase include hypotension; arrhythmias; bleeding, including GI bleeding, bleeding at puncture sites, and cerebral hemorrhage; and hypersensitivity reactions.

What to consider

- Monitor the patient's ECG for reperfusion arrhythmias.
- Monitor coagulation studies and assess the patient for bleeding. Avoid IM injections, invasive procedures, and nonessential handling of the patient.
- Heparin is usually administered during or after alteplase injection as part of the treatment regimen for acute MI or pulmonary embolism.
- Don't mix alteplase with other medications.

- Treatment with alteplase should be performed only in facilities that can provide appropriate evaluation and management of intracranial hemorrhage.
- Don't give anticoagulant or antiplatelet therapy for 24 hours when alteplase is used for acute ischemic stroke.
- Medications that antagonize platelet function (abciximab and dipyridamole) may increase the risk of bleeding if given before, during, or after alteplase therapy; avoid concomitant use.
- Discontinue the alteplase infusion immediately if signs or symptoms of bleeding occur and notify the prescriber.

Alteplase

- Produces local fibrinolysis in the area of recent clot formation, with limited systemic proteolysis
- Indications: acute myocardial infarction (MI), acute massive pulmonary embolism, and acute ischemic stroke
- For acute MI with ST-segment elevation—Give an accelerated infusion over 1½ hours. For patients greater than 67 kg, give an initial IV bolus of 15 mg IV and then administer 50 mg over the next 30 minutes and 35 mg over the next 30 minutes. The total dosage shouldn't exceed 100 mg. For patients less than or equal to 67 kg, give an initial IV bolus of 15 mg and then 0.75 mg/kg over the next 30 minutes followed by 0.5 mg/kg over the next 30 minutes.
- For acute ischemic stroke, give 0.9 mg/kg over 60 minutes; 10% of the total dose should be given as an IV bolus over the first minute.

Reteplase

Reteplase (recombinant, Retavase) is used to treat acute MI. It enhances cleavage of plasminogen to generate plasmin, which leads to fibrinolysis.

How to give it

Here's how to administer reteplase:

- Give reteplase as an IV double-bolus injection. First, give 10 units over 2 minutes; 30 minutes later, give a second dose of 10 units over 2 minutes.
- Remember to flush the IV line with normal saline solution before and after each bolus.

What can happen

Adverse reactions to reteplase include hypotension; arrhythmias; bleeding, including GI bleeding, bleeding at puncture sites, and cerebral hemorrhage; and hypersensitivity reactions.

What to consider

- Monitor the patient's ECG for reperfusion arrhythmias.
- Monitor coagulation studies and assess the patient for bleeding. Avoid IM injections, invasive procedures, and nonessential handling of the patient.
- Use caution when giving heparin, oral anticoagulants, or platelet inhibitors (abciximab, aspirin, or dipyridamole) with reteplase because these medications may increase the risk of bleeding.
- Reteplase may alter coagulation studies.
- Potency is expressed in units specific for reteplase and isn't comparable to other thrombolytic medications.
- Heparin and reteplase are incompatible in a solution.

Tenecteplase

Tenecteplase (TNKase) is used to treat acute MI. It's as effective as conventional fibrinolytics but differs in that it's given in a single-dose injection. Tenecteplase promotes plasmin activity to produce fibrinolysis. It targets established clots and, therefore, doesn't impair the natural clotting process throughout the body.

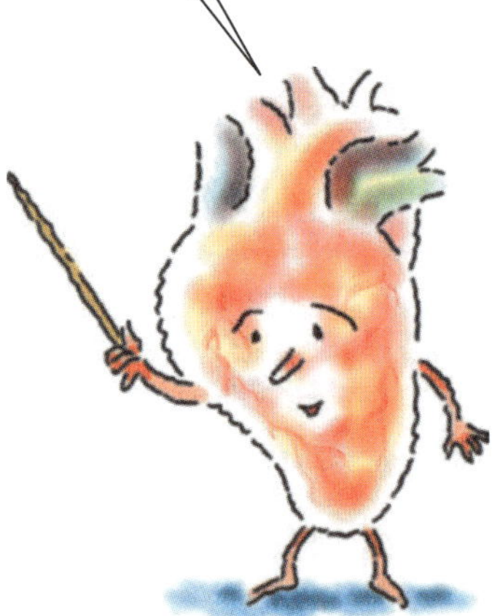

How to give it

Here's how to administer tenecteplase:

- Give as a 30- to 50-mg IV bolus injection over 5 seconds.
- Dosage is based on the patient's weight with a maximum total do age of 50 mg.

What can happen

Adverse reactions to tenecteplase include arrhythmias; hypotension; bleeding, including GI bleeding, bleeding at puncture sites, and cerebral hemorrhage; and hypersensitivity reactions.

What to consider

- Monitor the patient's ECG for reperfusion arrhythmias.
- Monitor coagulation studies and assess the patient for bleeding. (Tenecteplase may alter coagulation studies.) Avoid IM injections, invasive procedures, and nonessential handling of the patient.
- Use caution when giving heparin, oral anticoagulants, or platelet inhibitors (abciximab, aspirin, or dipyridamole) with reteplase because these medications may increase the risk of bleeding. (Discontinue concomitant heparin and antiplatelet therapy if bleeding occurs.)

Inotropics

Inotropic agents, which include the subcategories of chronotropics and dromotropics, influence the force of muscular contractions. Digoxin, inamrinone, and milrinone are discussed here. For information on dobutamine.

Positives and negatives are all positive

Inotropics are typically used in treating heart failure and have either positive or negative effects. For example, positive dromotropic agents influence the conductivity of cardiac muscle and action of cardiac nerves, while negative dromotropic agents slow the electrical impulse conduction through the nodal pathway (AV node).

Digoxin

Digoxin (Lanoxin) is an inotropic and antiarrhythmic used in heart failure, atrial fibrillation, atrial flutter, and PSVT. It depresses the SA node and increases the refractory period of the AV node. It also indirectly increases intracellular calcium by inhibiting sodium-potassium–activated adenosine triphosphatase.

How to give it

Here's how to administer digoxin:

- Give a loading dose of 10 to 12 mcg/kg (ideal body weight) IV or in divided doses over 24 hours. Follow with a maintenance dose determined by the patient's body weight and renal function.
- Don't mix digoxin with other medications or give in the same IV line.
- Digoxin orally: 10 to 15 mcg/kg loading dose followed by a maintenance dose of 3.4 to 5.1 mcg/kg daily.

What can happen

Adverse reactions to digoxin include an increased risk of arrhythmias, confusion, irritability, and vision changes (blurred vision, yellow-green halos around visual images).

What to consider

- Monitor the patient's heart rate and rhythm. Excessive slowing of the pulse rate (60 beats/minute or less) may be a sign of digoxin toxicity. Withhold the medication and notify the prescriber.
- Before giving a loading dose, obtain baseline data (heart rate, rhythm, blood pressure, and electrolyte levels).
- The therapeutic serum level of digoxin is 0.5 to 2 ng/mL based on the patient's body weight and response to the medication.
- Avoid electrical cardioversion with digoxin unless the patient's condition is life threatening; if necessary, use a lower current setting (10 to 20 joules).
- Don't give digoxin with dobutamine.
- Don't give digoxin with calcium salts because severe arrhythmias caused by the effects on cardiac contractility and excitability may occur.
- Don't give digoxin to patients with digoxin toxicity, AV block, profound sinus bradycardia, VT, atrial and junctional tachycardia, or PVCs.
- Use caution when giving digoxin with amiodarone, captopril, diltiazem, nifedipine (Procardia), quinidine, spironolactone (Aldactone), and verapamil because these medications increase digoxin levels.
- Digoxin immune Fab can be used to treat digoxin toxicity.

Milrinone lactate

Milrinone (Primacor) is used for the short-term management of severe heart failure. It produces inotropic action by increasing cellular levels of cAMP. Milrinone produces vasodilation through a direct relaxant effect on vascular smooth muscle.

How to give it

Here's how to administer milrinone lactate:

- Give an IV loading dose of 50 mcg/kg over 10 minutes followed by a maintenance infusion of 0.375 to 0.75 mcg/kg/minute not to exceed 1.13 mg/kg in a 24-hour period.
- Titrate infusion to hemodynamic response per facility protocol.

What can happen

The most common adverse reactions reported with milrinone include ventricular arrhythmias and headache.

What to consider

- Milrinone is prescribed primarily for patients who haven't responded to cardiac glycosides, diuretics, and other inotropic medications. The majority of the experience with milrinone has been in patients receiving digoxin and diuretics.
- Use hemodynamic monitoring to monitor the patient's heart rate, rhythm, function, and fluid balance.
- Utilize caution when weaning, milrinone has a longer half-life than other inotropes. (The half-life is 2.3 hours and the effect ceases 8 hours after termination of infusion.)

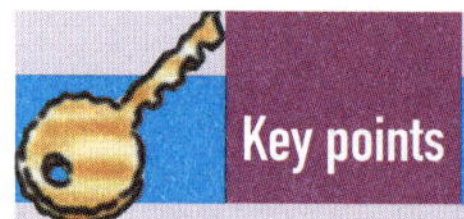

Milrinone lactate

- Produces inotropic action by increasing cellular levels of cyclic adenosine monophosphate; produces vasodilation through a direct relaxant effect on vascular smooth muscle
- Indications: for the short-term (48 hours) intravenous therapy of severe congestive heart failure patients in intensive care and coronary care units not responding to other therapy and for low-output states following cardiac surgery, including weaning from cardiopulmonary bypass pump
- Give an IV loading dose of 50 mcg/kg over 10 minutes followed by a maintenance infusion of 0.375 to 0.75 mcg/kg/minute not to exceed 1.13 mg/kg in a 24-hour period; titrate to clinical effect.

Nitrates

Nitrates are used to prevent or relieve angina and to reduce high blood pressure. (See *How antianginal agents relieve angina*.) The most commonly used nitrate is nitroglycerin.

Nitroglycerin

Nitroglycerin functions as an antianginal agent and vasodilator. It's used to treat suspected ischemic pain during the initial 24 to 48 hours in patients with acute MI complicated by heart failure, large anterior wall infarction, persistent or recurrent ischemia, hypertension, recurrent angina, persistent pulmonary congestion, or hypertensive urgency. Be cautious with nitroglycerine usage in patients taking phosphodiesterase inhibitors if they have taken sildenafil or vardenafil in the past 24 hours or tadalafil in past 48 hours; this can cause severe hypotension refractory to vasopressors.

To the rescue

Nitroglycerin relaxes the vascular smooth muscle of the venous and arterial beds, resulting in decreased myocardial oxygen consumption. It dilates coronary vessels, leading to the redistribution of blood flow to ischemic tissue.

Because peripheral vasodilation decreases venous return to the heart (preload), nitroglycerin also helps to treat pulmonary edema and heart failure. Arterial vasodilation decreases arterial impedance (afterload), thereby decreasing left ventricular workload and aiding the failing heart.

Key points

Nitroglycerin
- Antianginal and vasodilator
- Indications: ischemic pain, myocardial infarction, hypertension, angina, pulmonary congestion
- IV infusion at 10 mcg/minute increased by 10 mcg/minute until desired response occurs
- Sublingual route: 1 tablet (0.30 to 0.4 mg) and repeat every 5 minutes
- Aerosol spray: 0.5 to 1 second at 5-minute intervals, which provides 0.4 mg per dose

How to give it

Here's how to administer nitroglycerin:

- IV bolus (emergency route of choice)—Give an IV infusion at 10 mcg/minute increased by 10 mcg/minute every 5 to 10 minutes until the desired hemodynamic or clinical response occurs. Administration as an IV infusion requires special nonabsorbent tubing because regular plastic tubing may absorb up to 80% of the medication. Prepare the infusion in a glass bottle or container.
- Sublingual route—Give 1 tablet (0.3 to 0.4 mg); repeat every 5 minutes up to a total of three doses.
- Aerosol spray—Give a 0.5- to 1-second spray at 5-minute intervals (provides 0.4 mg per dose). The maximum dose is three sprays within 15 minutes.

What can happen

Adverse reactions to nitroglycerin include hypotension and headache. Medication toxicity may cause hypotension, persistent throbbing headache, palpitations, flushing of the skin, nausea and vomiting, bradycardia, heart block, tissue hypoxia, metabolic acidosis, and circulatory collapse; circulatory collapse or asphyxia may cause death.

What to consider

- In IV form, nitroglycerin is contraindicated in patients with cardiac tamponade, restrictive cardiomyopathy, or constrictive pericarditis.
- Use nitroglycerin cautiously in patients with hypotension or volume depletion.
- Ask about use of sildenafil citrate (Viagra) as concomitant use of nitroglycerin may cause hypotension.

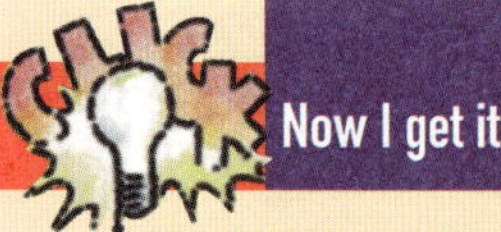

How antianginal agents relieve angina

Angina occurs when the coronary arteries—the heart's primary source of oxygen—supply insufficient oxygen to the myocardium. This increases the heart's workload, which in turn increases heart rate, preload (blood volume in ventricles at end of diastole), afterload (pressure in arteries leading from ventricles), and force of myocardial contractility. The antianginal agents (nitrates, beta-adrenergic blockers, and calcium channel blockers) relieve angina by decreasing one or more of these four factors. This illustration summarizes how antianginal agents affect the cardiovascular system.

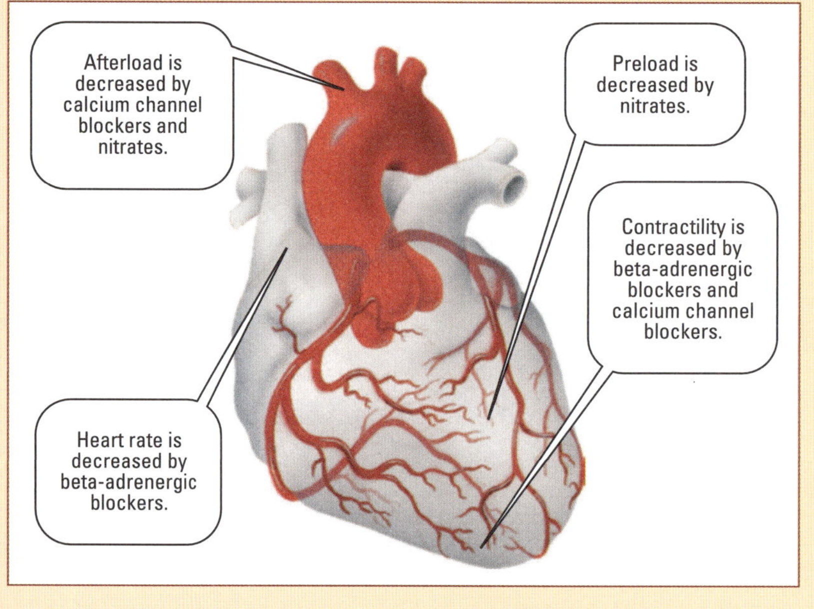

Vasodilating antihypertensive agents

Vasodilating antihypertensive agents include direct vasodilators (typically nitroprusside sodium and IV nitroglycerin) and calcium channel blockers (typically clevidipine and nicradipine). Direct vasodilators act on arteries, veins, or both and commonly produce adverse reactions related to reflex activation of the SNS. Calcium channel blockers produce arteriolar relaxation, which reduces the mechanical activity of vascular smooth muscle. These medications are usually used as adjuncts in treating hypertension rather than as primary agents.

Nitroprusside sodium is discussed below.

Nitroprusside sodium

Nitroprusside (Nipride) is a potent vasodilator used to treat hypertensive crisis. It's known to reduce afterload in heart failure, acute pulmonary edema, and acute mitral or aortic valve regurgitation. Nitroprusside acts directly on vascular smooth muscle, causing peripheral vasodilation.

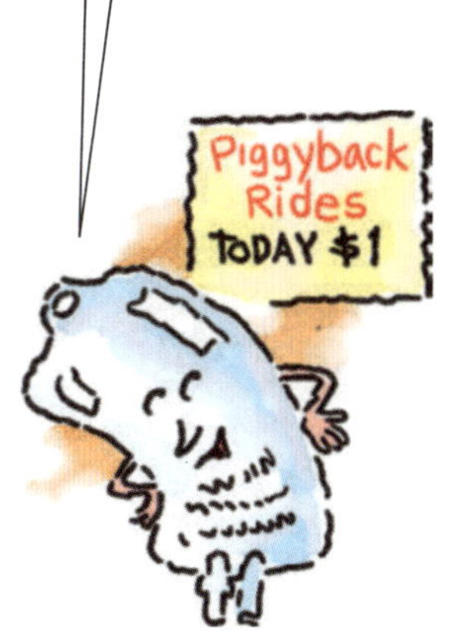

How to give it

Here's how to administer nitroprusside sodium:

- Begin an IV infusion of 0.1 mcg/kg/minute and titrate upward every 3 to 5 minutes to the desired effect (up to 5 mcg/kg/minute, but dosages up to 10 mcg/kg may be needed). Blood pressure should start decreasing within 1 to 2 minutes.
- Prepare nitroprusside using D_5W. Foil-wrap the IV solution (but not the tubing) because of light sensitivity. Fresh solutions have a faint brownish tint; discard after 24 hours.
- Remember to use an infusion pump when giving nitroprusside. Nitroprusside is best run piggyback through a peripheral line with no other medications. Don't adjust the rate of the main IV line while the medication is running because even small boluses can cause severe hypotension. Ideally, the patient should have an arterial line to continuously monitor blood pressure.

What can happen

Nitroprusside may cause cyanide toxicity, which can produce profound hypotension, metabolic acidosis, dyspnea, ataxia, and vomiting. Rapid infusion can also cause severe hypotension.

What to consider

- Monitor blood pressure closely while medication is infusing.
- Check serum thiocyanate levels every 72 hours (levels above 100 mg/mL are associated with cyanide toxicity).
- Don't give epinephrine with nitroprusside because this causes increased blood pressure.
- Use caution when giving other antihypertensives with nitroprusside because these medications may potentiate its effects.
- If symptoms of cyanide toxicity occur, stop the infusion and reevaluate therapy.
- Protect nitroprusside from light, as light can cause degradation of the medication.
- Placement of an arterial line is strongly recommended when using nitroprusside.

Nicardipine (Cardene) and clevidipine (Cleviprex) are both dihydropyridine calcium channel blockers. By inhibiting calcium influx in the arterial smooth muscle, a decrease in mean arterial blood pressure can occur by causing arterial dilation.

Clevidipine is a lipid-based emulsion, and nicardipine is a dextrose- and water-based formulation.

How to give it: Clevidipine (Cleviprex) is supplied as a lipid emulsion medication in a 50- to 100-mL vial. Start the infusion at 1 to 2 mg/hour, and titrate by doubling the dose at 90-second intervals until the goal blood pressure is reached. The maximum dose has not been studied, but the dose should generally be less than 21 mg/hour.

Nicardipine is started as an infusion at 5 mg/hour and titrated by 2.5 mg/hour every 5 to 15 minutes to achieve desired blood pressure goal. Maximum dose is 15 mg/hour.

The half-life of clevidipine is initially 1 minute; the terminal half-life is at 15 minutes.

The half-life of nicardipine is 3 to 45 minutes; the terminal half-life for extended infusions is up to 14 hours.

What can happen

Adverse reactions can be hypotension, atrial fibrillation, increased serum triglycerides, and hypersensitivity reaction to the medication from the egg or soybean content.

What to consider

- Clevidipine is a lipid-based solution so strict asepsis should be employed.
- Tubing change should occur every 12 hours or every time a new bottle is started.
- Lipase and triglycerides should be checked in cases of extended use.
- Cleviprex must be refrigerated.
- Do not confuse dosage of oral and IV preparations of nicardipine; they are substantially different.
- Limit drop in systolic blood pressure to 30 mmHg below baseline in patients with hypotension.
- Limit drop to 10% of baseline in patients with normotension.

Nitroprusside sodium

- A potent vasodilator indicated for hypertensive crisis
- Known to reduce afterload in heart failure, acute pulmonary edema, and acute mitral or aortic valve regurgitation
- Acts directly on vascular smooth muscle, causing peripheral vasodilation
- For hypertension, begin at 0.1 mcg/kg/minute and titrate upward every 3 to 5 minutes to desired effect (up to 5 mcg/kg/minute).
- Can cause cyanide toxicity; check serum thiocyanate levels every 72 hours; levels above 100 mcg/mL are associated with cyanide toxicity, which can produce profound hypotension, metabolic acidosis, dyspnea, ataxia, and vomiting; if such symptoms occur, stop infusion and reevaluate therapy.

Antidotes

Antidotes are used to reverse the effects of medications or situations in which the patient's life might be in danger. Among these are naloxone, digoxin immune Fab, flumazenil, and glucagon.

Naloxone hydrochloride

Naloxone is used as an antidote for respiratory and neurologic depression caused by opioid intoxication. In patients who have received an opioid agonist or other analgesic with opioid-like effects, naloxone antagonizes most of the effects, especially respiratory depression, sedation, and hypotension. The precise mechanism of action is unknown, but it's thought to involve competitive antagonism of more than one opiate receptor in the CNS. It is reasonable to administer naloxone to patients with known or suspected opioid use or addiction who present with respiratory depression or arrest.

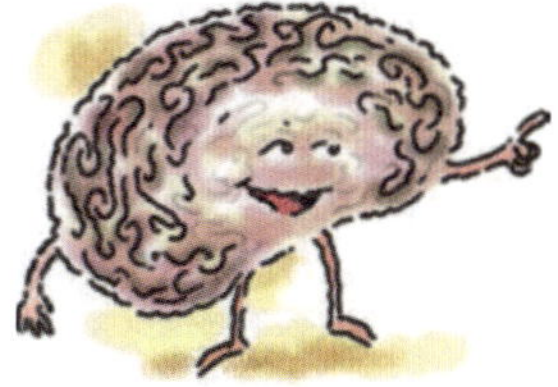

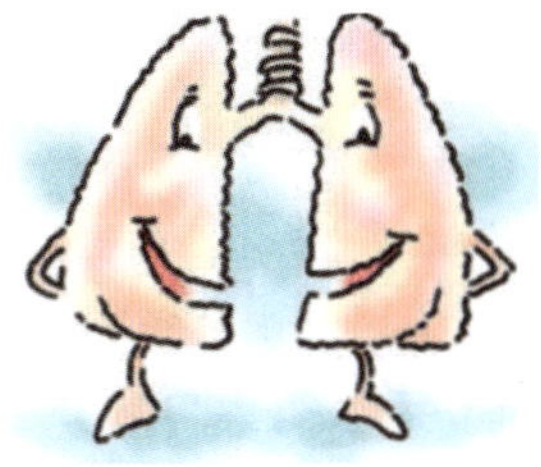

How to give it

Here's how to administer naloxone hydrochloride:

- Give 0.04 to 0.4 mg IV repeated every 2 to 3 minutes as needed; higher doses may be used for complete opioid reversal, and up to 10 mg can be administered over a short period (less than 10 minutes).
- For suspected opioid-addicted patients and postoperative opioid depression, use smaller doses and titrate the dosage until ventilations are adequate.
- Naloxone can be diluted in D_5W or normal saline solution; use within 24 hours after mixing for continuous infusion.

What can happen

Adverse reactions to naloxone include tachycardia, hypertension (with higher-than-recommended doses), hypotension, VF, and cardiac arrest.

What to consider

- Because the duration of activity with naloxone is shorter than that of most opioids, continued monitoring and repeated doses are usually necessary to manage acute opioid overdose in a nonaddicted patient. A continuous infusion may be indicated.
- Don't give naloxone with cardiotoxic medications because they may cause potentially serious cardiovascular effects, including ventricular arrhythmias.
- Withdrawal symptoms may occur in opioid-dependent patients with higher-than-recommended doses of naloxone.
- Naloxone isn't effective in treating respiratory depression caused by nonopioid medications.

Digoxin immune Fab

Digoxin immune Fab (Digibind) is an antibody fragment that prevents or reverses the toxic effects of cardiac glycosides. It's used for potentially life-threatening digoxin toxicity (life-threatening arrhythmias and hyperkalemia with a plasma level greater than 5 mEq/L).

A binding agreement

With digoxin immune Fab, specific antigen-binding fragments bind with free digoxin intravascularly or in extracellular spaces, making them unavailable for binding at their sites of action.

Medication tips
- Most emergency medications are given IV
- Elderly patients and patients with decreased renal or liver function may need smaller dosages.
- The first-line medications used most commonly in adult acute cardiac life support situations include epinephrine, atropine, amiodarone, adenosine, dopamine, beta-adrenergic blockers, and calcium channel blockers.
- Naloxone may be administered if opioid use is suspected as cause of respiratory depression or arrest.

How to give it

Here's how to administer digoxin immune Fab:

- For adults—Give a dose based on the ingested amount or serum level of digoxin.
- If cardiac arrest is imminent—Give rapidly by direct IV injection into the vein or use an IV line containing a free-flowing, compatible solution, using a 0.22-micron filter needle.

What can happen

Adverse reactions to digoxin immune Fab include heart failure, decreased cardiac output, hypokalemia, and rapid ventricular rate in patients with atrial fibrillation.

What to consider

- Digoxin levels greater than 2.5 ng/mL may be toxic. Ingestion of more than 10 mg of digoxin (in adults) or 4 mg (in children) at one time may cause cardiac arrest; therefore, use Digibind.
- Obtain serum digoxin levels 8 hours after the last dose to ensure accuracy.
- Closely monitor the patient's serum potassium level during and after medication administration.

Flumazenil

Flumazenil (Romazicon) is a benzodiazepine antagonist. It's used to treat the respiratory depression and sedative effects caused by pure benzodiazepine overdose. Flumazenil competitively inhibits the actions of benzodiazepines on the gamma-aminobutyric acid/benzodiazepine receptor complex.

How to give it

Here's how to administer flumazenil:

- The initial dosage is 0.2 mg IV over 15 seconds. If the patient doesn't reach the desired level of consciousness, give 0.3 mg IV over 30 seconds. If the patient is still not responding adequately, give 0.5 mg IV over 30 seconds; repeat 0.5-mg doses at 1-minute intervals until a cumulative dosage of 3 mg has been given. On rare occasions, a total dose of 5 mg may be necessary.

Contraindications and precautions for flumazenil

Flumazenil is contraindicated in patients who:

- have been given a benzodiazepine for a potentially life-threatening condition (such as to control intracranial pressure or status epilepticus)
- show signs of serious cyclic antidepressant overdose
- are at risk for mixed overdose (especially in cases when seizures are likely to occur).

Use flumazenil with caution in patients who:

- are at high risk for developing seizures
- are withdrawing from sedative-hypnotics
- are displaying some signs of seizure activity (such as myoclonus)
- may be at risk for unrecognized benzodiazepine dependence
- are experiencing alcohol or other medication dependencies because of the increased risk of benzodiazepine tolerance
- have a head injury.

- Sedation that persists after 5 minutes when a total of 5 mg has been given is unlikely to be caused by benzodiazepines. (See *Contraindications and precautions for flumazenil.*)
- If the patient becomes sedated again, the dosage may be repeated after 20 minutes; however, no more than 1 mg should be given at any one time.

What can happen

Adverse reactions to flumazenil include resedation, which may occur because the duration of flumazenil action is shorter than that of all benzodiazepines; agitation; dizziness; seizures; flushing; tachycardia; and hypertension.

What to consider

- Make sure the patient has a secure airway and IV access before administering flumazenil. Also make sure to wake the patient gradually.
- The provider should evaluate the risks versus benefits of administering flumazenil; it can lower the patient's seizure threshold and induce seizures.
- Monitor the patient closely for resedation after reversal of benzodiazepine effects. The duration of monitoring depends on the specific medication being reversed; for example, monitor the patient after long-acting benzodiazepines, such as diazepam (Valium), or after high doses of short-acting benzodiazepines such as midazolam.
- Monitor the patient's cardiac and respiratory status during medication use.
- Monitor for withdrawal symptoms after administering flumazenil to a patient with long-term benzodiazepine use.

Glucagon

Glucagon reverses low blood glucose levels. It's used as an adjuvant treatment of the toxic effects of calcium channel blockers or beta-adrenergic blockers. Glucagon promotes hepatic glycogenolysis and gluconeogenesis, raising serum glucose levels. It also relaxes GI smooth muscle and produces a positive inotropic and chronotropic myocardial effect.

How to give it

Here's how to administer glucagon:

- Give 1 mg IV over 2 to 5 minutes for treatment of hypoglycemia.
- For treatment of toxic effects of calcium channel blockers or beta-adrenergic blockers, give an initial IV dose of 3 mg to 10 mg over 3 to 5 minutes, followed by an infusion at 3 to 5 mg/hour, as needed.
- Remember that glucagon is incompatible with normal saline solution and other solutions with a pH of 3.0 to 9.5 because it may cause precipitation.

What can happen

- Adverse reactions to glucagon include vomiting and hypotension.

What to consider

- If a patient with hypoglycemia doesn't respond to glucagon, give IV dextrose.
- Glucagon may fail to relieve coma because of markedly depleted hepatic stores of glycogen or irreversible brain damage caused by prolonged hypoglycemia.
- Glucagon has been used as a cardiac stimulant in managing toxicity resulting from the use of beta-adrenergic blockers, quinidine, and tricyclic antidepressants.

Quick quiz

1. The patient's cardiac monitor reveals short runs of VT. He becomes symptomatic, and a bolus of amiodarone is ordered followed by a continuous infusion. What amount should you expect to administer?

A. 300-mg bolus followed by a 1-mg/minute continuous infusion for 6 hours

B. 300-mg bolus followed by a 0.5-mg/minute continuous infusion for 6 hours

C. 150-mg bolus followed by a 1-mg/minute continuous infusion for 6 hours

D. 150-mg bolus followed by a 0.5-mg/minute continuous infusion for 6 hours

Answer: C. For wide-complex tachycardia, give a rapid bolus infusion of 150 mg IV over the first 10 minutes (15 mg/minute) followed by a slow infusion of 360 mg IV over 6 hours (1 mg/minute). A maintenance infusion of 540 mg IV over 18 hours (0.5 mg/minute) may then be given.

2. Adenosine is administered:
   A. Slow IV push over 1 minute followed by a 20-mL saline flush
   B. Slow IV push over 2 minutes followed by a 20-mL saline flush
   C. Rapid IV push followed by a 20-mL saline flush
   D. Mixed in 50-mL bag of normal saline and infused over 10 minutes

Answer: C. Adenosine has a short half-life and must be administered rapidly followed by a 20-mL saline flush. Initial dosage is 6 mg, and if needed, a second (and third) dose of 12 mg may be given.

3. Indications for the administration of atropine sulfate include:
   A. symptomatic bradycardia and bradyarrhythmias.
   B. VF and atrial fibrillation.
   C. asystole and atrial fibrillation.
   D. third-degree heart block, PEA, and VT.

Answer: A. Atropine is an antiarrhythmic indicated for symptomatic bradycardia and bradyarrhythmias (junctional and escape rhythms). Dosage is 0.5 mg IV or IO push every 3 to 5 minutes with a maximum cumulative dosage of 3 mg.

4. The use of which medication may precipitate torsades de pointes?
   A. Procainamide
   B. Diltiazem
   C. Atenolol
   D. Atropine

Answer: A. Procainamide can precipitate torsades de pointes secondary to its prolonging effect on the QT interval.

5. The initial medication administered during Vtach or Vfib arrest and asystole and PEA is:
   A. sodium bicarbonate.
   B. atropine.
   C. adenosine.
   D. epinephrine.

Answer: D. Epinephrine is the initial medication administered during cardiac arrest caused by Vtach, Vfib, asystole, or PEA. Dosage is 1 mg (10 mL of 1:10,000 solution) IV or IO push every 3 to 5 minutes, with no maximum cumulative dose.

Scoring

☆☆☆ If you answered all five questions correctly, wow! Pharmacologically speaking, you're down with these medications.

☆☆ If you answered four questions correctly, hooray! Your knowledge is impressive.

☆ If you answered fewer than four questions correctly, give it another try! Just a small dose of review will prepare you for a perfect score next time.

Suggested references

ACLS for experienced providers; manual and resource text. (2017). American Heart Association.

Advanced cardiac life support: provider manual. (2020). American Heart Association.

AHA Council on Epidemiology and Prevention Statistics Committee and Stroke Statistics Subcommittee. (2018). Heart Disease and Stroke Statistics—2018 Update. *Circulation, 137*, e67–e492.

Attaran, R. R., & Ewy, G. A. (2010). Epinephrine in resuscitation: Curse or cure? *Future Cardiology, 6*(4), 473–482.

Farkas, J. (2015, October 25). 2015 ACLS Guidelines: What happened to VSE? *PulmCrit (EMCrit)*.

Fisk, C. A., Olsufka, M., Yin, L., McCoy, A. M., Latimer, A. J., Maynard, C., Nichol, G., Larsen, J., Cobb, L. A., Sayre, M. R. (2018). Lower dose epinephrine administration and out of hospital cardiac arrest outcomes. *Resuscitation, 124*, 43–48.

Hagihara, A., Hasegawa, M., Abe, T., Nagata, T., Wakata, Y., Miyazaki, S. (2012). Prehospital epinephrine use and survival among patients with out-of-hospital cardiac arrest (OHCA). *JAMA, 307*(11), 1161-1168.

Highlights of the 2020 American Heart Association Guidelines for CPR and ECC. (2020). American Heart Association.

Jacobs, I., Finna, J., Jelinek, G. A., Oxer, H. F., Thompson, P. L. (2011). Effect of adrenaline on survival in out of hospital cardiac arrest: A randomised double blind placebo controlled trial. *Resuscitation, 82*, 1138–1143.

Kempton, H., Vlok, R., Thang, C., Melhuish, T., & White, L. (2019). Standard dose epinephrine versus placebo in out of hospital cardiac arrest: A systematic review and meta-analysis. *The American Journal of Emergency Medicine*, 37(3), 511–517.

Olasveengen, T. M., Wik, L., Sunde, K., & Steen, P. A. (2012). Outcome when adrenaline (epinephrine) was actually given vs. not given—Post hoc analysis of a randomized clinical trial. *Resuscitation, 83*, 327–332.

Panchal, A. R., Bartos, J. A., Cabañas, J. G., Donnino, M. W., Drennan, I. R., Hirsch, K. G., Kudenchuk, P. J., Kurz, M. C., Lavonas, E. J., Morley, P. T., O'Neil, B. J., Peberdy, M. A., Rittenberger, J. C., Rodriguez, A. J., Sawyer, K. N., & Berg, K. M. (2020). Part 3: adult basic and advanced life support: 2020 American Heart Association guidelines for cardiopulmonary resuscitation and emergency cardiovascular care. *Circulation, 142*(16; suppl 2), S366–S468.

Perkins, G. D., Ji, C., Deakin, C. D., Quinn, T., Nolan, J. P., Scomparin, C., Regan, S., Long, J., Slowther, A., Pocock, H., Black, J. J. M., Moore, F., Fothergill, R. T., Rees, N., O'Shea, L., Docherty, M., Gunson, I., Han, K., Charlton, K., … Lall, R.; PARAMEDIC2 Collaborators. (2018). A randomized trial of epinephrine in out of hospital cardiac arrest. *The New England Journal of Medicine, 379*(8), 711–721.

Chapter 7

IV access and invasive techniques

Just the facts

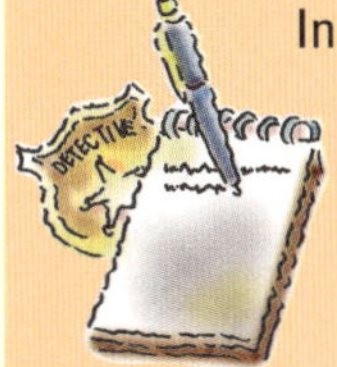

In this chapter, you'll learn:

- basics of IV access
- basics of intraosseous access
- use of different venipuncture devices
- techniques for successful peripheral and central IV access
- techniques for lifesaving emergency invasive procedures

IV access basics

An intravenous (IV) device is utilized to gain peripheral or central access to the patient's venous circulation. An IV device is inserted to:

- administer medications and fluids
- administer blood and blood products
- obtain blood for laboratory tests
- provide for insertion of a catheter into the central circulation for hemodynamic monitoring and electrical pacing

Choosing an access site

During resuscitation attempts, it is best to obtain venous access via the largest vein available that doesn't require interrupting resuscitation (such as the antecubital or femoral vein).

Choose wisely, my son

The site you choose for IV access is based on the patient's needs and condition. Factors include:

- availability and condition of peripheral veins
- duration for IV therapy or emergent indication
- volume and type of fluid to be administered
- indication for IV therapy

Veins used in IV therapy

This illustration shows the veins commonly used for peripheral IV and central venous therapy.

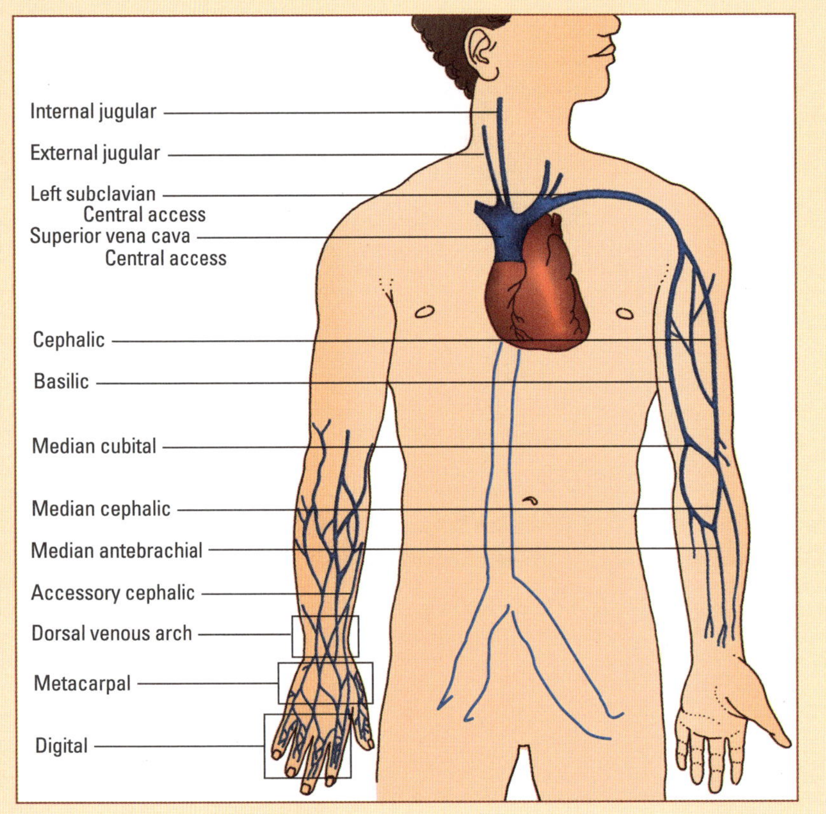

Here are some suggestions for selecting a vein:

- Keep in mind that the most prominent veins aren't necessarily the best veins; they may be sclerotic from previous use.
- Optimally, select a vein in the nondominant arm or hand.
- Avoid selecting a vein in an edematous or impaired arm, if possible.
- Never select a vein in the arm closest to an area that's surgically compromised, such as veins compromised by a mastectomy or by placement of dialysis access.
- For subsequent venipunctures, select sites above the previously used or injured vein.
- Always rotate access sites. (See *Veins used in IV therapy*.)

IV safety

Regardless of the site you choose, you must take precautions to ensure safety for yourself and your patient. These include:

- using standard precautions
- appropriately cleaning the selected site using an antiseptic solution
- engaging the needle safety if present
- disposing of needles appropriately
- changing the IV site every 3 days or according to your facility's policy
- evaluating the site for infiltration, extravasation, or thrombosis per facility policy and as needed
- gauze dressing changes every 2 days; semipermeable dressing (Tegaderm) changes every 7 days
- mainline IV tubing can be changed every 96 hours
- secondary or IV piggyback (IVPB) tubing can be changed every 24 hours
- blood tubing changes every 24 hours
- propofol and lipid-based solutions change every 6 to 12 hours or when new bottle is started

It's also important to change IV lines placed in the patient outside the hospital setting within 24 hours, if possible. Because these IV lines aren't usually inserted under ideal circumstances, they're more likely to cause infection or complications.

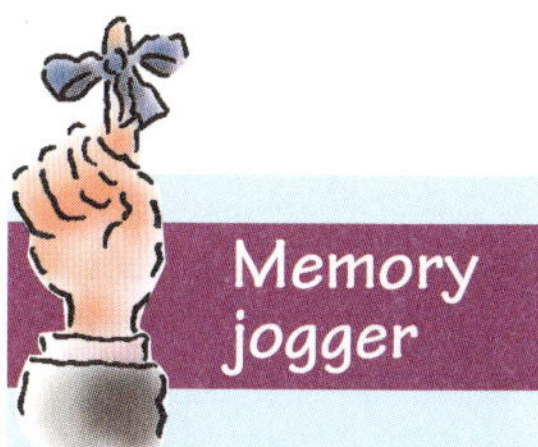

Memory jogger

In selecting the best site for venipuncture, remember the acronym **VIP**:

Vein

Infusion

Patient.

For the vein, consider its location, condition, and physical path along the extremity.

For the infusion, consider its purpose and duration.

For the patient, consider his or her degree of cooperation and compliance, along with preference. Also consider patient history.

Basic venipuncture devices

Two major types of venipuncture devices exist: over-the-needle catheters and winged steel needle sets. Which catheter you choose is based on what type of IV administration is needed or what equipment is available. Over-the-needle catheters are preferred for long-term therapy (such as in a hospital stay) and winged steel needles may be preferred for short-term therapy such as administering medication for a procedure. (See *Comparing basic venous access devices*.)

Over-the-needle catheters

The over-the-needle catheter can be used for long-term therapy and is often useful for an active or agitated patient.

Advantages of the over-the-needle catheter include the following:

- Inadvertent puncture of the vein is less likely than with a winged steel needle set.
- It is more comfortable for the patient.
- Easy check of blood return and prevention of air entering the vessel on insertion with units that have an attached syringe.

Comparing basic venous access devices

These illustrations show the differences between an over-the-needle catheter and a winged steel needle set.

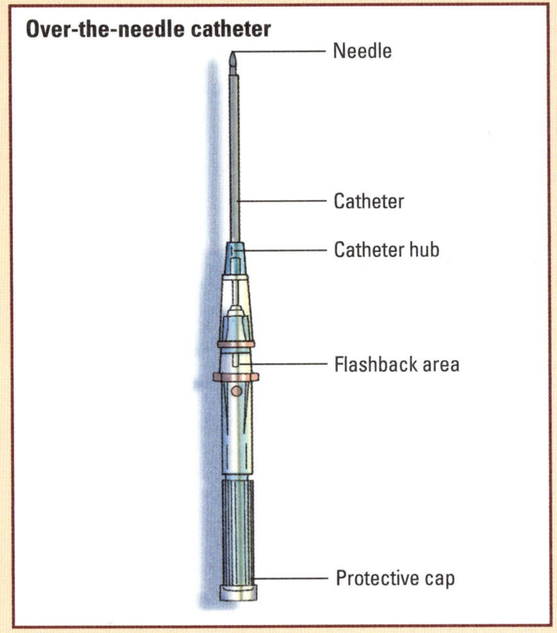

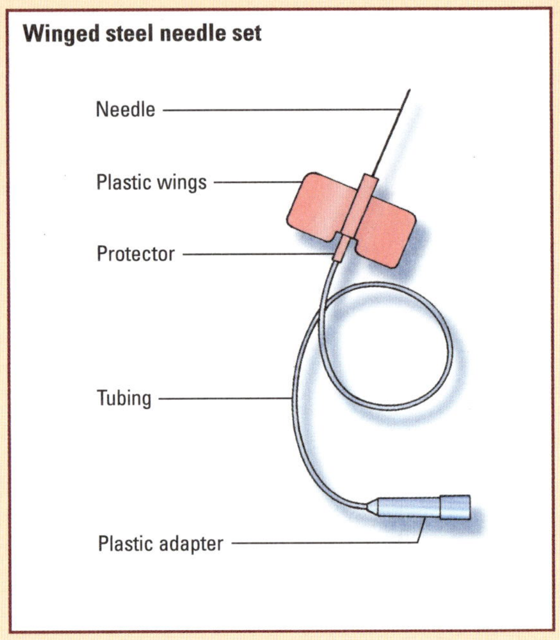

- Some devices have a needle safety feature to decrease chance of accidental needlestick.
- Attaching an activity-restricting device, such as an arm board, is rarely required.

One disadvantage of the over-the-needle catheter is that it requires more expertise to insert successfully. In addition, extra care is needed to ensure that both the needle and catheter are inserted into the vein.

Winged steel needle sets

The winged steel needle set is used for short-term IV therapy in a cooperative adult patient. It may also be used for therapy of any duration for an elderly patient with fragile or sclerotic veins.

Advantages of the winged steel needle set include the following:

- It is easier to insert because the needle is thin walled and extremely sharp.
- Inidcations are for short-term therapy or single-dose medication administration.
- A catheter that can be left in place is available in some units, such as an over-the-needle catheter.

The disadvantage of the winged steel needle set is that infiltration can easily occur if a rigid needle winged infusion device is used.

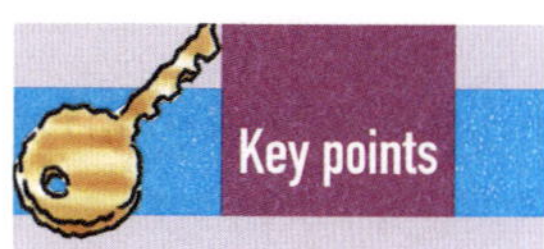

Peripheral IV lines
- Multiple sites available; may provide easy, rapid access
- Rapidly inserted by trained personnel
- Easily removed
- Access site may be inappropriate for administration of some medications
- Not appropriate for administration of hypertonic or irritating solutions
- May be easily dislodged

Establishing peripheral IV lines

Peripheral venipuncture sites—located on the dorsal and ventral surfaces of the upper extremities—include the antecubital, metacarpal (hand), cephalic, basilic, and median veins. The leg veins shouldn't be used routinely because of increased risk of thrombophlebitis, ulcers, and infection. The external jugular vein may also be used for rapid access in an emergency. Selection of an IV site depends on the type of fluid to be infused; the frequency and duration of the infusion; the patency and location of accessible veins; the patient's age, size, and physical condition; and patient preference (if possible). (See *Comparing peripheral venipuncture sites*.)

Advantages of a peripheral IV line include:
- rapid insertion by trained personnel
- easy access to veins and rapid administration of solutions, blood, and drugs
- continuous administration of drugs to produce rapid systemic changes
- easy to monitor

Disadvantages of a peripheral IV line include:
- associated risks of bleeding, infiltration, and infection due to being an invasive procedure
- limited time for safe use
- Associated with higher costs when compared too more than oral, subcutaneous, or IM therapy (See *Risks of peripheral IV therapy*.)

Upper extremity veins

The largest superficial veins of the arms are located in the antecubital fossa. Of these veins, the most commonly selected for IV access are the median cephalic and median basilic.

Up the ante for quick IV access

The antecubital fossa site is the recommended site for a rapid IV access because its veins are easily accessed. This site is optimal for patients in circulatory collapse or cardiac arrest because it does not impede CPR. The cephalic and basilic veins may also be accessible both above and below the antecubital fossa. If long-term therapy is anticipated, start with the most distal, adequate site possible, such as the dorsal hand veins. Don't use the distal cephalic vein above the thumb and the veins of the inner wrist, to avoid damaging nerves.

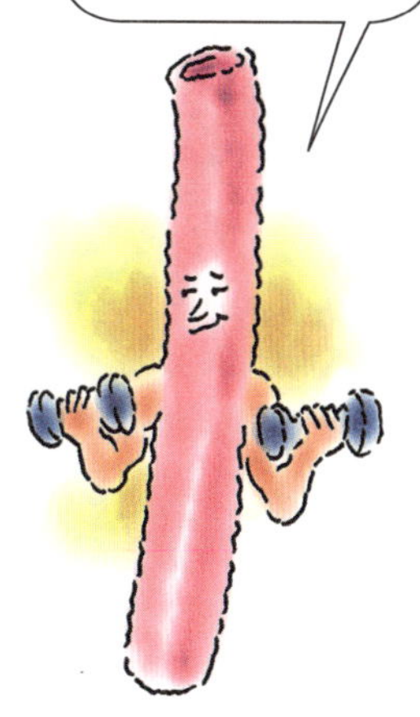

Comparing peripheral venipuncture sites

This chart includes some of the major advantages and disadvantages of several common venipuncture sites.

Site	Advantages	Disadvantages
Digital veins Run along the lateral and dorsal portions of the fingers	• May be used for short-term therapy • May be used when other means aren't available	• Splinting the fingers with a tongue blade is required, which decreases the patient's ability to use the hand • Uncomfortable for the patient • Significant risk of infiltration • Not used if veins in the dorsum of the hand are already used • Not useful for certain medication infusions such as dopamine
Metacarpal veins On the dorsum of the hand; formed by the union of digital veins between the knuckles	• Easily accessible • Lie flat on the back of the hand; more stable position • In an adult or large child, bones of the hand act as a splint	• Wrist movement decreased unless a short catheter is used • Painful insertion because of the large number of nerve endings in the hands • Phlebitis more common at the site • Not useful for certain medication infusions such as dopamine
Accessory cephalic vein Runs along the radial bone as a continuation of metacarpal veins of the thumb	• Large vein excellent for venipuncture • Readily accepts large-gauge needles • Doesn't impair mobility • May not require an armboard in an older child or adult	• Some difficulty positioning catheter flush with skin • Discomfort during movement due to device located at bend of wrist
Cephalic vein Runs along the radial side of the forearm and upper arm	• Large vein excellent for venipuncture • Readily accepts large-gauge needles	• Decreased joint movement due to proximity of the device to the elbow • Tendency of vein to roll during insertion
Median antebrachial vein Arises from the palm and runs along the ulnar side of the forearm	• Holds winged needles well • A last resort when no other means are available • High risk of infiltration in the area	• Painful insertion or infiltration damage is possible due to the large number of nerve endings in the area
Basilic vein Runs along the ulnar side of the forearm and upper arm	• Readily accepts large-gauge needles • Straight, strong vein suitable for large-gauge venipuncture devices • Ultrasound guidance may be required to access vein	• Uncomfortable position for the patient during insertion • Tendency of vein to roll during insertion • This vein usually lies deeper and may be more difficult to visualize

Comparing peripheral venipuncture sites *(continued)*

Site	Advantages	Disadvantages
Antecubital veins		
Located in the antecubital fossa (median cephalic, on radial side; median basilic, on ulnar side; median cubital, which rises in front of the elbow joint)	• Large veins; facilitate drawing blood • Often more visible or palpable when other veins won't dilate • May be used in an emergency or as a last resort	• Difficult to splint the elbow area with an arm board • Veins may be scarred if used frequently for obtaining blood

What you need

- IV start kit (available in some facilities)
- 2% chlorhexidine solution
- Gloves
- Tourniquet
- IV access device with safety shield
- Syringe with IV flush solution or IV solution with attached and primed administration set
- IV pole
- IV pump
- Transparent semipermeable dressing
- Catheter securement device or 1-inch hypoallergenic tape
- Sharps container

How it's done

- Perform hand hygiene and put on gloves.
- Select the site and place the arm in a dependent position if possible.
- Apply a tourniquet 4 to 6 (10 to 15 cm) above the intended puncture site to dilate the vein.
- Leave the tourniquet in place for no longer than 3 minutes. If you're unable to locate a vein and prepare the site in that time, release the tourniquet and reapply it after the site is prepared.
- Clean the site with the chlorhexidine solution using a back-and-forth scrubbing motion and allow it to dry.
- Ask the patient to open and close the fist a few times (if able) to enhance your visualization of the veins.
- Remove the cover from the access device and make sure the needle is smooth and intact.
- Stabilize the vein by stretching the skin taut below the intended insertion site.
- Ensure that the needle's bevel is facing up and then puncture the skin.

Risks of peripheral IV therapy

Complications from peripheral IV therapy may be local or systemic. This chart lists some common complications along with their signs and symptoms, possible causes, and nursing interventions, including preventive measures.

Signs and symptoms	Possible causes
Local complications	
Phlebitis	
• Tenderness at or above tip of device • Erythema at tip of catheter and along vein • Vein hard on palpation • Elevated temperature	• Poor blood flow around device • Friction from catheter movement along vein • Device left in vein too long or clot in cannula tip • Solution with high or low pH or high osmolarity
Infiltration	
• Swelling surrounding the IV site (may extend along entire limb) • Discomfort, burning, or pain at site • Feeling of tightness at site • Blanching at site • Absent blood backflow • Skin cool to the touch around IV site	• Device dislodged from vein or perforated vein
Catheter dislodgment	
• Catheter partly backed out of vein • Infiltrated tissue • Leaking of IV fluid at site	• Loosened tape or tubing accidently pulled, resulting in partial retraction of catheter
Occlusion	
• Infusion doesn't flow • Infusion pump alarm reads "occlusion" • Discomfort at insertion site	• IV flow interrupted • Intermittent device not flushed regularly • Blood backup in line • Hypercoagulable patient • Line clamped too long
Vein irritation or pain at IV site	
• Pain during infusion • Possible blanching if vasospasm occurs • Red skin over vein during infusion • Rapidly developing signs of phlebitis	• Solution with high or low pH or high osmolarity, such as 40 mEq/L of potassium chloride, phenytoin, and some antibiotics (vancomycin and nafcillin)
Severed catheter	
• Leakage from catheter shaft	• Faulty catheter • Catheter inadvertently cut by scissors or broken • Reinsertion of needle into catheter • Agitated patient

Nursing interventions	Prevention
• Remove device. • Apply warm pack. • Notify the practitioner. • Document your assessment of the patient's IV site, interventions, and patient response.	• Use a larger vein for irritating substances or restart with a smaller-gauge device to ensure adequate blood flow. • Secure the device to prevent dislodgment.
• Stop the infusion and remove the device. • Apply warm soaks to aid absorption. • Elevate the limb. • Periodically assess circulation by checking for pulse and capillary refill. • Restart infusion above the infiltration site or in another limb. • Document your assessment of the patient's IV site, interventions, and patient response.	• Assess the IV site per facility policy and as needed. • Use transparent dressing for easy visualization of site. • Immobilize the IV site if possible to avoid catheter movement. • Remind the patient to report discomfort, pain, or swelling.
• Remove device. • Restart infusion at a different site or in another limb. • Document your assessment of the patient's IV site, interventions, and patient response.	• Tape the device securely on insertion. • Immobilize the site if possible.
• Attempt flushing device using mild pressure; don't force. If unsuccessful, remove and restart at another site or in another limb. • Document your assessment of the patient's IV site, interventions, and patient response.	• Maintain the IV flow rate. • Flush promptly after intermittent piggyback administration. • Have the patient walk with his arm below heart level to reduce risk of blood backup.
• Decrease the flow rate, if possible. • Use an electronic flow device to achieve a steady, regulated flow. • Document your assessment of the patient's IV site, interventions, and patient response.	• Dilute solution before administration, if possible. • If long-term therapy of an irritating medication is planned, ask the practitioner to insert a central IV line.
• If the broken part is visible, attempt to retrieve it. If unsuccessful, immediately notify the practitioner. • If a portion of the catheter enters the bloodstream, place a tourniquet above the IV site to prevent progression of broken portion. Notify the practitioner and the radiology department. • Document your assessment of the patient's IV site, interventions, and patient response.	• Inspect catheter prior to insertion for signs of damage. • Avoid using scissors around an IV site. • Never reinsert a needle into the catheter. • Remove an unsuccessfully inserted catheter and needle together. • Immediately remove a damaged catheter.

(*continued*)

Risks of peripheral IV therapy *(continued)*

Signs and symptoms	Possible causes
Hematoma • Tenderness and swelling at venipuncture site • Bruising around site	• Vein punctured through ventral wall at time of venipuncture • Leakage of blood into tissue
Venous spasm • Pain along vein • Sluggish IV flow rate when clamp is completely open • Blanched skin over vein	• Severe vein irritation from certain drugs or fluids • Administration of cold fluids or blood • Very rapid flow rate (with fluids at room temperature)
Thrombosis • Painful, reddened, swollen, hard vein • Sluggish or stopped IV flow	• Injury to endothelial cells of vein wall, allowing platelets to adhere and thrombus to form
Thrombophlebitis • Severe discomfort • Reddened, swollen, and hardened vein	• Thrombosis and inflammation
Nerve, tendon, or ligament damage • Extreme pain (similar to electric shock when nerve is punctured) • Limb numbness and muscle contraction • Delayed effects, including paralysis, numbness, and deformity	• Improper venipuncture technique, resulting in injury to surrounding nerves, tendons, or ligaments • Tight taping or improper splinting with arm board

Nursing interventions	Prevention
• Remove the device. • Reinsert the device at a different site or limb. • Apply pressure and cold compresses to the affected area. • Recheck for bleeding. • Document your assessment of the patient's IV site, interventions, and patient response.	• Choose a vein that can accommodate the size of the intended venous access device. • Release the tourniquet as soon as you achieve successful insertion.
• Apply warm soaks over the vein and surrounding area. • Decrease the flow rate, if possible. • Document your assessment of the patient's IV site, interventions, and patient response.	• Use a blood warmer for blood or packed red blood cells when appropriate.
• Remove the device; restart the infusion in the opposite limb if possible. • Apply warm soaks. • Watch for IV therapy-related infection (thrombi provide an excellent environment for bacterial growth). • Notify the practitioner. • Document your assessment of the patient's IV site, interventions, and patient response.	• Use proper venipuncture techniques to reduce injury to the vein. • Assess the IV site per facility policy and as needed.
• Remove the device; restart the infusion in the opposite limb if possible. • Apply warm soaks. • Watch for IV therapy-related infection (thrombi provide an excellent environment for bacterial growth). • Notify the practitioner. • Document your assessment of the patient's IV site, interventions, and patient response.	• Assess the IV site per facility policy and as needed. • Remove the device at the first sign of redness and tenderness.
• Stop the procedure and notify the practitioner. • Document your assessment of the patient's IV site, interventions, and patient response.	• Know where the superficial nerves are and avoid placing an IV catheter close to their location. • Document your assessment of the patient's IV site, interventions, and patient response. • Don't repeatedly penetrate tissues with the venipuncture device. • Don't apply excessive pressure when taping. Don't encircle the limb with tape. • Pad the arm board and, if possible, pad the tape securing the arm board.

(*continued*)

Risks of peripheral IV therapy *(continued)*

Signs and symptoms	Possible causes
Systemic complications *Circulatory overload* • Jugular vein distention • Respiratory distress • Increased blood pressure • Crackles in the lungs • Positive fluid balance. (Intake is greater than output.)	• Flow rate too rapid • Miscalculation of fluid requirements • Infusion pump failure • Patient condition
Systemic infection (septicemia or bacteremia) • Fever, chills, and malaise for no apparent reason • Decreased blood pressure • Altered mental status • Immunocompromised patient	• Failure to maintain aseptic technique during insertion or site care • Severe phlebitis, which can set up ideal conditions for organism growth • Movement of access device, which can introduce organisms into bloodstream • Prolonged indwelling time of device
Air embolism • Respiratory distress • Weak pulse • Increased central venous pressure • Decreased blood pressure • Loss of consciousness	• Solution container empties; next container pushes air down line. • Disconnected lines allow air into system. • Failure of IV pump in-line air detector
Allergic reaction • Itching • Tearing eyes and runny nose • Bronchospasm and wheezing • Edema at IV site • Urticarial rash • Anaphylactic reaction, including flushing, chills, anxiety, agitation, generalized itching, palpitations, paresthesia, throbbing in ears, wheezing, coughing, seizures, and cardiac arrest	• Allergens such as medications

Nursing interventions	Prevention
• Raise the head of bed. • Administer oxygen as needed. • Slow or stop the infusion. • Notify the practitioner. • Obtain chest X-ray and administer medications (such as a diuretic) as ordered. • Document your assessment of the patient's condition, interventions, and patient response.	• Use an IV pump, volume-control set or rate minder for elderly or compromised patients. • Monitor the infusion flow rate frequently.
• Remove the device after another access has been established. • Notify the practitioner. • Administer medications and IV fluids as prescribed. • Obtain blood cultures and lactate level. • Monitor vital signs. • Assess for severe sepsis and provide interventions per facility policy. • Document your assessment of the patient's IV site and condition, interventions, and patient response.	• Use scrupulous aseptic technique when handling solutions and tubings, inserting the venipuncture device, and discontinuing the infusion. • Secure all connections. • Change the IV solutions, tubing, and access device per facility policy.
• Discontinue the infusion. • Place the patient in left lateral Trendelenburg's position to allow air to enter the right atrium. • Administer oxygen. • Notify the practitioner. • Document the patient's condition, your interventions, and patient response.	• Purge tubing or air completely before infusion. • Use an air detection device on the pump or an air-eliminating filter proximal to the IV site. • Maintain secure connections.
• Stop the infusion immediately. • Maintain IV access with a normal saline infusion. • Maintain a patent airway and assist with ventilations if needed. Perform CPR if indicated. • Notify the practitioner. • Administer antihistamine, corticosteroid, and antipyretic drugs as ordered. • Give aqueous epinephrine subcutaneously. • Document your assessment of the patient's condition, interventions, and patient response.	• Review the patient's allergy history before administering medications. Be aware of cross-allergies. • Assist with test dosing. • Monitor the patient carefully during the first 15 minutes of infusion when administering new drugs.

- Check the flashback chamber behind the hub for blood return, signifying that the vein is accessed.
- Advance the needle and hold it in place, if using a winged infusion set.
- Advance the catheter and remove the needle, if using an over-the-needle cannula. Place the needle in a sharps container.
- Remove the tourniquet and dispose.
- Flush with saline or attach the primed IV administration tubing and allow fluid to infuse. Note if there is any difficulty in flushing or IV fluid does not flow, as this may indicate a problem with the insertion.
- Secure the catheter with tape.
- Clean the surrounding area, and apply a catheter securement device and a transparent semipermeable dressing.
- Label the site and with the date and your initials.
- Document the procedure in the patient's electronic health record according to your facility's policy.

What to consider

- Remember that IV insertion at the antecubital fossa or dorsal veins may restrict movement in the active patient.
- Dorsal hand veins may be short and difficult to stabilize.
- If infiltration occurs, sites below the insertion site may be unusable.
- Accessing any peripheral vein may be difficult if the patient is in circulatory collapse.
- Drugs given peripherally take longer to reach central circulation during cardiac arrest. For this reason, follow administration with a 20-mL bolus of normal saline solution and raise the patient's arm during cardiopulmonary resuscitation (CPR).
- Hypertonic or irritating solutions shouldn't be administered through a peripheral vein because of damage to surrounding tissue if infiltration occurs.

External jugular vein

The external jugular vein is large and usually easy to access. It can be used when rapid IV access is needed, such as in patients in circulatory collapse or cardiac arrest when peripheral insertion isn't attainable. According to the Infusion Nurses Society (INS), external jugular IVs are considered peripheral; therefore, they can remain in place for the same amount of time as other peripheral IVs. The INS supports trained RNs with this insertion. Many facilities restrict cannulation of this site to physicians or trained advanced practice health care professionals, so be aware of your state board of nursings scope of practice and your local facility's policy.

What you need

- IV start kit (available in some facilities)
- 2% chlorhexidine solution
- Gloves
- IV access device with safety shield
- IV solution with attached and primed administration set
- IV pole
- Transparent semipermeable dressing
- Catheter securement device or 1-inch hypoallergenic tape
- Sharps container

How it's done

- Perform hand hygiene and put on gloves.
- Position the patient in Trendelenburg's position to enhance your visualization of the vein.
- Turn the patient's head to the opposite side of insertion.
- Clean the site with the chlorhexidine solution using a back-and-forth motion and allow to dry.
- Anesthetize the skin if the patient is awake.
- Remove the cover from the access device and make sure the needle is smooth and intact.
- Aim the needle toward the ipsilateral (same side) shoulder, making sure that the bevel is facing up.
- Stabilize the vein by holding the skin taut right above the clavicle.
- Insert the needle midway between the angle of the jaw and the midclavicular line.
- Check the flash-back chamber behind the hub for blood return, signifying that the vein has been accessed.
- Advance the catheter and remove the needle. Place the needle in a sharps container.
- Attach the primed IV administration tubing and allow fluid to flow. Note if the fluid does not flow freely, as this indicates a problem with the insertion.
- Secure the catheter with tape.
- Clean the area, apply a catheter securement device, and apply a transparent semipermeable dressing.
- Label the site with the date and your initials.
- Document the procedure in the patient's electronic health record according to your facility's policy.

What to consider

- IV insertion into the external jugular vein requires more skill than insertion into other peripheral veins and is usually performed by a trained practitioner.

- Infiltration of IV solutions at this site may affect the patency of the patient's airway.
- Movement of the patient's head may affect the flow of IV solutions.

Adjunctive devices for use in obtaining peripheral IV and central line access

For the general pediatric or adult populations, transillumination will not be helpful due to the amount of subcutaneous tissue. However, for patients with thin skin or minimal subcutaneous tissue, consider using transillumination devices to illuminate superficial veins. Avoid direct heat-producing devices such as certain flashlights.

For these patients, you can consider a near-infrared device (nIR). Available technology includes hands-free devices that capture an image of the veins and reflect it back to the skin's surface or to a screen. Use nIR light technology to assess peripheral venous sites and facilitate more informed decisions about vein selection (e.g., bifurcating veins, tortuosity of veins, palpable but nonvisible veins, location of venous valves). The use of nIR technology has been associated with enhanced first-time insertion success and decreased procedural time (compared to traditional visual assessment and palpation) in some populations, such as neonates.

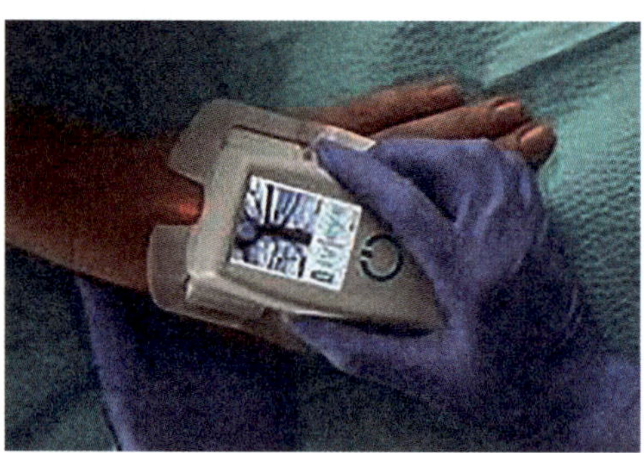

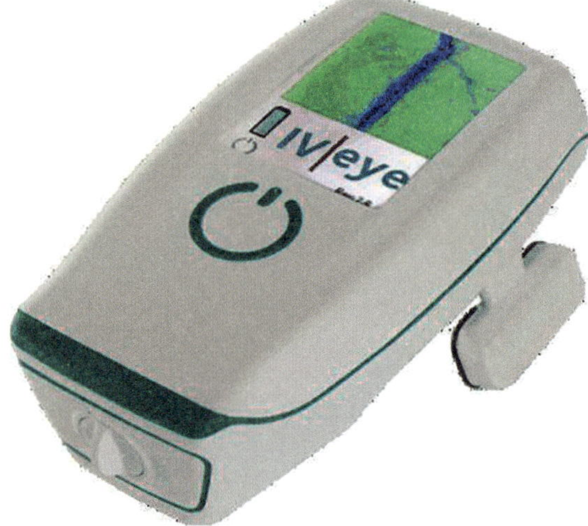

Ultrasound can also be utilized for peripheral IV access and has rapidly become a strong recommendation for usage in all central line placement to avoid pneumothoraxes and backwalling the vessel. It can also decrease the number of sticks and repositioning needed to locate access and cannulate the vessel.

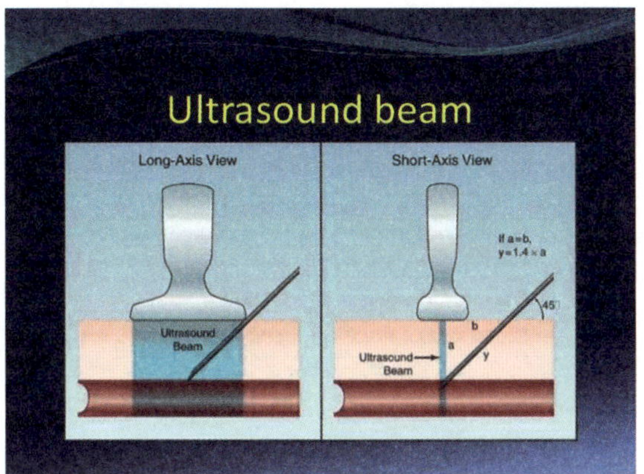

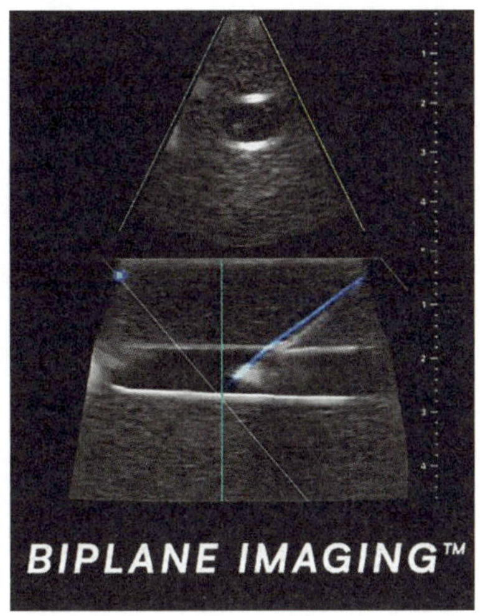

Establishing central IV lines

Here I am! Major Super Vein to help you gain central IV access.

The internal jugular, subclavian, and femoral veins can be used to establish a nontunneled central IV access during an emergency or when a patient's peripheral veins are inaccessible. This procedure is usually restricted to physicians or trained advanced practice health care practitioners. With central venous (CV) therapy, drugs or fluids are infused directly into a major vein. (See *Comparing CV insertion sites*.)

Central IV lines are used for:

- infusing large volumes of fluid and blood components
- multiple infusions

Comparing CV insertion sites

This chart lists the insertion sites for a central venous (CV) catheter and the advantages and disadvantages of each.

Site	Advantages	Disadvantages
Subclavian vein	• Easy and fast access • Easy to keep dressing in place • Allows for high fluid flow rate or rapid fluid infusion, which reduces the risk of thrombus	• Proximity to the subclavian artery (If artery is punctured during catheter insertion, hemorrhage can result.) • Difficult to control bleeding • Increased risk of pneumothorax • Need to interrupt CPR for insertion
Internal jugular vein	• Short, direct route to superior vena cava • Catheter stability, resulting in less movement with respiration • Decreased risk of pneumothorax	• Proximity to the common carotid artery (If artery is punctured during catheter insertion, uncontrolled hemorrhage, emboli, or impedance to flow can result.) • Difficult to keep the dressing in place • Close proximity to the trachea
Femoral vein	• Easy and fast access • No need to interrupt CPR to access • No risk of pneumothorax	• Less direct route • May have increased risk of infection due to location • Proximity to femoral artery and nerve • Site should be changed at first opportunity

- long-term IV therapy
- drawing blood samples
- establishing hemodynamic monitoring
- administering medications that may be irritating to peripheral veins or cause harm to tissues if infiltration occurs
- administering parenteral nutrition or chemotherapy.

The fewer, the better

Besides the uses already mentioned, another advantage of central IV access is that it reduces the need for repeated venipunctures. Fewer venipunctures decrease pain caused to the patient as well as lower the patient's anxiety level. It also helps preserve or restore the patient's peripheral veins.

However, using a CV catheter also has disadvantages and risks. A CV catheter:

- requires more time and skill to insert than a peripheral IV catheter and is usually inserted by a trained practitioner

- costs more to insert and maintain than a peripheral IV catheter
- carries a risk of pneumothorax during insertion or air embolism postinsertion (certain sites only)
- creates a source of infection, by either poor insertion technique or improper care and maintenance

Central IV access is contraindicated when the patient has scar tissue in the area or the configuration of their lung apices doesn't lend itself to inserting a subclavian subclavian central IV line. Use caution if central IV access will interfere with the patient's surgical site or other therapy or their lifestyle or daily activities. (See *Risks of CV therapy*.)

Central IV lines

- Access important in emergencies or when peripheral access inaccessible or inappropriate
- Inserted by a trained practitioner
- Appropriate for parenteral nutrition or irritating infusions, such as chemotherapy administration
- Allows for hemodynamic monitoring
- Appropriate for blood samples and multiple infusions
- More potential complications than with peripheral access

Internal jugular vein

The internal jugular vein is lateral and anterior to the common carotid artery. The right internal jugular vein is preferred for IV access because the right lung and pleura are lower and there's a fairly straight line to the superior vena cava. You don't have to visualize the internal jugular vein to access it.

Hypertonic? Irritating? This vein's for you!

Use the internal jugular vein when peripheral venous access is unsuccessful or you need to administer emergency medications. This access is also acceptable for administering hypertonic or irritating solutions and inserting catheters into the heart and pulmonary circulation for hemodynamic monitoring.

Fill it up! And check the fluids, please

The internal jugular vein allows direct access to central circulation. It is also an excellent means for rapid administration of large volumes of fluid. In addition, multiple blood samples can be withdrawn through the catheter. Most facilities require using an infusion pump for infusing fluids and medications through a central line.

What you need

- Two (14 or 16G) CV catheters (antimicrobial impregnated, if available)
- Central line introducer kit (available in most facilities)
- Sterile gown and gloves
- Maximum barrier kit or sterile towel and large sterile drape
- Masks with shields and cap

Risks of CV therapy

As with any invasive procedure, central venous (CV) therapy can have complications. This chart outlines how to recognize, manage, and prevent these complications.

Signs and symptoms	Possible causes
Pneumothorax, hemothorax, chylothorax, or hydrothorax	
• Chest pain • Dyspnea • Cyanosis • Decreased breath sounds on affected side • Tracheal deviation • With hemothorax, decreased hemoglobin because of blood pooling • Abnormal chest X-ray • Cardiac arrest	• Lung puncture by catheter during insertion or exchange over a guide wire • Large blood vessel puncture with bleeding inside or outside of the lung • Lymph node puncture with leakage of lymph fluid • Infusion of solution into chest area through infiltrated catheter
Air embolism	
• Respiratory distress • Weak pulse • Increased CV pressure • Decreased blood pressure • Churning murmur over precordium • Change in level of consciousness	• Intake of air into CV system during catheter insertion or tubing changes; inadvertent opening, cutting, or breaking of catheter • Inadvertent disconnection of tubing
Thrombosis	
• Edema at or below puncture site • Ipsilateral swelling of arm, neck, and face • Fever spike and malaise • Tachycardia • Pain	• Sluggish flow rate • Hematopoietic status of the patient • Repeated or long-term use of same vein • Preexisting cardiovascular disease • Irritation of vein lining during insertion
Local infection	
• Redness, warmth, tenderness, and swelling at insertion site • Possible exudate of purulent material • Local rash or pustules • Fever, chills, and malaise • Pain • Notify the practitioner, who may remove the catheter.	• Failure to maintain aseptic technique during catheter insertion or care • Wet or soiled dressing remaining on site • Immunosuppression • Irritated suture line

Nursing interventions	Prevention
• Notify the practitioner and stop the infusion. • Remove the catheter or assist with its removal, as ordered. • Administer oxygen, as ordered. • Set up for and assist with chest tube insertion. • Monitor vital signs and pulse oximetry. • Initiate CPR if indicated. • Document your interventions and patient response in the patient's electronic health record.	• Position the patient's head down, with a towel roll between his scapulae, to dilate and expose the internal jugular or subclavian vein as much as possible during catheter insertion. • Assess for early signs of fluid infiltration, such as swelling in the shoulder, neck, chest, and arm area. • Ensure immobilization of the patient during the procedure; active patients may need to be sedated or taken to the interventional radiology for CV catheter insertion. • Minimize patient activity after insertion. • Confirm CV catheter placement by X-ray before infusion of IV fluids.
• Clamp the catheter immediately. • Turn the patient on his left side with his head down so air can enter the right atrium. Maintain this position for 20 to 30 minutes or as ordered by the practitioner. • Don't have the patient perform Valsalva's maneuver. (A large intake of air will worsen the situation.) • Administer oxygen. • Monitor vital signs. including pulse oximetry. • Notify the practitioner. • Document your interventions and patient response in the patient's electronic health record.	• Purge all air from the IV tubing before connecting. • Teach the patient to perform Valsalva's maneuver during catheter insertion and tubing changes. • Use an infusion-control device with air detection capability. • Use Luer-lock tubing, tape connections, or use locking devices for all connections. • Use air-eliminating filters.
• Stop the infusion. • Notify the practitioner, who may remove the catheter. • Possibly, infuse a thrombolytic to dissolve the clot. • Verify thrombosis with diagnostic studies. • Don't use the limb on the affected side for subsequent venipuncture. • Document your interventions and patient response in the patient's electronic health record.	• Verify that the catheter tip is in the correct position before use.
• Evaluate site condition with every dressing change. Assess for signs of infection. • Monitor the patient's vital signs, including temperature, per facility policy and as needed. • Culture the site if drainage is present. • Provide proper maintenance and care per facility policy, maintaining aseptic technique. • Treat systemically, as ordered, with antibiotics or antifungals. • Notify the practitioner, who may remove the catheter. • Document your interventions and patient response in the patient's electronic health record.	• Maintain strict aseptic technique on insertion. • Provide proper maintenance and care per facility policy, maintaining aseptic technique. • Change a wet or soiled dressing immediately. • Use an antimicrobial patch at the insertion site.

(*continued*)

Risks of CV therapy *(continued)*

Signs and symptoms	Possible causes
Systemic infection	
• Fever and chills without other apparent reason • Leukocytosis and possible elevated lactate level • Nausea and vomiting • Malaise • Decreased blood pressure	• Contaminated catheter • Poor insertion technique or maintenance care • Long-term use of single IV access • Repeated contamination of dressing or insertion site, such as with copious oral or tracheal secretions • Immunosuppression

- Skin preparation kit with chlorhexidine sponges
- Alcohol pads
- 3-mL syringe with 25G needle
- 1% or 2% injectable lidocaine
- Suture material
- Three 10-mL syringes filled with normal saline solution
- Catheter securement device or sterile tape
- Antimicrobial patch
- Transparent semipermeable dressing

How it's done

Please note in an emergency situation, the following steps in the procedure may need to be altered.

- Explain the procedure to the patient and answer all questions. Obtain consent if able.
- Confirm the patient's identity using two identifiers and perform a "time-out" verification process according to the facility's policy, if not emergent.
- Perform hand hygiene.
- Place the patient in Trendelenburg's position to dilate the vein and reduce the risk of air embolism.
- Turn the patient's head in the opposite direction of the insertion site to make it more accessible and to prevent site contamination from airborne pathogens.

Nursing interventions	Prevention
• Draw blood cultures and lactate level. • Remove catheter after alternate IV access is obtained. • Evaluate for severe sepsis and provide interventions per facility protocol. • Treat the patient with fluids and an antibiotic regimen, as ordered. • Monitor the patient's vital signs closely. • Document your interventions and patient response in the patient's electronic record.	• Provide proper maintenance and care per facility policy, maintaining aseptic technique. • Use a 0.2-micron filter for infusions. • Keep the system closed as much as possible. • Change a wet or soiled dressing immediately. • Use an antimicrobial patch at the insertion site.

- Establish a sterile field on a bedside table, and then open the catheter and central line insertion tray. Be sure to label all medications, medication containers, and solutions on and off the sterile field.
- Put on a cap, mask, sterile gown, and gloves.
- Clean the area with the chlorhexidine sponge using a side-to-side motion for 30 seconds; allow the area to dry.

The practitioner:

- puts on a cap, mask, sterile gown, and gloves and then drapes the procedure area
- anesthetizes the area with 1% or 2% lidocaine
- locates the suprasternal notch and moves laterally until the clavicular head of the sternomastoid muscle is located. The carotid artery is identified by its pulse. The internal jugular vein runs lateral to the carotid artery
- inserts the needle with the bevel side up at the apex of the triangle formed by the two heads of the sternomastoid muscle and the clavicle (See *The central approach.*)
- maintains negative pressure on the syringe as the needle is advanced. The vein is normally ¾ to 1½" (2 to 4 cm) deep
- asks the awake patient to perform a Valsalva's maneuver after the vein is accessed and before the caps are attached. A Valsalva's maneuver increases the intrathoracic pressure, reducing the possibility of an air embolus. (See *Performing Valsalva's maneuver*.)
- confirms blood return in all ports, flushes them with normal saline solution, and sutures the catheter in place

- orders a chest X-ray to confirm placement of the line in the superior vena cava and evaluate for pneumothorax

After successful cannulation:

- apply an antimicrobial patch and transparent dressing according to the facility's policy. Label the dressing with the date, time, and your initials
- remove your gloves, perform hand hygiene, and document the procedure in the patient's electronic health record according to facility policy

Peak technique

The central approach

To perform the central approach for accessing the internal jugular vein, the practitioner:

- Places the patient in a supine position with his head turned toward the left side.
- Stands at the patient's head and locates the vessel.
- Inserts the needle into the internal jugular vein, keeping the bevel facing up.

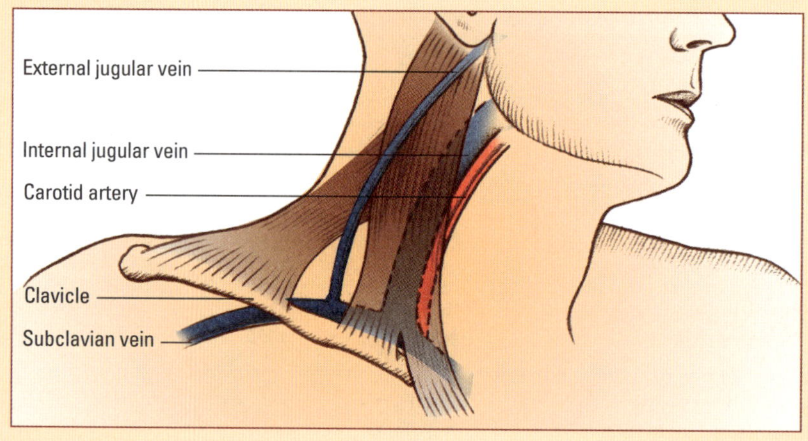

What to consider

- Accessing the internal jugular vein requires more skill than accessing peripheral veins and is usually performed by a trained practitioner.
- Every attempt should be made to avoid interrupting CPR.
- Nearby structures (carotid artery, apical pleura, lymphatic ducts, and nerves) can be damaged.
- Using the internal jugular vein carries a higher risk of complications than peripheral IV access.

Subclavian vein

The subclavian vein lies beneath the clavicle. It's frequently used for central venous access when peripheral venous access is unsuccessful. Generally, the subclavian vein is the preferred site, although during an emergency, the internal jugular or common femoral vein may be easier and quicker to access.

I'm pumped! According to my new contract, fluids infusing via a central line must now go through me!

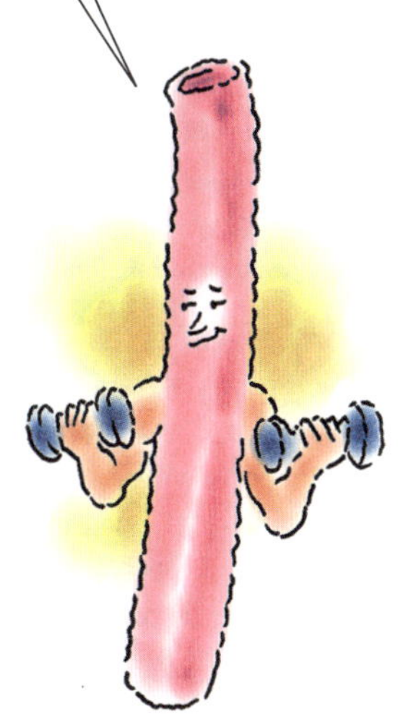

Nothing succeeds like access

The subclavian vein offers the opportunity to administer hypertonic or irritating solutions and for inserting catheters into the heart and pulmonary circulation for hemodynamic monitoring. More neck movement is possible with this site than with the internal jugular site.

What you need

- Two (14 or 16G) CV catheters (antimicrobial impregnated if available)
- Central line kit (available in most facilities)
- Sterile gown and gloves
- Maximum barrier kit or sterile towel and large sterile drape
- Masks with shields, cap
- Skin preparation kit with chlorhexidine sponges
- Alcohol pads
- 3-mL syringe with 25G needle
- 1% or 2% injectable lidocaine
- Suture material
- Three 10-mL syringes filled with normal saline solution
- Catheter securement device or sterile tape
- Antimicrobial patch
- Transparent semipermeable dressing
- Rolled bath towel

How it's done

Please note in an emergency situation, the following steps in the procedure may need to be altered.

- Explain the procedure to the patient and answer all questions. Obtain consent if able.
- Confirm the patient's identity using two identifiers and perform a "time-out" verification process according to the facility's policy if not emergent.
- Perform hand hygiene.
- Place the patient in Trendelenburg's position to dilate the vein and reduce the risk of air embolism.

Performing a Valsalva's maneuver

Use a Valsalva's maneuver as a diagnostic tool for patients with suspected heart abnormalities or as a treatment measure for patients with an abnormal heart rhythm.

How it's done

To perform Valsalva's maneuver, instruct your patient to:

- forcibly exhale while keeping his mouth and nose closed, and bear down (as if having a bowel movement)
- blow against an aneroid pressure measuring device (manometer) and maintain a pressure of 40 mm Hg for 30 seconds

What happens

Performing a Valsalva's maneuver causes specific changes in blood pressure and the rate and volume of blood returning to the heart. Characteristic heart sounds that indicate a heart abnormality can be auscultated during the maneuver. When performed by patients with a rapid arrhythmia, the maneuver may cause the heart to change its rhythm and slow its rate.

What to consider

Valsalva's maneuver shouldn't be performed by patients who have:

- severe coronary artery disease
- experienced a recent heart attack
- a severe reduction in blood volume.

Possible complications include:

- dizziness or syncope
- detachment of blood clots
- abnormal ventricular rhythm
- cardiac arrest

- Place a rolled towel under the patient's opposite shoulder to extend his neck, making anatomic landmarks more visible.
- Turn the patient's head in the opposite direction of the insertion site to make it more accessible and to prevent site contamination from airborne pathogens.
- Establish a sterile field on a bedside table, and then open the catheter and central line insertion tray. Be sure to label all medications, medication containers, and solutions on and off the sterile field.
- Put on a cap, mask, sterile gown, and gloves.
- Clean the area with the chlorhexidine sponge using a side-to-side motion for 30 seconds; allow the area to dry.

The practitioner:

- puts on a cap, mask, sterile gown, and gloves and then drapes the procedure area
- anesthetizes the area with 1% or 2% lidocaine
- locates the suprasternal notch and moves laterally until the clavicular head of the sternomastoid muscle is located. The carotid artery is identified by its pulse. The internal jugular vein runs lateral to the carotid artery
- inserts the needle with the bevel side inferior to the clavicle at the deltopectoral groove
- maintains negative pressure on the syringe as the needle is advanced. A guide wire is introduced and the catheter is threaded over the guide wire

- asks the awake patient to perform a Valsalva's maneuver, which increases the intrathoracic pressure, reducing the possibility of an air embolus. (See *Performing Valsalva's maneuver*.)
- confirms blood return in all ports, flushes them with normal saline solution, and sutures the catheter in place
- orders a chest X-ray to confirm placement of the line in the superior vena cava and evaluate for pneumothorax

After successful cannulation:

- apply an antimicrobial patch and transparent dressing according to the facility's policy. Label the dressing with the date, time, and your initials
- remove your gloves, perform hand hygiene, and document the procedure in the patient's electronic record according to facility policy

What to consider

- Accessing the subclavian vein requires more skill than is needed to access peripheral veins. (This procedure is performed by a trained practitioner.)
- Every attempt should be made to avoid interrupting CPR.
- Nearby structures (carotid artery, apical pleura, lymphatic ducts, and nerves) can be damaged.
- Using the subclavian vein carries a higher risk of complications than peripheral access.
- Using the subclavian vein carries a higher risk of pleural puncture than the internal jugular vein.
- Hematomas may not be readily visible and aren't easily compressible.

Femoral vein

The femoral vein lies medial to the femoral artery below the inguinal ligament. Use the femoral vein only as a temporary access when you need rapid IV access, primarily for patients in circulatory collapse or cardiac arrest.

It's a wonderful site

You don't need to interrupt CPR when accessing the femoral vein. Also, you may easily access the femoral vein when peripheral veins have collapsed. In addition, a long catheter can be passed through this site above the diaphragm to access the central circulation.

What you need

- Two (14 or 16G) CV catheters (antimicrobial impregnated if available)

- Central line introducer kit (available in most facilities)
- Sterile gown and gloves
- Maximum barrier kit or sterile towel and large sterile drape
- Masks with shields, cap
- Skin preparation kit with chlorhexidine sponges
- Alcohol pads
- 3-mL syringe with 25G needle
- 1% or 2% injectable lidocaine
- Suture material
- IV solution with attached and primed administration set
- Infusion pump
- Three 10-mL syringes filled with normal saline solution
- Antimicrobial patch
- Transparent semipermeable dressing

How it's done

Please note in an emergency situation, the following steps in the procedure may need to be altered.

- Explain the procedure to the patient and answer all questions. Obtain consent if able.
- Confirm the patient's identity using two identifiers, and perform a "time-out" verification process according to the facility's policy if not emergent.
- Place the patient in a supine position with his hip on the desired side in a neutral or slightly externally rotated position.
- Establish a sterile field on a bedside table, and then, open the catheter and central line insertion tray. Be sure to label all medications, medication containers, and solutions on and off the sterile field.
- Put on a cap, mask, sterile gown, and gloves.
- Clean the area with the chlorhexidine sponge using a side-to-side motion for 30 seconds; allow the area to dry.

The practitioner:

- puts on a cap, mask, sterile gown, and gloves and then drapes the procedure area
- anesthetizes the area with 1% or 2% lidocaine
- locates the femoral artery by palpating the femoral artery pulse. The femoral vein will lie just medial to the pulsation
- attaches a 10-mL syringe to the needle. The needle is aligned with the vein and is pointed toward the patient's head
- inserts the needle with the bevel up at a 45-degree angle to the skin
- maintains negative pressure on the syringe until blood appears
- lowers the needle to be more parallel with the patient's leg and then advances catheter
- confirms blood return in all ports, flushes them with normal saline solution, and then sutures the catheter in place

After successful cannulation:

- apply an antimicrobial patch and transparent dressing according to your facility's policy. Label the dressing with the date, time, and your initials
- remove your gloves, perform hand hygiene, and document the procedure in the patient's electronic health record according to facility policy

What to consider

- Complications include excess bleeding (especially if the artery was traumatized), pseudoaneurysm, significant hematoma, arteriovenous fistula, venous thromboembolism, and leg ischemia.
- More skill is required to access the femoral vein. (This procedure is performed by a trained practitioner.)
- The femoral vein may be difficult to locate if the femoral artery pulse isn't palpable.
- The femoral artery may not be readily apparent in a patient in cardiac arrest because of low arterial pressure.
- Keeping dressings clean and the catheter secure in this area may be difficult.
- Any central line placed under emergent, non-sterile conditions must be replaced within 24 hours. It should be considered a "dirty" line.

CLABSI/CRBSI

Central line–associated bloodstream infection (CLABSI) or central line–related bloodstream infection (CRBSI) is potentially significant complications that can occur with central line insertion and utilization. The nurses should familiarize themselves with the following:

- The Centers for Disease Control and Prevention (CDC) prefers the term CLABSI, whereas the Infectious Disease Society of America (IDSA) prefers the term CRBSI. The two terms can be used interchangeably.
- CLABSI/CRBSI is a laboratory-confirmed bloodstream infection (not related to infection at another site) that develops within 48 hours of a central line placement.
- CLABSI/CRBSI is associated with a high-cost burden; it accounts for an estimated $46,000 per case.
- An estimated 250,000 bloodstream infections occur each year (most with central line devices in place).
- In the United States, the rate of infection in the ICU is 0.8 per 1000 central line dates.
- CLABSI/CRBSI is associated with 28,000 deaths each year and costs over $2 billion per year.
- Femoral lines are associated with the highest risk.
- Subclavian sites are associated with the lowest risk; they are recommended by both the CDC and IDSA are the preferred site to use.

- Costs associated with CLABSI/CRBSI are no longer reimbursable by Medicare or Medicaid.
- Rates of infection are publicly reported and can affect hospital reimbursement rates.
- These infections can be fatal despite treatment.

Interventions for reducing CLABSI/CRBSI rates:

- Use an insertion checklist.
- Remove or discontinue line as soon as no longer needed.
- Use a strict aseptic technique with a maximal sterile barrier.
- Avoid routine post-IV antibiotic utilization.
- Use 2% chlorhexidine in skin preparation.
- Have appropriate hand hygiene.
- Use ultrasound guidance to minimize complications.
- Subclavian sites are preferred for IV access.
- Replace central lines placed during emergencies within 24 to 48 hours.
- Consider using specialized vascular access teams.
- Use closed-circuit pressure tubing.
- Use dedicated central lines for total parenteral nutrition.
- Adequately disinfect access ports prior to accessing them.
- Remember that nonfunctional or clotted lines are at increased risk of contribution to infection.

Establishing intraosseous access

During emergency situations, when rapid venous access is difficult or impossible, intraosseous (IO) access is the recommended alternative for the safe and effective short-term delivery of fluids, medications, or blood. IO is access into the bone marrow and is appropriate for all age groups. Anything that can be given IV can be given via the IO route with comparable absorption and effectiveness. Medications administered by the IO route are more predictable compared to drugs given via endotracheal tube. IO access can also be used to obtain blood samples for laboratory analysis. In addition, CPR doesn't have to be interrupted to establish an IO access.

Unshockable!

With shock conditions, blood is shunted away from the peripheral vessels and to the central circulation, often making peripheral IV access difficult or impossible. In contrast, the highly vascular, non-compressible intraosseous space within bone remains unchanged during shock. With IO access, the venous sinusoids within the bone provide access to the circulation during emergency treatment. During cardiac arrest, establishing an IO access may be quicker than establishing either central or peripheral venous access.

IO access is commonly undertaken via the anterior surface of the tibia. Alternative sites include the iliac crest, spinous process, distal femur, humoral head and, rarely, the upper anterior portion of the sternum. This procedure is performed by specially trained personnel if it is within their scope of practice. An IO needle can be inserted using manual technique or through the use of a special bone injection device—sometimes termed an IO "gun." (See *Understanding intraosseous infusion.*)

IO access is contraindicated in patients with osteogenesis imperfecta, osteoporosis, and ipsilateral fracture because of the potential for subcutaneous extravasation. IO access is also contraindicated through an area of cellulitis or an infected burn because of the increased risk of infection.

What you need

- Bone marrow biopsy needle or specially designed IO infusion needle (cannula and obturator) or bone injection device
- Antiseptic pads
- Antiseptic ointment
- Sterile gauze pads
- Sterile gloves

Understanding intraosseous infusion

With an intraosseous infusion, the bone marrow serves as a noncollapsible vein; thus, fluid infused into the narrow cavity rapidly enters the circulation by way of an extensive network of venous sinusoids. Here, the needle is shown positioned in the patient's tibia.

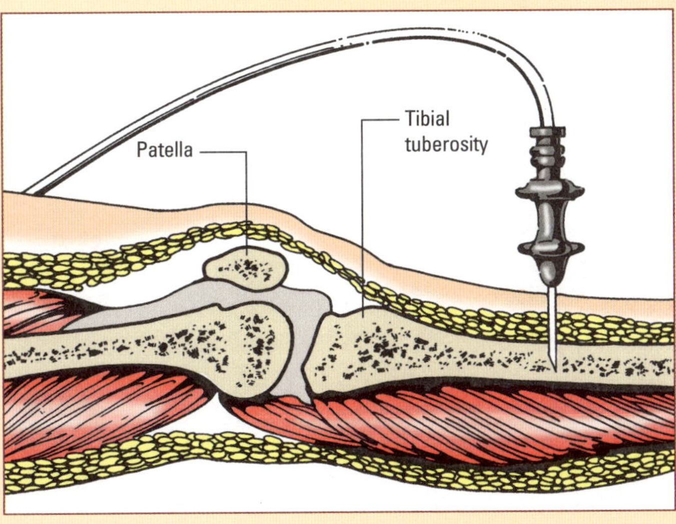

- Sterile drape
- A 10-mL syringe with flush solution
- IV fluids and tubing
- 1% or 2% lidocaine
- A 3- to 5-mL syringe
- Tape
- Sterile occlusive dressing
- Sterile marker and sterile labels
- Sedative, if prescribed

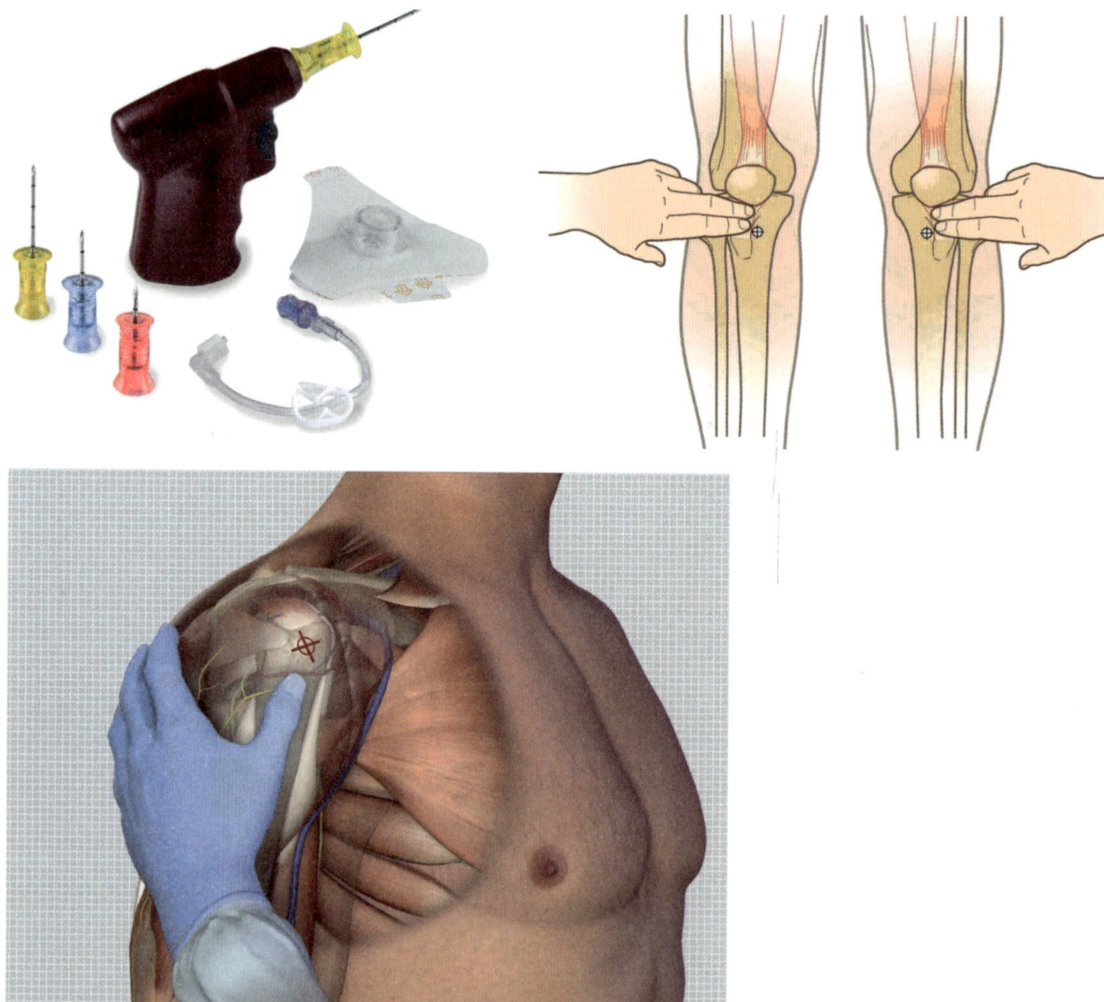

*EZ IO is now FDA approved for patients ≥ 12 years old, the device may be extended for up to 48 hours in the U.S. when alternate intravenous access is not available or reliably established, remaining IO devices are approved for 24hrs.

How it's done

Please note in an emergency situation, the following steps in the procedure may need to be altered.

- Confirm the patient's identity using two patient identifiers according to your facility's policy.
- Explain the procedure to the patient or family and answer all questions. Ensure that the patient or family understands the procedure and a consent form has been signed, if possible.
- Tell the patient which bone site will be accessed. Inform them that they will receive a local anesthetic (check for allergies) and will feel pressure from needle insertion.
- Perform hand hygiene.
- Administer a sedative, if prescribed, before the procedure following safe medication administration practices.
- Position the patient based on the selected puncture site.
- Perform hand hygiene again and put on sterile gloves.
- Clean the puncture site with an antiseptic pad using sterile technique and allow it to dry.

The practitioner:

- covers the area with a sterile drape
- anesthetizes the infusion site
- inserts the infusion needle through the skin and into the bone at an angle of 10 to 15 degrees from vertical, advancing it with a forward and backward rotary motion through the periosteum until the needle penetrates the marrow cavity. Alternatively, the bone insertion device is used to deliver the needle. The needle should "give" suddenly as it enters the marrow and should stand erect when released
- removes the obturator from the needle and attaches a 10-mL syringe, aspirating some bone marrow to confirm needle placement and then flushes with normal saline solution

After successful cannulation:

- attach IV tubing to the cannula to allow infusion of medications and IV fluids
- clean the infusion site with antiseptic pads; then, secure the site with tape and a sterile gauze dressing
- monitor the patient's vital signs and check the infusion site for bleeding and extravasation
- remove and discard your gloves, perform hand hygiene, and document the procedure in the patient's electronic health record according to the facility's policy

What to consider

- An IO infusion should be discontinued as soon as conventional vascular access is established (within 2 to 4 hours, if possible, and no more than 24 hours). Insertion of IO is very typically tolerated in the awake patient; however, it is the infusion into the space that causes pain. Lidocaine 40mg given via IO slowly over 120 seconds let dwell for 60 seconds and then followed with 5-10mls of saline flush prior to utilization can alleviate pain. Prolonged infusion significantly increases the risk of infection.
- After the needle has been removed, apply firm pressure to the site for 5 minutes and place antiseptic ointment and a sterile occlusive dressing over the injection site.
- IO flow rates are determined by needle size and flow through the bone marrow. Fluids should flow freely if needle placement is correct and infusion pumps should be used. However, a pressure infuser may be required for fluid resuscitation.
- Possible complications of IO infusion include extravasation of fluid into subcutaneous tissue resulting from incorrect needle placement, subperiosteal effusion resulting from failure of fluid to enter the marrow space, and clotting in the needle resulting from delayed infusion or failure to flush the needle after placement. Other complications include subcutaneous abscess, osteomyelitis (rarely), and epiphyseal injury.

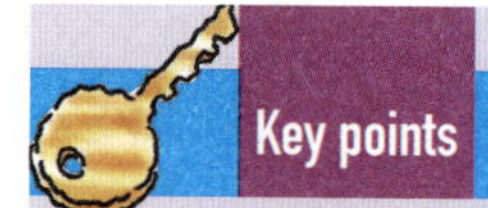

Intraosseous infusions

- During emergencies, intraosseous (IO) infusions may be quicker to start than peripheral or central line infusions.
- IO access can be used to obtain laboratory samples.
- IO infusions can be used for any IV medications, fluids, or blood products.
- IO infusions provide more predictable dosing than medication doses administered via an endotracheal tube.
- An IO access should be used only for 24 hours.

Flow rates

- Humeral: 6.3L/hour (medications reach the heart in 3 seconds)
- Tibial: 1L/hour (fluids via pressurized flow)
- FAST1™ sternal IO: 80mls/minute (via gravity tubing)

Other invasive techniques

Emergency invasive techniques, such as pericardiocentesis and needle thoracostomy, are sometimes needed to restore cardiac function or treat cardiac arrest. A trained practitioner should perform these procedures, with the nurse assisting. While there are risks to invasive techniques, the ultimate advantage is that the procedure may save the patient's life, therefore outweighing the risk of complications that may occur.

Pericardiocentesis

Pericardiocentesis is the aspiration of fluid or blood with a needle from the pericardial sac surrounding the heart. It's indicated to

Peak technique

Aspirating pericardial fluid

To perform pericardiocentesis, the practitioner inserts a needle with a syringe through the chest wall into the pericardial sac (as shown below). Electrocardiogram (ECG) monitoring, with a leadwire attached to the needle and electrodes placed on the limbs (right arm [RA], left arm [LA], and left leg [LL]), helps ensure proper placement and avoid damage to the heart.

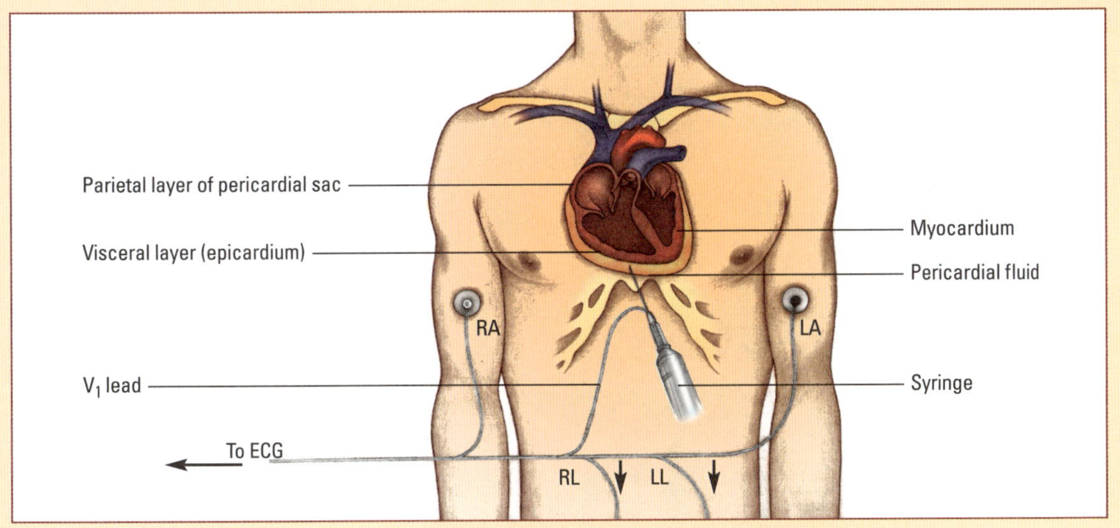

relieve cardiac tamponade (fluid or blood in the pericardial sac) or to obtain fluid for diagnostic studies. (See *Cardiac tamponade*.) Pericardiocentesis is contraindicated in cardiac tamponade without evidence of hemodynamic instability; surgical treatment is safer. Cardiac tamponade should be evaluated as a cause of cardiac arrest.

Complications of pericardiocentesis include:

- cardiac arrhythmias
- puncture of the heart or its vessels
- inadvertent introduction of air into the heart chambers
- hemothorax
- pneumothorax
- hemorrhage from myocardial or coronary artery puncture or laceration

Cardiac tamponade

Pericardiocentesis may be used to treat cardiac tamponade, a condition in which fluid or blood fills the pericardial sac causing a decrease in ventricular filling.

Causes

- Trauma and cardiac surgery
- Infection
- Neoplastic disease
- Myocardial infarction or rupture
- Uremia
- Collagen-vascular disease
- Cardiopulmonary resuscitation
- Radiation or medication reactions
- Perforation of the heart or its vessels by a vascular catheter

Signs and symptoms

- Hypotension (due to decreased ventricular filling and decreased contractility of the heart)
- Jugular vein distention
- Muffled heart sounds
- Pulsus paradoxus (a decline greater than 10 mm Hg in systolic pressure with normal inspiration)
- Dyspnea or cyanosis
- Signs of shock
- Decreasing voltage of electrocardiogram complexes

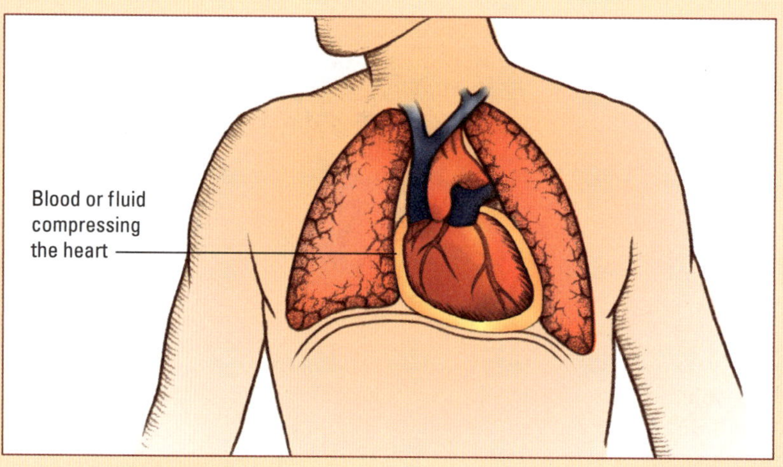

What you need

- Electrocardiogram monitor and pulse oximeter
- Resuscitative equipment
- Sterile alligator clip connected to V_1 lead
- Sterile 14G, 16G, and 18G 4″ or 5″ cardiac needles
- 20- to 60-mL syringe with luer-lock tip and three-way stopcock
- Antiseptic solution (2% chlorhexidine-based)
- Syringe with 1% or 2% lidocaine for local anesthesia
- Sterile gloves and gown
- Maximum barrier kit or sterile drapes

- Caps, masks with shields
- Sterile 4″ × 4″ dressing and gauze pads
- Tape
- Sterile marker, labels, and specimen container

How it's done

- Confirm the patient's identity using two patient identifiers according to the facility's policy.
- Explain the procedure to the patient, if possible. Answer all questions. Ensure that a consent is signed, if possible.
- Administer an IV bolus of normal saline solution to transiently increase filling pressures while preparing to perform pericardiocentesis, if appropriate.
- Create a sterile field on a bedside table. Label all medications, medication containers, and solutions on and off the sterile field.
- Place the patient in a supine position or elevate his head 60 degrees and attach cardiac monitoring leads.
- Perform hand hygiene (this applies to both the practitioner and the nurse) and put on caps, masks, sterile gowns and gloves.
- Conduct a "time-out" per facility policy.

The practitioner:

- cleans the area (left fifth intercostal space) with antiseptic solution and drapes the procedure area
- anesthetizes the area with 1% lidocaine
- attaches the 50-mL syringe to one end of the three-way stopcock and the cardiac needle to the other. The V_1 lead of the electrocardiogram may be attached to the hub of the aspirating needle using the alligator clips. Monitor for electrocardiogram (ECG) changes.
- inserts the needle perpendicular to the patient's chest into the pericardial sac and aspirates fluid. (Removing as little as 5 to 10 mL of fluid can improve cardiac performance.) (See *Aspirating pericardial fluid.*)
- removes the needle after pericardial fluid is withdrawn

After successful pericardiocentesis:

- resume CPR if needed
- send the fluid to the laboratory for analysis
- apply pressure to the site with sterile gauze pads for 3 to 5 minutes
- place a sterile dressing over the site and tape it securely
- remove personal protective equipment, perform hand hygiene, and obtain a postprocedure chest X-ray
- document the procedure in the patient's electronic health record

What to consider

- Procedure may be performed as part of resuscitative measures. CPR must be paused during the procedure.

- Continually monitor the patient's cardiac rhythm, vital signs, and oxygen saturation level during and after the procedure. If the needle touches the epicardium, ST-segment elevation may occur.
- Removal of fluid from the pericardial sac may produce immediate improvement in the patient's symptoms. Grossly, bloody fluid aspirate may indicate inadvertent puncture of a cardiac chamber.
- Blood obtained from the pericardial space won't clot. (Blood is defibrinated from agitation during myocardial contraction; in addition, this blood will have a lower hematocrit than venous blood.)
- Be alert to the possibility that emergency thoracostomy may be needed. Prepare the patient for surgery if necessary.

Needle thoracostomy

Needle thoracostomy, or needle decompression, may be necessary during a cardiac arrest to treat a tension pneumothorax (caused by air entering the pleural space) by removing air from the pleural space, relieving pressure on the lungs, heart, trachea, and great vessels. When a tension pneumothorax occurs, needle thoracostomy must be performed as soon as possible to improve oxygenation, ventilation, and cardiac function and stabilize the patient until a chest tube is inserted.

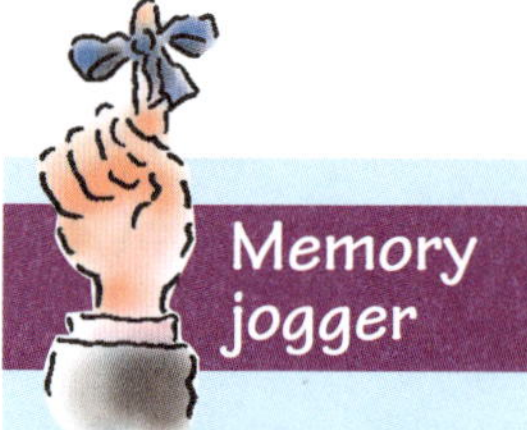

Use the acronym **ACT** to remember the signs and symptoms of tension pneumothorax so that you can "act" fast to protect your patient:

Acute respiratory distress

Chest wall motion that's asymmetrical

Tracheal shifting.

Give me a sign

Signs and symptoms of tension pneumothorax include:

- drop in oxygen saturation
- dyspnea, tachypnea, and absent breath sounds on the affected side
- chest pain and tachycardia diaphoresis
- jugular vein distention
- deviated trachea (away from the affected side) (Mainly an xray finding)
- precipitous loss of blood pressure and loss of peripheral pulses
- initial hypertension, followed by hypotension
- hyperresonance on injured side
- increasing difficulty when using a bag valve mask device to manually ventilate an intubated patient

Damage control

Complications of needle thoracostomy include damage to vessels or nerves or pleural infection. If the patient has a simple pneumothorax, needle thoracostomy converts it to an open pneumothorax. If the patient had no pneumothorax, needle thoracostomy produces a pneumothorax.

What you need

- Antiseptic solution
- 14G catheter with a one-way valve
- Sterile gloves
- 4 × 4 gauze dressing and tape

How it's done

- Confirm the patient's identity using two patient identifiers according to the facility's policy.
- Explain the procedure to the patient and answer all questions, if possible. Tell him he may feel some discomfort and a sensation of pressure when the needle is inserted. Ensure a signed consent, if able.
- Obtain baseline vital signs and assess respiratory function.
- You may give a sedative as ordered, if time permits.
- Perform hand hygiene and put on personal protective equipment.
- Elevate the head of the bed and expose the patient's entire chest.
- Conduct a "time-out" before starting the procedure, according to facility policy.
- Create a sterile field on a bedside table. Label all medications, medication containers, and solutions on and off the sterile field.
- Perform hand hygiene (this applies to both the practitioner and the nurse) and put on caps, masks, sterile gowns and gloves.

Peak technique

Landmarks for needle thoracostomy

Needle thoracostomy is an emergency procedure performed when the patient has hemothorax or tension pneumothorax. Typically, a trained practitioner accesses the second intercostal space (midclavicular line) on the affected side if a tension pneumothorax is suspected and the fifth intercostal space on the affected side if hemothorax is suspected.

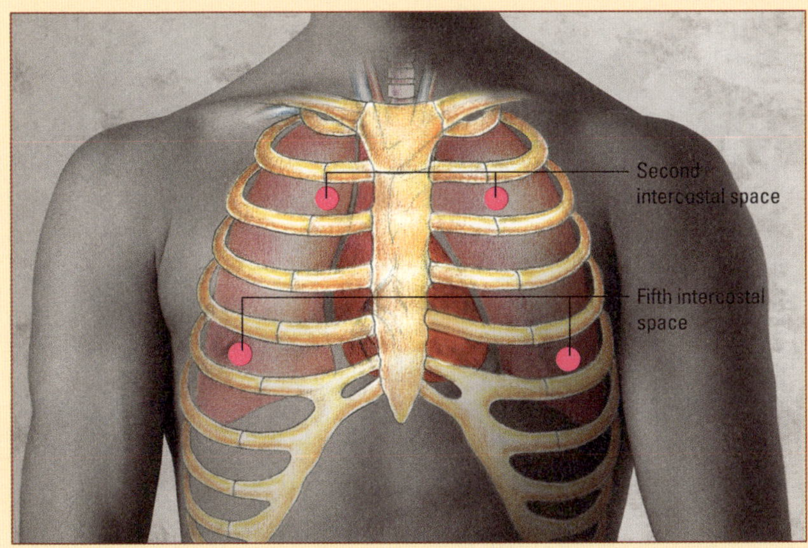

- Remind the patient not to cough, breathe deeply, or move suddenly during the procedure to avoid puncture of the visceral pleura or lung.

The practitioner:

- cleans the area (second intercostal space) with antiseptic solution and drapes the procedure area
- anesthetizes the area with 1% lidocaine
- inserts the needle into the second intercostal space in the midclavicular line, just above the top of the third rib on the injured side; alternatively, he may insert the needle into the fifth intercostal space in the midaxillary line on the injured side. (See *Landmarks for needle thoracostomy*.)
- listens for the air to escape
- removes the needle and attaches the one-way valve to the catheter. The valve prevents air from entering the pleural space and allows air inside the pleural space to escape. The catheter may be left in place until a chest tube is inserted
- orders a chest X-ray to evaluate pneumothorax

After successful needle thoracostomy:

- resume CPR if needed
- secure the flutter valve with the 4 × 4 gauze dressing and tape
- remove personal protective equipment, perform hand hygiene, and document the procedure in the patient's electronic health record per facility policy

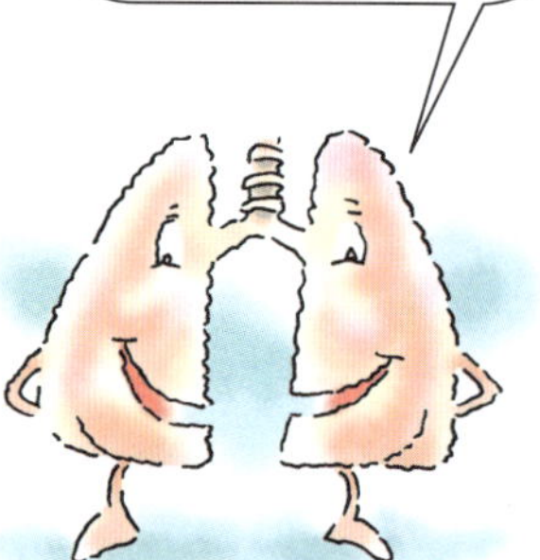

What to consider

- Monitor the patient's vital signs, cardiac rhythm, and oxygenation saturation during and after the procedure.
- Provide supplemental oxygen.
- Prepare the patient for chest tube insertion.

Quick quiz

1. CPR is being performed on Mr. White after he collapsed at his doctor's office. Paramedics are unsuccessful at obtaining a peripheral IV for medication and fluid administration. The best alternative intervention for the paramedic is:
   - A. intraosseous access.
   - B. endotracheal tube use.
   - C. central line access via subclavian vein.
   - D. central line access via internal jugular vein.

Answer: A. Insertion of an intraosseous catheter is recommended if peripheral access cannot be obtained.

2. You're performing CPR on a patient with a peripheral IV line in the antecubital vein. Which intervention would best help get medications to the central circulation?

A. Increase the rate of chest compressions for 1 to 2 minutes after medication administration.
B. Give a 20-mL bolus of normal saline solution and raise the arm.
C. Give all IV medications over 1 to 2 seconds.
D. Pause respirations during IV medication administration.

Answer: B. Medications administered peripherally take a longer time to reach the central circulation than do those given through a central vein. To assist drugs in reaching the central circulation sooner, give a 20-mL bolus of normal saline solution and raise the arm after medication administration.

3. After inserting a subclavian line, it's necessary to obtain a chest X-ray to:

A. confirm correct placement.
B. identify hematomas.
C. rule out air embolism.
D. check for fluid overload.

Answer: A. A chest X-ray can confirm that the subclavian line catheter tip is in the superior vena cava. If the catheter tip is in the right atrium or ventricle instead, it may cause cardiac arrhythmias or perforation. A chest X-ray is also ordered to check for pneumothorax—a complication of CV therapy.

4. The preferred peripheral access site for a patient in cardiac arrest is the:

A. external jugular vein.
B. most distal site (usually the hand).
C. antecubital fossa.
D. saphenous vein.

Answer: C. During cardiac arrest, peripheral veins in the upper extremities are preferred. The largest and easiest to access are typically those in the antecubital fossa.

5. Immediate treatment for cardiac tamponade involves:

A. pericardiocentesis.
B. emergency thoracotomy.
C. needle thoracostomy.
D. emergency pericardial window.

Answer: A. The immediate, lifesaving treatment for cardiac tamponade is pericardiocentesis. Surgery may be necessary after the procedure to fully correct the condition.

Scoring

☆☆☆ If you answered all five questions correctly, spectacular! You've accessed a perfect score.

☆☆ If you answered four questions correctly, way to go! You're in a very therapeutic range.

☆ If you answered fewer than four questions correctly, nice effort! After a quick review, you'll be "pumped" for a perfect score next time.

Suggested references

Adams, A., & Zaryske, G., (2022). External jugular vein peripheral intravenous catheters: An emergency nurse's guide. *Journal of Emergency Nursing, 48*, 303–309. https://doi.org/10.1016/j.jen.2022.01.009

American Heart Association. (2015). *Highlights of the 2015 American Heart Association guidelines update for CPR and ECC.* Dallas, TX: Author.

Anson, J. A. (2014). Vascular access in resuscitation: Is there a role for the intraosseous route? *Anesthesiology, 120,* 1015–1031 doi: https://doi.org/10.1097/ALN.0000000000000140

Buetti, N., Marschall, J., Drees, M., Fakih, M. G., Hadaway, L., Maragakis, L. L., Monsees, E., Novosad, S., O'Grady, N. P., Rupp, M. E., Wolf, J., Yokoe, D., & Mermel, L. A. (2022) Strategies to prevent central line-associated bloodstream infections in acute-care hospitals: 2022 update. *Infection Control & Hospital Epidemiology, 43*(5), 553–569. doi: 10.1017/ice.2022.87

Frank, R. L. (2015). Peripheral venous access in adults. In A. B. Wolfson (Ed.) *UpToDate.* Retrieved from www.uptodate.com

Gorski, L. A., Hadaway, L., Hagle, M. E., Broadhurst, D., Clare, S., Kleidon, T., Meyer, B. M., Nickel, B., Rowley, S., Sharpe, E., & Alexander, M. (2021). Infusion therapy standards of practice, 8th Edition. *Journal of Infusion Nursing, 44*(1S), S1–S224. doi: 10.1097/NAN.0000000000000396

Haddadin, Y., Annamaraju, P., & Regunath, H. (2022 January). Central line associated blood stream infections. [Updated 2022 May 29]. In StatPearls [Internet]. *StatPearls* Publishing. https://www.ncbi.nlm.nih.gov/books/NBK430891

Heffner, A. C., & Androes, M. P. Overview of central venous access. In A. B. Wolfson, et al. (Eds.) *UpToDate.* Retrieved from www.uptodate.com

Retrieved from October 1, 2022. https: Arrow® EZ-IO® System | US | Teleflex

TEAM Rapid Response. (2015). *Rapid guide to IV starts, 3e.* Rapid Response Publishing/Kindle eBook.

Chapter 8

Treatment algorithms

Just the facts

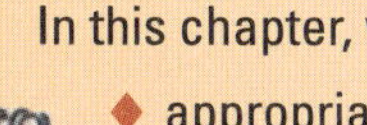

In this chapter, you'll learn:

- appropriate use of treatment algorithms
- classifications of intervention recommendations

Understanding algorithms

Algorithms are memory aids that quickly summarize the key information about a particular topic. The algorithms discussed in this chapter were created by the American Heart Association (AHA) for use when treating patients in emergency situations. When used properly, they can point you quickly to an assessment (observation) or intervention (action) step and serve as a treatment approach for a broad range of patients. The algorithms can also be helpful, concise tools to assist with studying for the advanced cardiovascular life support (ACLS) certification.

Remember the golden rule

Keep these points in mind when using treatment algorithms:

- They tend to oversimplify the complex processes of assessment and intervention.
- They can't replace clinical understanding and critical thinking.

Remember that in any patient care situation, the rule is always to treat the patient, not the algorithm. Aim to remain flexible because the patient may require care not covered by an algorithm. Never let an algorithm limit your treatment of the patient.

Multitasking matters

Although algorithms appear sequential, they aren't. Most resuscitations require multiple, simultaneous assessments and interventions. It isn't unusual to "jump" between several algorithms during a cardiac arrest, depending on the patient's rhythm, vital signs, level of consciousness (LOC), and response to treatment. For this reason, treatment recommendations are based on current research findings. The ultimate goal of treatment is the return of spontaneous circulation (ROSC). The AHA and the American College of Cardiology issue an evidence-based classification of intervention recommendations based on the risk-benefit ratio. (See *Classification of intervention recommendations*.)

Classification of intervention recommendations

The American Heart Association and the American College of Cardiology have issued an evidence-based classification of recommendations for treatment interventions. The classification is as follows:

- Class I, STRONG—The action is beneficial and is recommended.
- Class IIa, MODERATE—The action can be beneficial and is reasonable to perform.
- Class IIb, WEAK—The action's usefulness is uncertain, but it may be reasonable to consider.
- Class III, NO BENEFIT—The action is not beneficial and shouldn't be performed.
- Class IV, NO BENEFIT-HARM—The action is potentially harmful and shouldn't be performed.

Source: American Heart Association.

Adult BLS health care provider algorithm

The adult basic life support (BLS) health care provider algorithm begins with a basic step-by-step assessment, which applies to all adult patients and is recommended as the initial step in all ACLS situations. It emphasizes high-quality cardiopulmonary resuscitation (CPR) and early defibrillation. This approach helps keep team members organized and is useful before, during, and after resuscitation. Follow the BLS health care provider algorithm whenever you find a person collapsed. The AHA has a visual representation of a BLS health care provider algorithm that can be viewed at https://cpr.heart.org/en/resuscitation-science/cpr-and-ecc-guidelines/algorithms.

Back to basics

Remember these basic concepts when using the BLS health care provider adult cardiac arrest algorithm:

- When a patient is in cardiac arrest, cerebral resuscitation is of utmost importance.
- When caring for a patient, always maintain standard precautions. This requires, at minimum, gloved hands and possibly an airway barrier device for CPR.
- Reassess the patient at regular 2-minute intervals to see what effect your actions have had and adjust later actions accordingly.

The BLS health care provider adult cardiac arrest algorithm is divided into the initial finding and circulation, airway, breathing, and defibrillation assessments and actions.

Using basic life support skills

- Establish responsiveness of collapsed patient. Call for help.
- Check for a pulse (no longer than 10 seconds). At the same time, assess for breathing or only gasping.
- If no pulse, provide effective chest compressions (hard and fast).
- Open and maintain a patent airway.
- Give two breaths over 1 second each to produce a visible chest rise.
- Using a defibrillator or an automatic external defibrillator, defibrillate as soon as possible.
- If patient's condition is the result of possible opioid overdose, administer naloxone, if available.

Initial finding

The initial finding occurs when you find a patient has collapsed, possibly as a result of cardiac arrest. Although cardiac arrest is a likely cause, people lose consciousness for many reasons. Before approaching a patient, ensure that the scene of the collapse is safe.

When you find a patient who has collapsed, follow these steps:

- Assess responsiveness by shaking the patient and shouting "Are you OK?" Assessing responsiveness is always the first step because a patient may only be sleeping or may have fainted.
- If the patient is responsive (they arouse), you should observe them and support their airway, breathing, and circulation. Accessing help, such as the emergency medical service (EMS) (if out of the hospital) or rapid response team (if in hospital), is still warranted for follow-up because the responsive patient may still require oxygen, an IV line, or medications to maintain stability.
- If the patient isn't responsive (doesn't arouse), call "911" or activate the in-hospital "cardiac arrest" emergency response system. If someone is available, ask them to get help and to bring you an AED or defibrillator, if possible.
- After you've called for help, begin the adult BLS sequence of steps.

Circulation

Assess the patient's circulation by feeling for a carotid pulse for at least 5 seconds but no longer than 10 seconds. If the patient is breathing and has a pulse, place him in a side-lying position and stay with him until help arrives. If a pulse is present, but the patient is not breathing, provide rescue breathing by delivering one breath every 5 to 6 seconds (10 to 12 breaths/minute). Monitor the patient by checking his pulse every 2 minutes and wait for help to arrive.

If you are unable to detect a pulse (or are not certain) within 10 seconds, give 30 compressions followed by two breaths. The compression rate should be 100 to 120/minute. Push hard and fast. The depth of compressions should be at least 2 inches (5 cm) but not deeper than 2.4 inches (6 cm). Allow the chest to recoil after each compression to allow the heart to fill with blood. Avoid leaning on the patient's chest. Continue this for five cycles (about 2 minutes) before rechecking for a pulse. Minimize interruptions in chest compressions to no more than 10 seconds at a time. You should be providing compressions at least 60% of the time spent in resuscitation of the patient.

Airway

Make sure the patient has a patent airway. To open their airway, open their mouth using the head-tilt, chin-lift maneuver. As a health care provider, if you suspect neck injury, use the jaw thrust maneuver. If there is anything in the patient's mouth or throat that you can remove easily, do so.

Breathing

If the patient isn't breathing adequately, provide breaths using a barrier device, such as a pocket face mask (with a one-way valve) or bag valve mask device. For rescue breathing (patient has a pulse but is not breathing), give one breath every 5 to 6 seconds (10 to 12 breaths/minute). Each breath should be delivered over 1 second and should produce a visible chest rise. Avoid overventilation because this may cause the patient to vomit and may also decrease blood return to the heart. During CPR, use a compression-to-ventilation rate of 30 chest compressions to two breaths, pausing compressions to deliver breaths. When an advanced airway is placed, give one breath every 6 seconds without pausing compressions.

Defibrillation

Early recognition and rapid defibrillation of ventricular fibrillation (VF) and pulseless ventricular tachycardia (VT) are key actions for improving cardiac arrest survival. When an AED or defibrillator arrives on the scene, use it right away to identify if the patient needs a shock. If a shockable rhythm is identified, the rescuer defibrillates the patient and immediately resumes CPR, continuing for 2 minutes. Then, the patient is checked for a shockable rhythm again. This cycle is repeated until the patient has a return of spontaneous circulation (regains a pulse), or ACLS providers take over.

Adult cardiac arrest algorithm

The cardiac arrest algorithm covers the actions you'll need to perform when treating VF, pulseless VT, asystole, and pulseless electrical activity (PEA). Surviving these lethal rhythms depends upon effective BLS, ACLS, and post–cardiac arrest care. The AHA has a visual representation of a cardiac arrest algorithm that can be viewed at https://cpr.heart.org/en/resuscitation-science/cpr-and-ecc-guidelines/algorithms.

VF or pulseless VT

VF is the most common rhythm causing cardiac arrest and rapid defibrillation is key to survival.

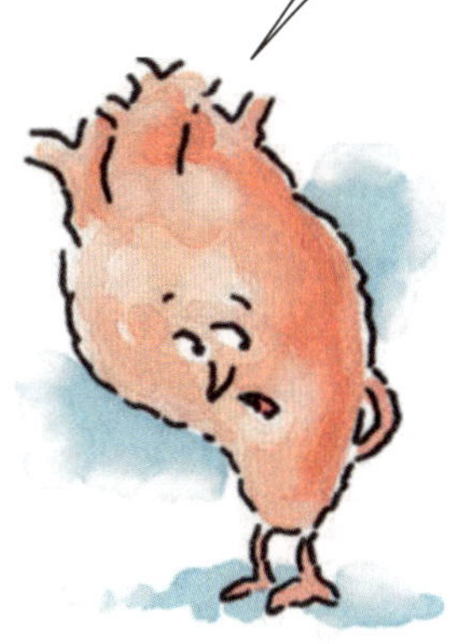

First steps

Begin treatment of a collapsed patient by following the algorithm for BLS.

Defibrillation

Once a defibrillator is available, attach it to the patient and confirm VF or VT. Defibrillate the patient with 360 joules if you're using a monophasic defibrillator or 120 to 200 joules if you're using a biphasic defibrillator. If you're using an AED, follow the prompts to shock the patient.

After you shock the patient, immediately resume CPR for five cycles and then recheck his rhythm. If VF or pulseless VT persists, defibrillate the patient again or as prompted by the AED. (See *Scenario:Adult cardiac arrest.*)

Team arrival

While CPR and defibrillation continues, the ACLS team should begin the following actions:

- Place the patient on a cardiac monitor (if they aren't already) to monitor their cardiac rhythm.
- Establish IV access as efficiently as possible without interrupting ACLS.
- If you're unable to establish IV access, then place an intraosseous (IO) access (bone marrow cavity is accessed). IO access enables fluid and medication delivery similar to that of central venous access.
- If unable to obtain adequate chest rise with bag-valve-mask ventilations, secure an advanced airway. Choose an airway that's within your ability to insert based on your scope of practice. Compressions should be interrupted for no more than 10 seconds during insertion of any type of advanced airway.
- Once the patient has an advanced airway, make sure that the airway device is appropriately placed and functional by listening for breath sounds, observing for chest rise and $ETCO_2$ monitoring. Administer one breath with 100% oxygen every 6 seconds while compressions are given without pauses. Continuous waveform capnography is recommended for confirmation and monitoring of ET tube placement and the quality of compressions. With high-quality compressions, $ETCO_2$ readings should be between 10 and 20 mm Hg.
- Following the treatment algorithms, administer medications as indicated and as the patient's condition permits.

Medications

If VF or pulseless VT persists after you defibrillate the patient, administer:

- epinephrine—give 1 mg by IV or IO push; repeat every 3 to 5 minutes.

If VF or VT still persists, consider administering an antiarrhythmic drug:

- amiodarone (Cordarone), first-line drug—Give 300 mg rapidly IV or IO push, diluted in 20 to 30 mL of dextrose 5% in water (D_5W); if VF recurs, give a second dose of 150 mg by rapid IV or IO push; maximum cumulative daily dose is 2.2 g
- lidocaine—Give 1 to 1.5 mg/kg by IV or IO push, with repeat doses of 0.5 to 0.75 mg/kg at 5 to 10 minute intervals for a total of 3 mg/kg
- magnesium sulfate—Give 1 to 2 g IV or IO diluted in 10 mL of D_5W or normal saline over 5 to 20 minutes to treat torsades de pointes or patients known or suspected to have hypomagnesemia.

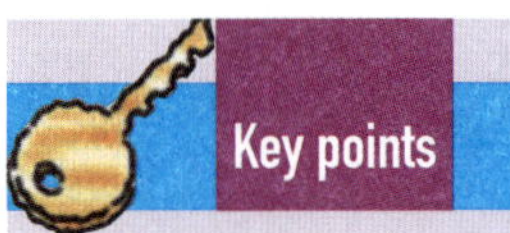

Using the adult cardiac arrest algorithm

- Begin cardiopulmonary resuscitation, provide oxygen, and attach defibrillator.
- Determine rhythm.
- Provide defibrillation for ventricular tachycardia/fibrillation as soon as possible, if indicated.
- Establish IV or IO access.
- Administer epinephrine.
- Consider advanced airway placement.
- Continue CPR and defibulate again.
- Administer antiarrhythmic.
- Continue CPR and defibulate again.
- Identify and treat reversible causes of asystole or pulseless electrical activity.
- If return of spontaneous circulation occurs, provide post–cardiac arrest care.

Checks and balances

Recheck the patient's rhythm on the monitor and recheck his pulse every 2 minutes. If VF or VT persists, repeat the "CPR-defibrillation-drug" cycle (continue CPR during drug administration) until a change in rhythm occurs. If you successfully defibrillate the patient, administer an infusion of the antiarrhythmic you administered during resuscitation.

Asystole

Ventricular asystole usually signals confirmation of death rather than a treatable rhythm. However, you may mistake fine VF for asystole, or a monitor error may have occurred. For this reason, you must confirm the presence of asystole in two leads.

First steps

As with any possible cardiac arrest situation, begin with the initial assessment.

If the patient does not have a pulse, initiate CPR immediately and follow the adult cardiac arrest algorithm.

Defibrillation

Defibrillation isn't recommended for asystole because there is no cardiac activity to stop with the shock.

Medications

Epinephrine is the only drug of choice for treating asystole. Administer 1 mg by IV or IO push every 3 to 5 minutes. If asystole persists after 20 to 25 minutes of high-quality CPR and no improvement, consider terminating resuscitative efforts.

Additional interventions

Make sure to identify and treat reversible causes, if possible. Causes of asystole are similar to those which cause PEA and will be discussed at the end of that section.

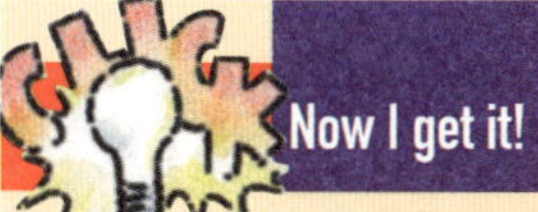

Scenario: Adult cardiac arrest

Mrs. B. is a 78-year-old woman admitted to the hospital with a diagnosis of heart failure. She's presently on a medical-surgical floor, preparing for discharge to home. While making morning rounds, the nurse finds Mrs. B. unresponsive. She takes the following actions:

- Calls for help as she assesses for breathing. A "code blue" (for cardiac arrest team) is called by another team member. The emergency cart is brought to the room.
- Palpates the carotid artery (for no more than 10 seconds) for a pulse. No pulse is found so she starts compressions at a rate of 100 to 120/minute.
- Another team member opens the patient's airway and provides breaths (at a ratio of 30 compressions/2 breaths) using a bag valve mask device and 100% oxygen. The patient's chest is noted to rise with each ventilation.

The code team arrives and performs the following actions:

- Attaches the "hands free" defibrillator pads and assesses the patient's cardiac rhythm. *Ventricular fibrillation (VF) is identified.*
- Charges the biphasic defibrillator to 200 joules and calls out. "Turn the oxygen off" and then "All clear." *After visual confirmation, that the oxygen source is removed from the patient and no personnel are touching the patient or bed, the SHOCK is delivered.*
- Resumes CPR immediately for five cycles or 2 minutes, at a rate of at least 100 to 120 compressions per minute and a compression depth of at least 2 to 2.4 inches. *A recorder is documenting all interventions, times, and patient response.*
- Establishes IV or IO access (if not already present).
- Reassesses the rhythm. *VF continues and another shock is delivered, with CPR immediately resumed.*
- Administers epinephrine 1 mg IV or IO push.
- Reassess the rhythm after 2 minutes and identifies sinus tachycardia on the monitor.
- Assesses the patient's carotid artery and finds a palpable pulse.
- Inserts an advanced airway, *if the patient is not breathing*, and manually ventilates the patient with a bag valve mask device and 100% oxygen to improve oxygenation.
- Obtains the patient's vital signs and oxygen saturation and monitors the cardiac rhythm.
- Follows steps in the adult post–cardiac arrest algorithm (see *Adult post–cardiac arrest algorithm*).

PEA

PEA isn't a rhythm on its own but it's characterized by electrical activity with little to no mechanical activity. It's identified when there's a cardiac rhythm on the monitor but the patient has no detectable pulse. Cardiac ultrasound studies show that the heart may actually be contracting during PEA but is too weak to produce a viable pulse.

First steps

Begin treatment by following the adult cardiac arrest algorithm. Resuscitation of the patient in PEA is more successful if the underlying cause is rapidly identified and treated.

Treating underlying causes of PEA

PEA is treated like asystole. After you've started CPR and assessed that the patient is in PEA, administer epinephrine (1 mg) every 3 to 5 minutes. Next, you must think about possible causes and promptly treat them.

Follow the five H's and T's

The underlying causes of PEA/asystole that may be possible to reverse include:

- hypovolemia
- hypoxia
- hydrogen ion acidosis
- hyperkalemia or hypokalemia
- hypothermia
- toxins (drug overdose)
- tamponade (cardiac)
- tension pneumothorax
- thrombosis (coronary)
- thrombosis (pulmonary)

Hypovolemia

Treat hypovolemia with a bolus infusion of fluid or blood products, as appropriate. If you note an obvious cause of fluid depletion, attempt the appropriate intervention. For example, if the patient was hemorrhaging from an identified site, apply pressure to the site to stop the bleeding.

Hypoxia

Hypoxia implies that the patient's airway and breathing aren't secure or adequate. Treat hypoxia with proper ventilation and oxygenation. If unable to provide adequate breaths with a bag valve mask, an advanced airway, such as an endotracheal (ET) tube, may need to be inserted. If an ET tube is already in place, be sure to confirm accurate placement. Don't forget to monitor pulse oximetry and $ETCO_2$.

Hydrogen ion (acidosis)

Providing adequate ventilation and oxygenation most effectively treats acidosis resulting from cardiac arrest. Since CO_2 is an acid, increasing the amount exhaled during ventilations will quickly drop the acidity of the blood. To do so, hyperventilate the patient by administering 2 to 4 breaths/minute more than you normally would. Routine use of sodium bicarbonate isn't recommended for patients in cardiac arrest because it diminishes the chance of successful defibrillation. Give sodium bicarbonate (1 mEq/kg) only in special situations to treat pre-existing metabolic acidosis, hyperkalemia, or tricyclic antidepressant overdose.

Hyperkalemia or hypokalemia

Treatment of potassium imbalance depends on the severity of the patient's condition. For severe hyperkalemia, give regular insulin with 50% dextrose solution, calcium, loop diuretic to shift potassium into the cells. Give furosemide to promote diuresis and potassium excretion. For hypokalemia, administer an IV or IO potassium supplement infusion at a rate of 10 to 20 mEq/hour. Since potassium cannot be given IV or IO push, this is not a quick solution for PEA/asystole resulting from hypokalemia.

Hypothermia

Continue resuscitation efforts while attempting to rewarm the patient suffering from moderate to severe hypothermia. Rewarming can be accomplished with the use of warm IV fluids, warming blankets, warm humidified oxygen, and warming packets applied to pulse points. When the patient's body temperature reaches 86°F (30°C), ACLS measures are more successful. Institute interventions to prevent additional heat loss.

Toxins (drug overdose)

Commonly, tricyclic antidepressants, beta-adrenergic blockers, calcium channel blockers, and digoxin can cause PEA. Focus on clearing the drug from the patient's system. You may use an antidote to combat the effects of the overdosed drug. Contact your local poison control agency for guidelines on treating overdose or poisoning, if needed. Support hemodynamic functioning while initiating other therapies, for example, performing dialysis if the drug can't be cleared by the patient's renal system.

Tamponade (cardiac)

Perform pericardiocentesis to treat cardiac tamponade. This will remove the fluid that is compressing the heart from the pericardial space and allow the patient's heart to expand and fill more effectively.

Tension pneumothorax

A tension pneumothorax may be suspected if there is resistance to ventilations, decreased oxygen saturation despite oxygenation, and there are absent breath sounds on one side of the chest. Adequate ventilation and oxygenation are crucial for successful resuscitation. If not corrected, tension pneumothorax can be fatal. A needle thoracostomy is performed to treat tension pneumothorax quickly.

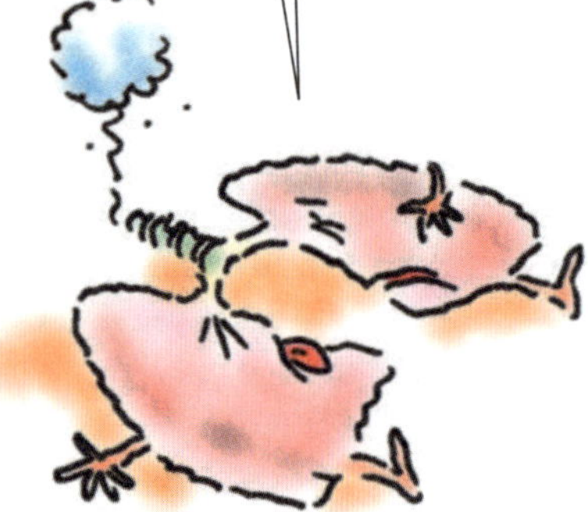

Thrombosis (coronary)

Coronary thrombosis is considered an acute coronary syndrome (ACS). To treat an ACS, see *Acute coronary syndromes algorithm*. As this cause of PEA/asystole commonly requires PCI, rapid intervention is not always possible.

Thrombosis (pulmonary)

After resuscitation, a pulmonary thrombosis may be treated by administering thrombolytics, surgical embolectomy, or percutaneous mechanical embolectomy. These treatments may not be readily available to reverse PEA/asystole.

Adult immediate post–cardiac arrest care algorithm

The goals of immediate post–cardiac arrest care after the return of spontaneous circulation (ROSC) include optimizing tissue perfusion, restoring metabolic homeostasis and supporting organ function, implementing goal-directed care, identifying and treating the causes of arrest, and objectively assessing the prognosis for recovery. Targeted treatment during the postresuscitation period increases the likelihood that the patient will survive neurologically intact. This care should be multidisciplinary, structured, and delivered in a consistent manner. The AHA has a visual representation of a post-cardiac arrest care algorithm that can be viewed at https://cpr.heart.org/en/resuscitation-science/cpr-and-ecc-guidelines/algorithms.

Optimizing tissue perfusion

Optimizing tissue perfusion requires adequate oxygenation and ventilation. Immediate interventions to achieve this include the following:

- Inserting an advanced airway if needed to optimize oxygenation and ventilation. After confirming proper placement, the airway should be secure and monitored. A chest X-ray is the gold standard for placement confirmation.
- Optimizing mechanical ventilation and titrating oxygen to the lowest level necessary to maintain an oxygen saturation of at least 94%.
- Using continuous waveform capnography to monitor and achieve target carbon dioxide levels (35 to 40 mm Hg).
- Avoiding excessive ventilation.

Treating hypotension

Once oxygenation and ventilation is addressed, look to maintain or restore hemodynamic stability. Interventions to achieve this include the following:

- Obtaining and monitoring vital signs frequently. Obtain blood pressure readings by manual BP cuff or arterial pressure line.
- Administering a fluid bolus of 1 to 2 L of normal saline or lactated Ringer's solution for hypotension (systolic BP less than 90 mm Hg or mean arterial pressure less than 65).
- Administering vasopressor infusion (such as norepinephrine, epinephrine, or dopamine) if hypotension persists after fluid bolus.

Supporting organ function

After cardiac arrest, organ function needs to be evaluated, supported, and monitored. Interventions to achieve this include:

- implementing cardiac monitoring and continuously evaluating cardiac rhythm for abnormalities to provide early treatment
- obtaining a 12-lead electrocardiogram to assess for myocardial ischemia or damage
- obtaining cardiac makers, including troponin levels
- transporting patient for coronary angiography if ST elevation myocardial infarction (MI) is present or if patient is hemodynamically unstable without ST elevation (and a cardiovascular lesion is suspected) or acute MI
- maintaining normothermia or mild hypothermia
- obtaining and monitoring electrolyte levels and blood urea nitrogen and creatinine levels to treat kidney abnormalities.

Implementing goal-directed care

Targeted temperature management (TTM) is a goal-directed care that has been identified as best practice for optimal neurologic recovery post–cardiac arrest. To qualify for TTM, the patient must have ROSC within 60 minutes of cardiac arrest and remain unconscious (not following commands). Interventions to achieve this include the following:

- Evaluating the patient for inclusion in therapy. Follow facility policy for inclusion and exclusion criteria.
- Initiating cooling as quickly as possible, with the goal of achieving the target cooling temperature within 6 hours of ROSC. Follow facility policy for target temperature (between 32°C and 36°C). Once achieved, temperature should be maintained for at least 24 hours.
- Following facility policy for rewarming and normothermia, as well as monitoring criteria (labs, bedside shivering assessment, etc.). Active fever should be prevented in comatose patients after TTM procedure is completed.
- Prognosis of neurologic outcomes should not occur until 72 hours after return of normothermia.

Identifying and treating reversible causes of arrest

Identifying the underlying cause of cardiac arrest will help direct postresuscitation care—from administering appropriate medications, fluids, and antidotes to performing diagnostic tests and procedures to help stabilize organ function, prevent complications, and improve survival. Interventions to achieve this include the following:

- Obtain appropriate laboratory studies (such as serum electrolyte, magnesium, and calcium levels; arterial blood gas analysis; CBC with differential; glucose level; renal and liver function tests; coagulation profile; and toxicologic screens).
- Correct electrolyte imbalances.
- Obtain chest X-ray, computed tomography (CT) scan, and other diagnostic tests to identify tension pneumothorax and pulmonary embolism.
- Correct hypothermia with warming techniques.
- Consider fibrinolytic therapy to treat pulmonary embolism.

Adult bradycardia algorithm

Bradycardia is considered a resting heart rate less than 60 beats/minute. In some patients, a heart rate less than 60 beats/minute may be physiologically normal. Generally, when bradycardia causes signs and symptoms, the ventricular rate is less than 50 beats/minute. The AHA has a visual representation of an adult bradycardia algorithm that can be viewed at https://cpr.heart.org/en/resuscitation-science/cpr-and-ecc-guidelines/algorithms.

Treatment

Begin assessing the patient for a pulse, an adequate airway, breathing effort, and stability of vital signs.

First steps

In your assessment, look for signs and symptoms associated with bradycardia. Remember that sometimes patients don't experience any ill effects from bradycardia. For example, trained athletes have much slower heart rates and tolerate them without difficulty.

Signs associated with bradycardia may include:

- hypotension and shock (systolic blood pressure less than 90 mm Hg and poor perfusion)
- acute heart failure
- increased ventricular ectopy (PVCs).

Symptoms may include:

- chest pain
- shortness of breath
- decreased or altered level of consciousness.

Identify and treat the underlying cause

Implement ECG monitoring, identify the bradycardic rhythm, and look for the underlying cause of the patient's symptoms. Identification of the cause of bradycardia will direct treatment. For example, bradycardia caused by another condition such as hypoxemia will respond to treatment of the hypoxemia (provision of adequate ventilation and oxygenation). While attempting to identify the cause of the bradycardia (such as AMI or drug overdose), maintain the patient's airway, provide oxygen and assist with ventilation if needed. Obtain IV access. Monitor vital signs and pulse oximetry. Obtain a 12-lead ECG but don't delay treatment to do so.

Medications

If the bradycardia persists despite treatment of the suspected cause and the patient is hemodynamically stable, consider administering atropine 1 mg by IV push every 3 to 5 minutes, for a total of 3 mg. Atropine will decrease vagal tone and increase the heart rate. Assess the patient's response after each dose. Be aware that patients with transplanted hearts don't respond to atropine because their hearts

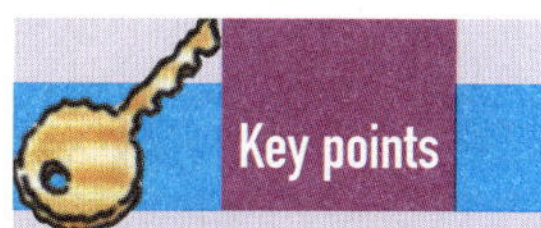

Using the adult bradycardia algorithm

- Assess appropriateness for clinical condition.
- In symptomatic patients, heart rate is generally less than 50 beats/minute.
- Identify and treat underlying cause, if possible.
- Administer atropine if needed.
- If atropine is ineffective, administer an epinephrine or dopamine infusion or use transcutaneous pacing if available.
- Consider expert consultation and transvenous pacing.

have been denervated. These patients may need a transcutaneous pacemaker or a catecholamine infusion instead.

If atropine is ineffective or the patient becomes unstable, consider initiating an epinephrine infusion (2 to 10 mcg/minute), a dopamine infusion (2 to 10 mcg/kg/minute), or application of a transcutaneous pacemaker. Expert consultation should be obtained and a transvenous pacemaker may be necessary.

Adult tachycardia algorithm (with pulse)

A heart rate over 100 beats/minute is considered tachycardia. Tachycardia can stem from many factors, such as hypovolemia, pain, fever, and anxiety. If the heart rate is less than 150, consider and treat the cause. The tachycardia is generally more significant and likely to be caused by an arrhythmia when the ventricular rate is 150 beats/minute or more. Tachycardia may be classified in different ways, based on the appearance of the QRS complex. General classifications include narrow complex tachycardia and wide-complex tachycardia.

Narrow complex tachycardia (QRS of less than 0.12 second) includes:

- sinus tachycardia
- atrial fibrillation
- atrial flutter
- AV nodal re-entry
- accessory pathway–mediated tachycardia
- atrial tachycardia
- multifocal atrial tachycardia
- junctional tachycardia

Wide-complex tachycardia (QRS greater than or equal to 0.12 second) includes:

- ventricular tachycardia
- supraventricular tachycardia with aberrancy
- aberrant conduction
- pre-excitation syndrome

You must determine the type of tachycardia that the patient is experiencing and identify if they have impaired cardiac function to treat the rhythm appropriately. The AHA has a visual representation of an adult tachycardia (with a pulse) algorithm that can be viewed at https://cpr.heart.org/en/resuscitation-science/cpr-and-ecc-guidelines/algorithms.

Treatment

Begin by following the BLS health care provider algorithm and then assess the patient for stability. Maintain a patent airway with adequate ventilation; provide oxygen as appropriate. Evaluate and identify the cardiac rhythm while monitoring the patient's blood pressure and oximetry. Assess the patient's IV access, if present, or insert an IV catheter. Obtain an ECG. Attempt to identify and treat the underlying cause.

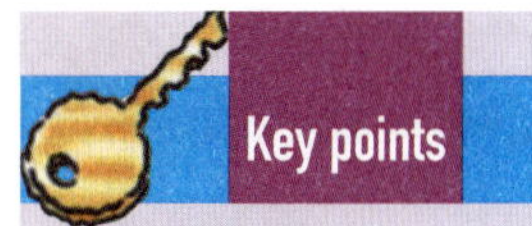

Using the adult tachycardia (with pulse) algorithm

- Assess appropriateness for clinical condition.
- Treat underlying causes for tachyarrhythmia, if possible.
- Ask the patient to perform a vagal maneuver (bearing down).
- Administer adenosine if rhythm is regular and monomorphic.
- Administer antiarrhythmic, beta blocker, or calcium channel blocker as appropriate for identified rhythm.
- Perform synchronized cardioversion if the rhythm is regular and monomorphic.

First steps

If the patient is stable and the QRS complex is 0.12 second or less, obtain expert consultation. A vagal maneuver (such as bearing down) may be attempted. If the vagal maneuver is unsuccessful, adenosine (if rate is regular), beta blocker or calcium channel blocker may be administered to help slow the rhythm and allow it to spontaneously convert.

Medications

Medication administration is based on the type of tachycardia that the patient is experiencing.

For a tachyarrhythmia that is regular with a QRS complex of 0.12 second or less, consider administering adenosine (Adenocard) 6 mg by rapid IV push (over 2 seconds or less) followed by a normal saline solution flush. If the rhythm doesn't slow and convert, consider giving adenosine 12 mg by rapid IV push. Then, consider obtaining expert consultation and possibly administering a calcium channel blocker such as diltiazem (Cardizem) or a beta-adrenergic blocker such as labetalol (Trandate).

For a tachyarrhythmia with a wide QRS complex (0.12 second or greater), consider giving adenosine 6 mg by rapid IV push but only if the rhythm is regular and monomorphic assumed to be SVT with aberrant conduction down a bundle branch. Other antiarrhythmic infusions to consider, with expert consultation, include amiodarone, procainamide, and sotalol: Give amiodarone 150 mg by IV bolus over 10 minutes followed by an amiodarone infusion. Alternatively, you may give procainamide 20-50 mg/minute IV for a maximum dose of 17 mg/kg or sotalol 1.5 mg/kg over 5 minutes. Both procainamide and sotalol should be avoided if the patient has a prolonged QT interval as both have the ability to further prolong the QTI.

If the patient is unstable (experiencing chest pain, shortness of breath, altered LOC, low blood pressure), perform synchronized cardioversion. Synchronization (shock that is delivered with the QRS complex) is important so that the energy isn't delivered during the vulnerable period of ventricular repolarization. Different rhythms require different energy levels for synchronized cardioversion:

- SVT and atrial flutter: 50 to 100 joules
- VTach with a pulse: 100 joules
- atrial fibrillation: 120 to 200 joules

If the first shock isn't successful in cardioverting the rhythm, repeat the shock at a higher Joule amount (increase in a stepwise fashion).

Acute coronary syndromes algorithm

Acute myocardial infarction (MI), ST-segment elevation MI (STEMI), non-STEMI, and unstable angina are each considered an ACS. Rupture or erosion of plaque—an unstable and lipid-rich substance—initiates nearly all ACSs. This rupture results in platelet adhesions, fibrin clot formation, and activation of thrombin, causing a thrombus.

Set the stage

However it happens (thrombus, vessel spasm, or plaque erosion), three stages occur when a vessel is occluded—ischemia, injury, and infarct.

- Ischemia: Blood flow and oxygen demand are out of balance; ECG changes show ST-segment depression or T-wave changes. (Ischemia can be resolved by improving oxygen flow or reducing oxygen needs.)
- Injury: Ischemia is prolonged enough to damage the affected area of the heart, which alters repolarization of the cells. This shows as ECG changes or ST-segment elevation of at least 1 mm (usually in two or more anatomically contiguous leads). This is what is known as a STEMI (ST elevation myocardial infarction). Keep in mind that a patient with a bundle-branch block has an altered shape to their ST segment, and it may be difficult to determine if there is ST-segment elevation. Assume that a patient with a new LBBB has ST-segment elevation and treat accordingly.
- Infarct: Death of myocardial cells occurs; ECG changes may reveal abnormal Q waves. (Q waves are considered abnormal when they appear greater than or equal to 0.04 second wide and their depth is greater than 2 mm.)

Damage by degrees

The degree of blockage and the time that the affected vessel remains occluded are major determinants for the type of infarct that occurs. The amount of damage to the myocardium depends on several factors:

- the area of the heart supplied by the affected vessel (see *Viewing the coronary vessels*)
- the demand for oxygen in the affected area of the heart
- the collateral circulation in the affected area of the heart. (Collateral circulation is an alternate circulation that develops when blood flow to tissue is blocked and rerouted.)

Viewing the coronary vessels

This illustration shows the major coronary vessels that may be affected during myocardial infarction.

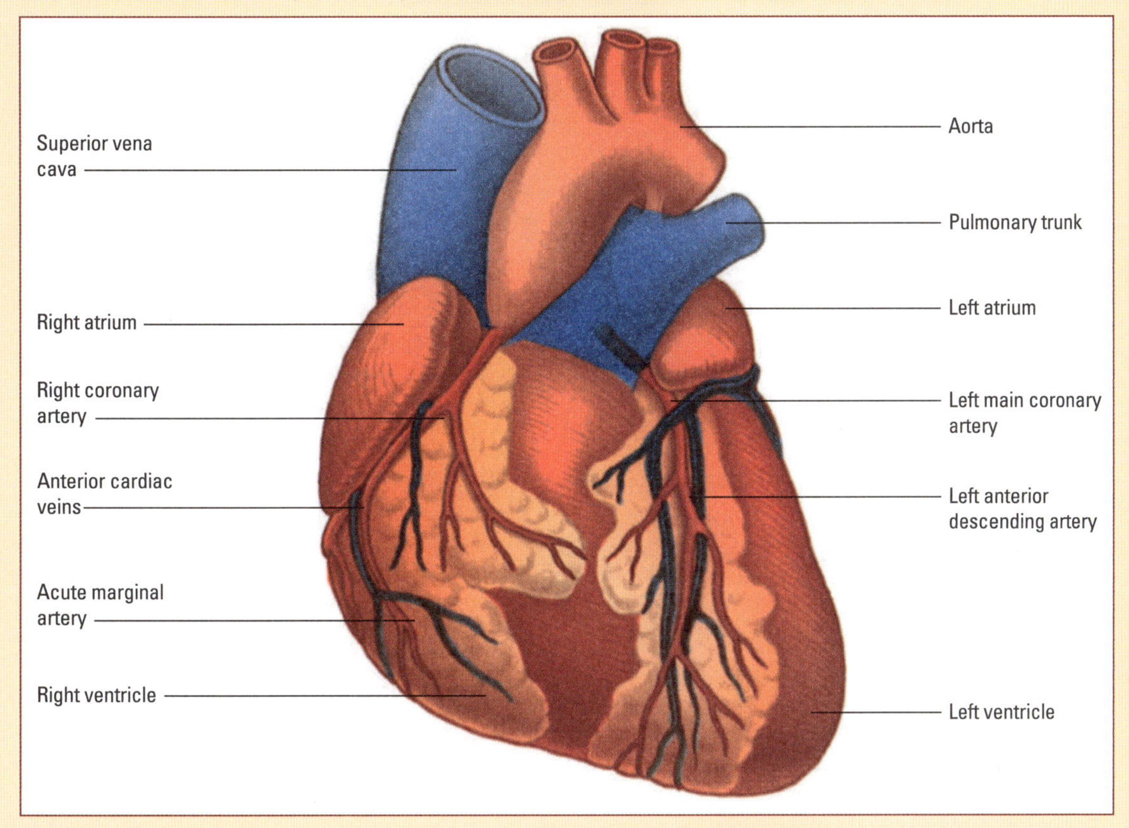

No laughing matter

Patients typically describe these symptoms when experiencing acute ischemia and MI:

- uncomfortable pressure, squeezing, pain, or fullness in the center of the chest lasting several minutes (usually longer than 15 minutes); this pain is often unrelieved by rest or nitroglycerin
- pain radiating to the shoulders, neck, arms, or jaws or pain in the back between the shoulder blades (women may complain of abdominal pain)
- fatigue, light-headedness, fainting, sweating, nausea, and shortness of breath, accompanied by a feeling of impending doom

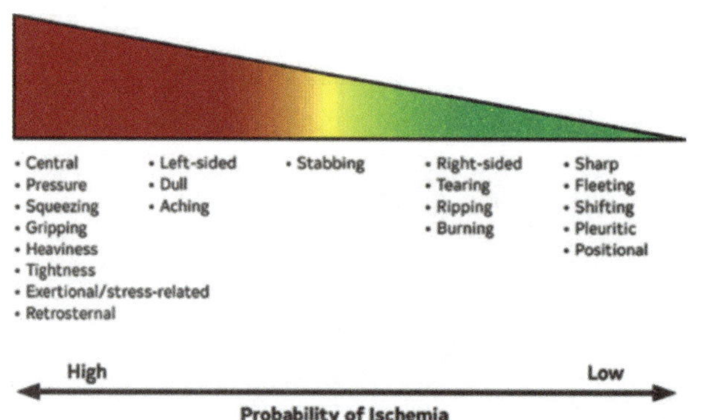

(Reprinted from Gulati M., Levy P. D., Mukherjee D., et al. (2021). 2021 AHA/ACC/ASE/CHEST/SAEM/SCCT/SCMR Guideline for the evaluation and diagnosis of chest pain: A report of the American College of Cardiology/American Heart Association Joint Committee on Clinical Practice Guidelines. *Circulation, 144*, e368–e454. Figure 2.)

Unusual or isolated symptoms may be seen more commonly in diabetics, older patients, and women. Patients at risk for ischemia fall into high-, intermediate-, and low-risk categories. (See *Risk factors for ischemia.*)

Using the acute coronary syndromes algorithm

- Immediate 12-lead electrocardiogram (ECG).
- Use ECG to identify type of syndrome: STEMI (ST elevation myocardial infarction) or new left bundle-branch block, unstable angina/non-STEMI (ST depression or dynamic T-wave inversion), and normal or nondiagnostic ECG.
- Administer oxygen, aspirin, nitroglycerin, and morphine as indicated.
- Assess and complete checklist for possible fibrinolytic treatment.
- Optimally, door to fibrinolytic treatment is less than 30 minutes from first medical contact.
- Optimally, door to balloon (percutaneous coronary insertion) is less than 90 minutes from first medical contact.

Treatment

Treatment goals for the patient experiencing an ACS include:

- reducing the amount of myocardial necrosis if the infarction is ongoing
- preventing major adverse cardiac events (nonfatal MI and death)
- treating life-threatening complications of ACS, such as unstable arrhythmias, cardiogenic shock, pulmonary edema, and mechanical complications from acute AMI

Prehospital screening, including a 12-lead ECG, should be done by EMS personnel and transmitted to the receiving facility, if possible, to determine if a patient is a candidate for thrombolytic therapy. Prehospital treatment includes aspirin and nitrates unless contraindicated or already taken by the patient. Morphine may possibly be given if chest pain doesn't respond to nitrates.

PCI preference

Performing percutaneous coronary intervention (PCI), which may decrease or limit the amount of necrosis, is the preferred treatment. Fibrinolytics aren't effective in patients who do not have a clot as the cause of their MI. In many instances, PCI is superior to fibrinolytic administration because treatment can be initiated to treat the specific cause of vessel occlusion. The restoration of vessel patency occurs in more than 90% of patients, leading to reduced mortality and reinfarction rates. Ideally, PCI will be started within 90 to 120 minutes of first medical contact; however, it can occur up to 12 hours after symptom onset. Fibrolytics can be used if PCI will be delayed. PCI can be safely performed after fibrinolytic administration. Glycoprotein IIb/IIIa inhibitors, heparin, and aspirin are often given during PCI to treat thrombus because these drugs affect platelet formation, decreasing platelet adhesion and infarct size.

Use the acute coronary syndromes algorithm to quickly classify patients so you can direct treatment appropriately. Base your treatment on ECG findings and the patient's status. The AHA has a visual representation of an acute coronary syndromes algorithm that can be viewed at https://www.ahajournals.org/doi/full/10.1161/circulationaha.110.971028.

First steps

Begin your assessment immediately when a patient complains of chest pain. Obtain a 12-lead ECG within the first 10 minutes if possible, because it's a crucial component in determining if myocardial ischemia is present. After the ECG is interpreted, your treatment plan can be formulated. Administer oxygen, aspirin, nitroglycerin, and morphine, as needed, to treat acute ischemia. Classify the patient as having ST-segment elevation or new left bundle-branch block (LBBB), ST-segment depression or dynamic T-wave inversion, or nondiagnostic or normal ECG.

Other actions include obtaining serial cardiac markers (including troponin), electrolyte levels, coagulation studies, repeat 12-lead ECG, chest X-ray, and continuous ST-segment monitoring (if available).

ST-segment elevation or new LBBB

Treat patients with an ST-segment elevation greater than or equal to 1 mm in two or more leads or with LBBB for acute MI (STEMI). More than 90% of patients who present with an ST-segment elevation greater than or equal to 1 mm will develop new Q waves and have positive serum cardiac markers.

Treatment options include:

- reperfusion therapy (with a goal of door to balloon [PCI] in 90 minutes and door to needle [fibrinolysis] in 30 minutes)
- beta-adrenergic blockers within 24 hours post diagnosis
- prasugrel, ticagrelor, or clopidogrel
- anticoagulation therapy such as aspirin.

ST-segment depression or dynamic T-wave inversion

Suspect ischemia with findings of ST depression greater than 1 mm, marked symmetrical T-wave inversion in multiple precordial leads, and dynamic ST-T changes with pain. Patients who display persistent symptoms and recurrent ischemia, diffuse or widespread ECG abnormalities, heart failure, and positive serum markers are considered at high risk for further heart damage.

Treatment options include:

- antiplatelet inhibitors such as asprin and a platelet P2y12
- anticoagulation therapy
- beta blockers
- statins
- nitroglycerin
- elective cardiac catheterization when the patient's condition is stable

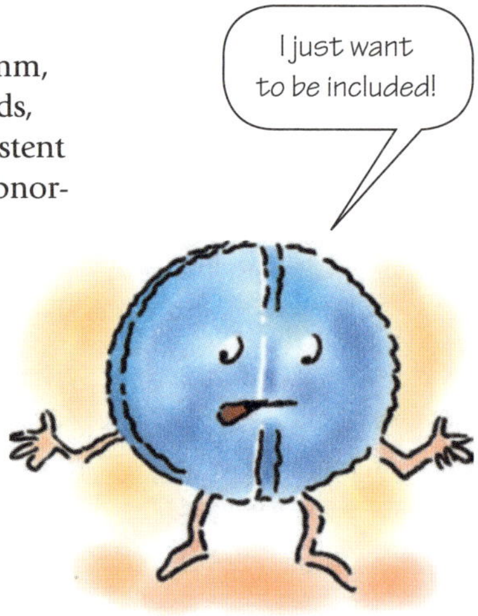

Normal or nondiagnostic ECG

A normal ECG won't show ST changes or arrhythmias. A nondiagnostic ECG may show an ST depression of 0.5 to 1 mm or a T-wave inversion or flattening in leads with dominant R waves. If further assessment is warranted, perform cardiac stress testing and echocardiography. Manage as high-risk patients who have ECG changes, positive serum markers, or positive findings on any functional studies.

Treatment for the patient is individualized; however, you should include aspirin in all treatment plans.

Treatment

The 2015 AHA guidelines recommend that the order of treatment for every patient experiencing acute ischemia and MI is oxygen, aspirin, nitroglycerin, and morphine.

Oxygen

Administer oxygen by nasal cannula or mask to anyone experiencing chest discomfort who is dyspneic, has an oxygen saturation of less than 94%, or has signs of heart failure or shock. The type and amount of oxygen you need to administer are determined by the patient's oxygen saturation. Measure pulse oximetry, if possible, and maintain oxygen saturation at more than 92%.

Aspirin

Aspirin is considered a class I action in the treatment of a patient with MI. Give aspirin 160 to 325 mg by mouth as soon as possible, if the patient hasn't already taken it and does not have a true aspirin allergy. Chewed aspirin is absorbed the fastest and is preferred.

Nitroglycerin

Sublingual nitroglycerin is the initial treatment for a patient with suspected ischemic chest pain. Nitrates decrease preload and afterload, reducing the heart's oxygen requirements. Don't give nitrates to patients with severe hypotension (less than 90 mm Hg systolic or 30 mm Hg or more below baseline), extreme bradycardia (heart rate less than 50 beats/minute), tachycardia in the absence of heart failure, or right ventricular infarction or patients who have taken medication for erectile dysfunction in the last 24 hours.

Sublingually speaking

Give nitroglycerin 0.3 to 0.4 mg sublingually up to three times at 5-minute intervals as long as the patient's blood pressure is stable (usually systolic greater than 90 mm Hg). If nitroglycerin will be continued, use the IV route because it allows for ongoing titration.

Morphine

Morphine should be avoided if possible unless pain is not tolerated and unresponsive to nitrates with acute MI. Morphine has been associated with increased mortality. Pain affects heart rate, contractility, and systolic blood pressure, which adversely increases myocardial oxygen demand. Give 2 to 4 mg initially by IV push with repeat doses of 2 to 4 mg every 5 to 10 minutes until the patient indicates pain relief. Be sure to evaluate the patient's pain response and his vital signs. Remember to frequently monitor his respiratory rate, oxygen saturation, and blood pressure because morphine can cause respiratory depression and hypotension.

Ongoing care

Obtain the patient's vital signs, oxygen saturation, brief and targeted history, 12-lead ECG, and IV access, and assess whether they're a candidate for thrombolytic therapy or PCI. Remember to focus on rapid but accurate diagnosis.

Double duty

While assessment is underway, you may perform simultaneous treatment. This includes oxygen and medication administration. You can start adjunctive therapy while reperfusion strategies are being considered.

Adjunctive therapies include:

- beta-adrenergic blockers (decrease the workload of the heart)
- IV nitroglycerin (dilates coronary arteries, improves preload and afterload)

- antiplatelet therapy
- anticoagulation therapy
- angiotensin-converting enzyme inhibitors (block conversion of angiotensin; should be given within 24 hours of symptoms)

Reperfusion strategies include:

- PCI, which includes angioplasty with or without stents
- cardiothoracic bypass surgery
- fibrinolytic therapy

Acute stroke algorithm

Acute stroke is a sudden impairment of cerebral circulation in one or more of the blood vessels supplying the brain. Stroke interrupts or diminishes oxygen supply and commonly causes serious damage or necrosis in brain tissues. The AHA has a visual representation of an adult-suspected stroke algorithm that can be viewed at https://www.ahajournals.org/doi/10.1161/CIRCULATIONAHA.110.971044.

Playing the odds

About 87% of strokes are ischemic, resulting from thrombus formation in a blood vessel supplying the brain or from embolism (typically from the heart or carotid artery). The remainder of strokes is hemorrhagic, resulting from the rupture of a cerebral artery or aneurysm.

The sooner, the better

The sooner normal blood flow is restored to the brain after a stroke, the better the patient's chance for recovery. A catch phrase that is commonly used is "time is brain." Therefore, prompt recognition and treatment of stroke can limit the extent of damage and significantly improve the patient's outcome. The National Institutes of Neurological Disorders and Stroke has established guidelines for the completion of interventions beginning from the time the patient is first suspected of suffering from a stroke.

What's the risk

A stroke is caused by a blocked or interrupted supply of blood to the brain. The risk of stroke is increased in patients with a history of:

- transient ischemic attacks (TIAs)
- atherosclerosis
- hypertension
- arrhythmias
- diabetes mellitus

- heart disease
- cigarette smoking or exposure to secondhand smoke
- hormonal contraceptive use
- personal or family history of stroke
- hypercoagulative state
- sickle cell disease
- carotid artery disease
- viral infections that cause inflammation such as Covid-19
- obesity
- physical inactivity
- heavy alcohol use
- use of illicit drugs, such as cocaine
- obstructive sleep apnea
- high cholesterol
- age over age 55
- male gender
- ethnicity (African Americans have greater risk)

What to look for

Signs and symptoms of stroke vary with the vessel affected (and, consequently, the portion of the brain it supplies), severity of damage, and extent of collateral circulation that develops to help the brain compensate for decreased blood supply.

Common signs and symptoms of stroke include the sudden onset of:

- facial droop affecting one side of the face
- hemiparesis on the affected side to unilateral or bilateral paralysis of the extremities
- unilateral sensory defect (such as numbness, tingling, or abnormal sensation), typically on the same side as the hemiparesis or hemiplegia
- slurred or indistinct speech or the inability to speak or understand speech
- loss of half of the field of vision to the same side in both eyes, double vision, or transient vision loss in one eye (usually described as a shade coming down)
- mental status changes or loss of consciousness (particularly if associated with at least one of the above symptoms)
- severe headache (seen with hemorrhagic stroke)

What to do

For all patients with signs and symptoms of stroke:

- Note the time of symptom onset, if possible.
- Maintain a patent airway and adequate oxygenation (oxygen saturation greater than 94%).

- Monitor for and treat hypoglycemia or marked hyperglycemia (serum glucose level of 80-179 mg/dl).
- Monitor blood pressure and manage it based on these considerations:
  - If the patient is a candidate for fibrinolytic therapy, achieve and maintain a blood pressure below 185 mm Hg systolic or 110 mm Hg diastolic to minimize the risk of bleeding complications.
  - If the patient isn't a candidate for fibrinolytic therapy, treat only a severely elevated blood pressure (systolic blood pressure greater than 220 mm Hg, diastolic blood pressure greater than 120). Inducing lower perfusion pressures may increase ischemia and worsen the stroke.
- STAT noncontrast CT or brain MRI
- STAT labs and ECG
- Fluid management
- Fever control with IV acetaminophen

It's important to maintain a patent airway and adequate oxygenation when treating a patient with signs and symptoms of stroke.

Stroke Chain of Survival

Similar to adult chain of survival for victims of cardiac arrest, the stroke chain of survival links actions to hasten the recognition and treatment of suspected stroke victims. The links depict rapid recognition of stroke symptoms (by family or bystanders), rapid EMD dispatch, rapid EMS transport and communication with receiving facility, and rapid diagnosis and treatment on arrival.

Additionally, the AHA highlights eight steps of care (called the 8 D's) to guide treatment of stroke victims in a timely manner to help minimize brain injury and maximize recovery.

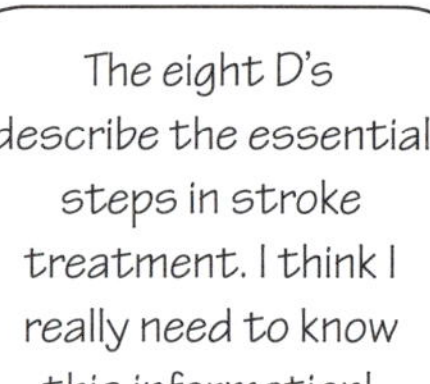

The 8 D's include:

- detection
- dispatch
- delivery
- door
- data
- decision
- drug/device
- disposition

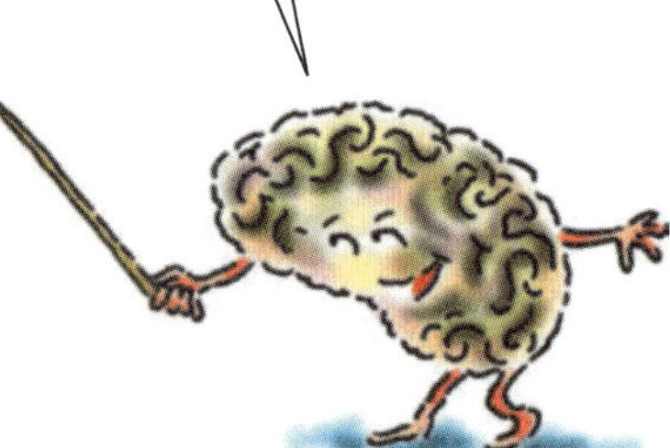

Detection

Early detection of the signs and symptoms of stroke may improve patient outcome. A patient presenting with signs of stroke, such as facial droop, difficulty talking or altered responsiveness, or limb weakness, may be experiencing a stroke. Help should be called immediately in order to provide the earliest care to the patient.

Dispatch

A patient with suspected stroke receives the same priority as a patient experiencing an acute myocardial infarction (MI). The 911 dispatcher is trained to ask specific questions of the caller to determine what type of emergency is occurring and alerts the EMS team as to how to respond.

Delivery

EMS responders will perform a quick assessment to rapidly confirm the signs and symptoms of stroke. They will perform a capillary glucose test to determine if the patient is suffering from hypoglycemia, which often presents with the same symptoms as stroke. A prehospital stroke assessment, such as the Cincinnati Prehospital Stroke Scale, is often used to assess for stroke. (See *Cincinnati Prehospital Stroke Scale.*)

EMS responders will ensure a patent airway and oxygenation and determine cardiac rhythm. Additionally, it is important for the responders to ascertain onset time of symptoms, if possible, to assist with determining eligibility for fibrinolytics.

The patient should then be transported to a stroke-prepared hospital, primary stroke center, or comprehensive stroke center as studies show that patients admitted to dedicated stroke centers have improved outcomes. Facilities with established stroke programs have protocols that establish a diagnosis of stroke and provide interventions quickly. Communication with the facility prior to arrival alerts the stroke team and hastens care on arrival.

Door

As soon as the patient arrives at the receiving facility, rapid assessment (within 10 minutes) should occur. The patient should be evaluated for signs and symptoms of stroke and onset time of symptoms established to determine if he's a candidate for fibrinolytic therapy. The stroke team should be activated if a suspected stroke is confirmed.

A secondary assessment is performed and the patient stabilized, as needed. Here are the steps that should occur:

- Ensuring that the patient has a pulse. Providing CPR is pulse is absent
- Assessing and maintaining the patient's airway and breathing Providing oxygen therapy as needed to maintain saturation greater than 94%
- Assessing blood pressure and instituting cardiac monitoring to evaluate cardiac rhythm
- Establishing IV access if not already in place
- Obtaining laboratory specimens for testing (including blood glucose level, CBC, and coagulation studies)

- Obtaining a 12-lead electrocardiogram (ECG)
- Assessing the patient's neurologic status to determine the extent of his deficits using a standardized tool such as the NIH Stroke Scale (see *NIH Stroke Scale*)
- Obtaining a CT scan without contrast medium within 25 minutes of the patient's arrival to the facility (the results should be available within 45 minutes of patient arrival to determine whether a subarachnoid hemorrhage is present)

Just to be sure

During the first few hours after an ischemic stroke, the CT scan may not show signs of ischemia. Those with a subarachnoid hemorrhage will have a normal CT scan only about 5% of the time. If you suspect a subarachnoid hemorrhage despite a normal CT scan, a lumbar puncture should be performed. Fibrinolytic therapy is contraindicated in patients who have experienced a subarachnoid hemorrhage. If the patient has a brain hemorrhage and a neurosurgical team isn't available, he may need to be transferred to another facility that offers the appropriate neurologic support.

Data

Data, such as assessment, vital signs, ECG, laboratory results, and CT scan findings, help the stroke team determine the best treatment plan for the patient. Additional data needed for complete evaluation of the patient include review of patient history and medications to determine if criteria for thrombolytics are met or if exclusions exist.

Decision

The decision of the type of treatment needed is based on the assessment parameters and the patient's situation and type of injury.

- Fibrinolytic therapy is indicated for acute ischemic stroke if it can be initiated within the first 3 hours of symptom onset. For some patients, the window of time for treatment may be extended to 4 ½ hours.
- Emergency angiography may be necessary if the patient has a subarachnoid hemorrhage.
- If an aneurysm is present, treatment may include aneurysm clipping, coiling, or exclusion, administering nimodipine, and correcting hyponatremia and water loss (if diabetes insipidus develops).
- If intracerebral hemorrhage is present, treatment may include preventing continued bleeding and managing intracranial pressure (ICP) and, possibly, neurosurgical decompression.
- Supportive care is provided for all patients.
- Elevate head of bed 30 degrees in the case of a hemorrhagic stroke. Start on statin medication.

Cincinnati Prehospital Stroke Scale

The Cincinnati Prehospital Stroke Scale is a simplified scale for evaluating patients with suspected stroke derived from the National Institutes of Health Stroke Scale. Use this scale to evaluate facial palsy, arm weakness, and speech abnormalities. An abnormality in any one of the categories below indicates that the probability of stroke is 72%.

Facial droop
Tell the patient to show his teeth or smile. If a stroke has occurred, one side of his face may not move as well as the other side.

Normal response

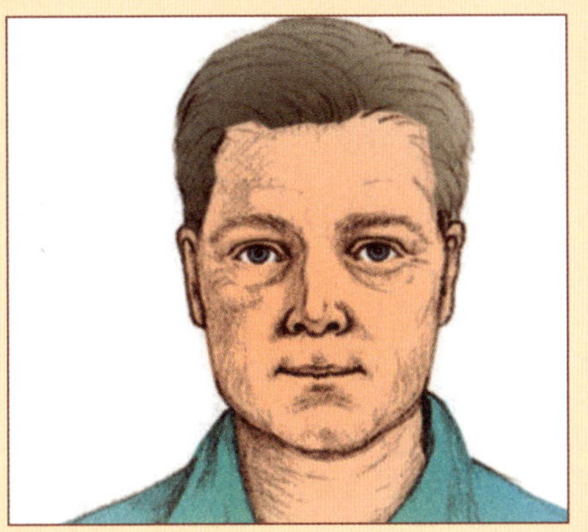

Facial droop on right side of face

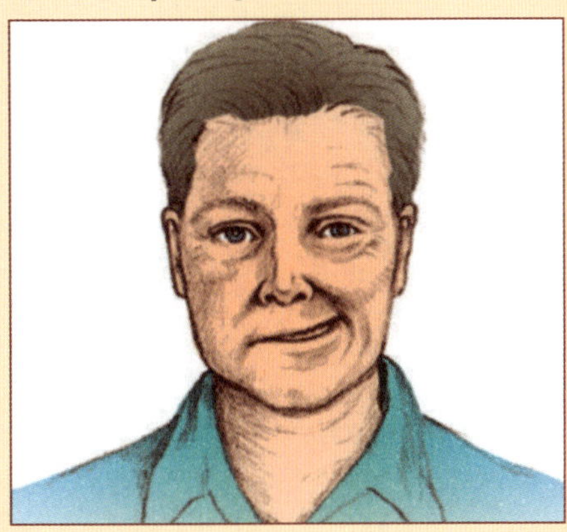

Arm drift
Tell the patient to close her eyes and hold both arms straight out in front of her for 20 seconds. If the patient has had a stroke, one arm may not move or will drift down compared with the other arm.

Normal response

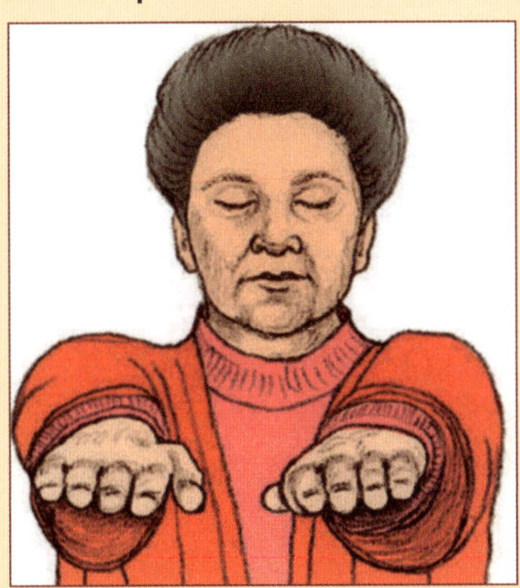

One-sided motor weakness in right arm

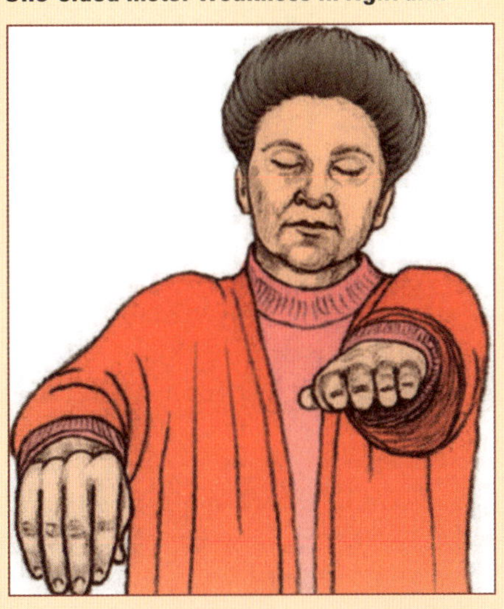

Abnormal speech
Have the patient say, "You can't teach an old dog new tricks." If they have had a stroke, they may use the wrong words, slur the words, be unable to speak at all, or not understand what you are asking.

Drug

Fibrinolytics are the drug therapy of choice, but the patient must meet certain criteria to be considered for this type of treatment. Medication should be initiated within 60 minutes of the patient's arrival to the facility. (See *Who's suited for fibrinolytic therapy?*)

Maybe, maybe not

Hypertension is commonly seen in stroke patients and may resolve without treatment. If the blood pressure is high and does not resolve on its own, medication may need to be administered. Caution should be applied when giving antihypertensive medications because hypotension may result, which can further impair cerebral perfusion. Blood pressure should not be dropped more than 15% in 24 hours.

Push or drip? It's all good!

Appropriate antihypertensives for the stroke patient include labetalol (Trandate), nicardipine (Cardene), or clevidipine (Cleviprex).

- Administer labetalol 10 to 20 mg by IV push over 1 to 2 minutes; may repeat once.
- Start nicardipine infusion at 5 mg/hour and titrate by 2.5 mg/hour every 5 to 15 minutes (maximum, 15 mg/hour).
- Initiate clevidipine at 1 to 2 mg/hour titrate every 90 seconds (max dose is 21 mg/hour. Titrate slower (every 5 to 10 minutes) as you get close to goal blood pressure.

Disposition

The stroke patients should be admitted to a specialized stroke unit or critical care unit quickly (within 3 hours of arrival is recommended). Studies show that care delivered in a stroke unit has more positive effects and optimizes patient outcomes.

What else to consider

- If seizures occur, maintain safety and administer anticonvulsants.
- If cerebral edema is present (clinically significant in only 10% to 20% of stroke patients), provide measures to reduce ICP, such as:
    - elevating the head of the bed 20 to 30 degrees
    - modestly restricting fluids
    - providing oxygenation and ventilation support to avoid hypoxemia and hypoventilation and inducing hyperventilation if indicated
    - initiating hyperosmolar therapy by giving mannitol (Osmitrol) (effects usually occur about 20 minutes after administration).

Who's suited for fibrinolytic therapy?

Not every stroke patient is a candidate for fibrinolytic therapy. Each patient must be evaluated to see whether he meets the established criteria.

Criteria that must be present

- Acute ischemic stroke associated with significant neurologic deficit
- Onset of symptoms less than 3 hours (or 4 ½ hours for selected patients) before treatment begins
- Age 18 or older

Criteria that must *not* be present

- Evidence of intracranial or subarachnoid hemorrhage during pretreatment evaluation
- Blood glucose level less than 50 mg/dL
- Intracranial neoplasm, arteriovenous malformation, or aneurysm
- History of intracranial hemorrhage
- History of recent (within 3 months) intracranial or intraspinal surgery, serious head trauma, or previous stroke
- Active bleeding
- Noncompressible arterial puncture within past week
- Known bleeding diathesis, involving but not limited to:
  - current use of oral anticoagulants and international normalized ratio greater than 1.5 or prothrombin time greater than 15 seconds
  - current use of direct thrombin inhibitors or direct factor XA inhibitors with elevated sensitive laboratory tests
  - receipt of heparin within 48 hours before the onset of stroke and having a partial thromboplastin time greater than the upper normal limit
  - platelet count less than 100,000/μL
- Uncontrolled hypertension at time of treatment greater than (185 mm Hg or diastolic greater than 110 mm Hg)
- Computed tomography scan shows multilobar infarction

Criteria that shouldn't be present

- Seizure at stroke onset with postseizure neurological impairments
- GI or urinary tract hemorrhage within 21 days
- Major surgery or trauma within 14 days
- Acute myocardial infarction within 3 months
- Only minor or rapidly improving signs and symptoms of stroke
- Pregnancy

Eligibility criteria for the treatment of acute ischemic stroke with intravenous thrombolysis (recombinant tissue plasminogen activator) or tPA

Inclusion criteria

- Clinical diagnosis of ischemic stroke causing measurable neurologic deficit
- Onset of symptoms <4.5 hours before beginning treatment; if the exact time of stroke onset is not known, it is defined as the last time the patient was known to be normal or at neurologic baseline
- Age ≥18 years

(continued)

Who's suited for fibrinolytic therapy? *(continued)*

Exclusion criteria

- Patient history
- Ischemic stroke or severe head trauma in the previous 3 months
- Previous intracranial hemorrhage
- Intra-axial intracranial neoplasm
- Gastrointestinal malignancy
- Gastrointestinal hemorrhage in the previous 21 days
- Intracranial or intraspinal surgery within the prior 3 months
- Clinical
- Symptoms suggestive of subarachnoid hemorrhage
- Persistent blood pressure elevation (systolic ≥185 mm Hg or diastolic ≥110 mm Hg)
- Active internal bleeding
- Presentation consistent with infective endocarditis
- Stroke known or suspected to be associated with aortic arch dissection
- Acute bleeding diathesis, including but not limited to conditions defined under "hematologic"
- Hematologic
- Platelet count <100,000/mm3*
- Current anticoagulant use with an INR >1.7 or PT >15 seconds or aPTT >40 seconds*
- Therapeutic doses of low molecular weight heparin received within 24 hours (e.g., to treat VTE and ACS); this exclusion does not apply to prophylactic doses (e.g., to prevent VTE)
- Current use (i.e., last dose within 48 hours in a patient with normal renal function) of a direct thrombin inhibitor or direct factor Xa inhibitor with evidence of anticoagulant effect by laboratory tests such as aPTT, INR, ECT, TT, or appropriate factor Xa activity assays
- Head CT
- Evidence of hemorrhage
- Extensive regions of obvious hypodensity consistent with irreversible injury

Warnings

- Only minor and isolated neurologic signs or rapidly improving symptoms
- Serum glucose <50 mg/dL (<2.8 mmol/L)
- Serious trauma in the previous 14 days
- Major surgery in the previous 14 days
- History of gastrointestinal bleeding (remote) or genitourinary bleeding
- Seizure at the onset of stroke with postictal neurologic impairments†
- Pregnancy
- Arterial puncture at a noncompressible site in the previous 7 days
- Large (≥10 mm), untreated, unruptured intracranial aneurysm
- Untreated intracranial vascular malformation
- Additional warnings for treatment from 3 to 4.5 hours from symptom onset
- Age >80 years
- Oral anticoagulant use regardless of INR
- Severe stroke (NIHSS score >25)
- Combination of both previous ischemic stroke and diabetes mellitus (UpToDate, 2022) Inclusion criteria

COVID-19 changes

COVID-19 has affected the way we approach CPR and ACLS. With suspected/known patients with COVID-19, all health care providers must use N95 masks and eye shields, gloves, and impermeable gowns. Rapid initiation of chest compressions increases the success rate of CPR, so it should not be delayed for the donning of protective personal equipment (PPE). Health care providers likely will already have masks on, so chest compressions should be initiated while waiting for personnel with appropriate PPE to arrive. A surgical mask can be placed over the patient's airway while waiting for airway management. There must be high-efficiency particulate absorbing (HEPA) filters on the exhaust valve of a bag valve mask for ventilation or an inline HEPA filter for other inserted airways such as ET tube or supraglottal airways. The 2020 CPR and ACLS guidelines should be followed according to the appropriate algorithms; COVID-19 does not change anything except for the above personal protection measures.

(Hsu et al., 2021)

Quick quiz

1. When treating a patient in asystole, it's important to:
   A. request a transcutaneous pacemaker.
   B. confirm the rhythm in a second lead.
   C. administer atropine 1 mg IV push.
   D. determine an underlying cause.

Answer: B. You must confirm the rhythm in two leads before initiating CPR because it's possible to have a false diagnosis of asystole. Also be sure to assess the patient.

2. What's the initial treatment for a patient found to be in VF?
   A. Lidocaine 1 mg/kg by IV push or IO
   B. Epinephrine 1 mg by IV push or IO
   C. Rapid defibrillation at 150 to 200 joules (biphasic energy)
   D. CPR for 5 minutes, followed by defibrillation at 360 joules

Answer: C. Rapid defibrillation of VF as soon as possible significantly increases the chances of a patient's survival to hospital discharge.

3. A patient is experiencing a regular wide-complex rhythm (0.12 second or more) of 250 beats/minute with diaphoresis, blood pressure of 80/50, and decreased LOC. You should:
   A. defibrillate at 200 joules.
   B. administer lidocaine 1 mg by IV push.
   C. administer amiodarone 300 mg by IV push.
   D. perform synchronized cardioversion at 100 joules.

Answer: D. These symptoms describe an unstable patient. Perform immediate synchronized cardioversion using 100 joules.

4. A patient is brought to the ED after a motor vehicle accident. They are unresponsive and EMS personnel are performing CPR. The patient has an endotracheal tube in place and has IV access. You place them on the monitor and the rhythm displays junctional tachycardia at a rate of 120 beats/minute. They have no discernible pulse. Which intervention is appropriate?

A. Adenosine 6 mg IVP followed by a flush
B. Sodium bicarbonate 1 mEq/kg by IV push
C. Fluid bolus infusion
D. Warming procedures

Answer: C. Your patient has a heart rhythm but no pulse. This is known as PEA. As a victim of a MVA, bleeding may be causing hypovolemia, which is a possible cause of PEA. You can rapidly infuse a fluid challenge while considering other causes and preparing epinephrine for administration.

5. A patient is in the intensive care unit after aortic aneurysm repair. They suddenly develop atrial fibrillation at a rate of 180 beats/minute. What medication should you consider using to convert the rhythm?

A. Amiodarone
B. Epinephrine
C. Atropine
D. Lidocaine

Answer: A. You can use amiodarone to convert atrial fibrillation for both the normal heart and the impaired heart.

Scoring

☆☆☆ If you answered all five questions correctly, congratulations! Your score is a clear sign of your success.

☆☆ If you answered four questions correctly, good work! Your knowledge of algorithms is flowing nicely.

☆ If you answered fewer than four questions correctly, it's no emergency! A quick review will point you to a perfect score next time.

Suggested references

American Heart Association (2020). *Advanced cardiovascular life support provider manual*, E-book edition.

American Heart Association. (2020). *Algorithms*. Retrieved from American Heart Association CPR & First Aid Emergency Cardiovascular Care: https://cpr.heart.org/en/resuscitation-science/cpr-and-ecc-guidelines/algorithms

American Heart Association and American College of Cardiology Foundation. (2021). *2021 AHA/ACC/ASE/Chest/SAEM/SCCT/SCMR guidelines for the evaluation and diagnosis of chest pain*. Elsevier.

Elmer, J., & Rittenberger, J. C. (2022, August 18). *Initial assessment and management of the adult post-cardiac arrest patient.* Retrieved from UpToDate: https://www.uptodate.com/contents/initial-assessment-and-management-of-the-adult-post-cardiac-arrest-patient#H9724120

Mount, D. B. (2022, August 17). *Treatment and prevention of hyperkalemia in adults.* Retrieved from UpToDate: https://www.uptodate.com/contents/treatment-and-prevention-of-hyperkalemia-in-adults?search=treatment%20of%20sever%20hyperkalemia&source=search_result&selectedTitle=1~150&usage_type=default&display_rank=1#H6

Oliveira-Filho, J., & Mullen, M. T. (2022, April 26). *Initial assessment and management of acute stroke.* Retrieved from UpToDate: https://www.uptodate.com/contents/initial-assessment-and-management-of-acute-stroke?search=acute%20stroke%20management&source=search_result&selectedTitle=1~150&usage_type=default&display_rank=1#H2191640006

Simmons, M., & Breall, J. (2022, July 21). *Overview of acute management of Non-ST-elevation acute coronary syndromes.* Retrieved from UpToDate: https://www.uptodate.com/contents/overview-of-the-acute-management-of-non-st-elevation-acute-coronary-syndromes?search=NSTEMI%20treatment&source=search_result&selectedTitle=1~142&usage_type=default&display_rank=1#H7

UpToDate. (2022). *Eligibility criteria for the treatment of acute ischemic stroke with intravenous thrombolysis (recombinant tissue plasminogen activator or tPA).* Retrieved from UpTo Date: https://www.Eligibility criteria for the treatment of acute ischemic stroke with intravenous thrombolysis (recombinant tissue plasminogen activator or tPA)uptodate.com/contents/image?imageKey=NEURO%2F71462&topicKey=NEURO%2F1126&search=acute%20stroke%20man

Zimetbaum, P. J. (2020, April 10). *Wide complex tachycardia: Causes, epidemiology, and clinical manifestations.* Retrieved from UpToDate: https://www.uptodate.com/contents/wide-qrs-complex-tachycardias-causes-epidemiology-and-clinical-manifestations?sectionName=Physical%20examination%20findings&search=wide%20complex%20tachycardia%20tachycardia&topicRef=920&anchor=H125977428&source=see_link#

Chapter 9

Critical situations

Just the facts

In this chapter, you'll learn:

- emergency care for pregnant women in cardiac arrest
- emergency care for patients in cardiac arrest caused by trauma
- special measures required for submersion or drowning victims
- treatment for victims of electric shock, lightning strike, or hypothermia
- emergency interventions to treat toxicologic emergencies, near-fatal asthma, and anaphylaxis

A look at critical situations

You may encounter critical situations in which it's difficult to apply the guidelines presented in an advanced cardiovascular life support (ACLS) treatment algorithm. Situations such as these require the health care provider to quickly assess the situation and potentially modify treatments to improve patient outcomes. These situations include pregnancy, trauma, submersion or drowning, electric shock or lightning strike, hypothermia, toxicologic emergencies, near-fatal asthma, and anaphylaxis. In addition, life-threatening electrolyte disturbances are frequently associated with critical situations, including cardiac arrest. Severe electrolyte disturbances may cause cardiac arrest and may complicate resuscitation efforts during cardiac arrest from other causes. (See *Managing electrolyte disturbances associated with cardiac arrest.*)

As with all emergencies, investigation into the background of the situation or the mechanism of the injury may be essential prior to treating the patient. For example, treatment measures in toxicologic emergencies are easier to provide if knowledge of the specific drug or substance ingested is provided as it helps to determine antidotal treatment.

In critical situations, you'll need to quickly assess the situation and modify treatment algorithm guidelines to provide the most effective treatment for your patient.

Cardiac arrest during pregnancy

Cardiovascular and respiratory systems are altered significantly during pregnancy. As a result, a pregnant woman is more susceptible to the effects of cardiovascular and respiratory difficulties.

When treating a pregnant patient, remember that circulating blood volume, cardiac output, heart rate, oxygen consumption, and minute ventilation increase during pregnancy. Systemic and pulmonary vascular resistance, pulmonary functional residual capacity, and colloid oncotic pressure decrease during pregnancy.

Treatment for two

Keep in mind that you need to consider optimal care for the mother and the fetus when managing cardiac arrest in a pregnant patient. If the mother isn't doing well, the fetus will also be affected. The key to resuscitation of the fetus is resuscitation of the mother because the two are inseparable in this situation.

What causes it

Cardiac arrest in a pregnant patient is typically caused by precipitating events that may be indirectly attributed to the physiologic changes that occur during pregnancy.

These include the following:

- bleeding/disseminated intravascular coagulation
- venous thromboembolism
- cardiac disease (heart failure, MI, aortic dissection, cardiomyopathy)
- trauma
- hypertension (preeclampsia, eclampsia)
- amniotic fluid embolism
- placenta abruptio, previa
- complications of tocolytic (anticontraction) therapy, such as arrhythmias, MI, or heart failure
- anesthetic complications, including spinal shock
- uterine atony
- sepsis

When treating a pregnant patient in cardiac arrest, remember that you're really caring for two patients—the mother and the fetus.

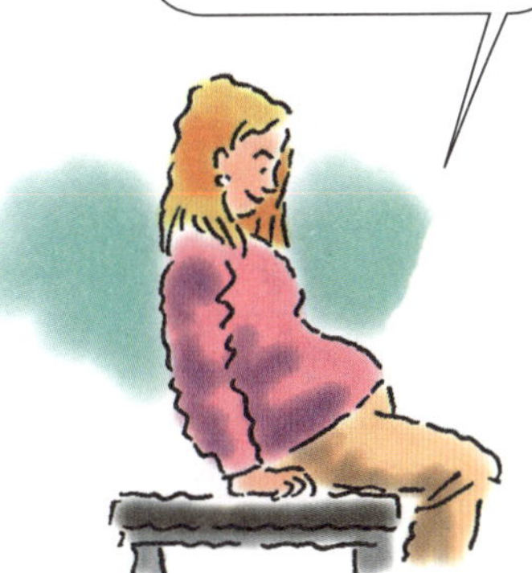

What to look for

Signs of cardiac arrest include the following:

- loss of consciousness
- inadequate or absent breathing
- absence of a pulse

How it's treated

Treatment of a pregnant woman during cardiac arrest involves assessment of the patient as well as the fetus. Size of the fetus may require some adjustments to delivery of care.

Position supposition

First, take note of the patient's position. When a pregnant patient is in a supine position, the pressure of the uterus on abdominal blood vessels (particularly the inferior vena cava) can inhibit venous return and filling of the abdominal aorta. This can inhibit cardiac output during compressions. For this reason, if the fundus is at or above the level of the umbilicus, a pregnant patient requires manual displacement of the uterus to the left when placed in a supine position, if possible.

Circulation

You may need to perform chest compressions slightly higher on the sternum (slightly above the center) of a patient in advanced pregnancy to accommodate the shifting of abdominal contents toward the patient's head.

When replacing fluid volume, remember that there's a normal increase in blood volume of up to 50% during pregnancy. In addition, you must monitor blood supply to the neonate to maintain stability. Optimally, establish IV access above the diaphragm.

Airway

Secure the airway early in the resuscitation effort. Airway securement and management of a pregnant patient may be more difficult than with a nonpregnant patient due to anatomic and physiologic changes that occur during pregnancy. Also, fetal status should be considered during intubation attempts.

Breathing

Be aware that the gravid uterus pushes up on the diaphragm and may decrease ventilatory volume, which makes providing positive pressure ventilation difficult. As during any resuscitation, make sure that there's adequate chest rise when providing ventilations. Be sure to provide good ventilations with 100% oxygen and bag valve mask device before intubation. Monitor oxygenation with pulse oximetry and utilize continuous waveform capnography whenever possible.

Defibrillation

Defibrillation requirements are unchanged when resuscitating a pregnant woman. If internal or external fetal monitors are in use, remove them before defibrillating.

Differential diagnosis

In certain situations, an emergency cesarean delivery may be indicated. This may increase the chance of survival for the mother and fetus when performed within 5 minutes of the cardiac arrest because blood supply to the fetus becomes rapidly hypoxic and acidotic. Points to consider when making this decision include the following:

- the patient's response to appropriate basic life support (BLS) and ACLS treatment
- the presence of an inevitably fatal injury or condition in the patient
- the possible benefit of a cesarean delivery to the mother (Removing the fetus and the placenta benefits the mother even if the fetus is too small to compress the inferior vena cava.)
- gestational age and viability of the fetus
- time that has elapsed between collapse of the mother and possible removal of the fetus
- availability of personnel able to perform a cesarean delivery and to support the mother and neonate after the procedure

After a cesarean delivery has been performed, provide supportive measures to the mother and neonate, as indicated, to promote their chance of survival.

What to consider

- If persistent arrest is due to an immediately reversible problem (such as excessive anesthesia or analgesia or bronchospasm), cesarean delivery isn't indicated.
- If standard BLS and ACLS measures fail and there's a chance that the fetus is viable, consider immediate perimortem cesarean delivery.

Cardiac arrest as a result of trauma

The treatment of a trauma patient experiencing cardiac or respiratory arrest is complex. Your prime consideration should be the patient's need for rapid transport to a facility capable of managing his condition rather than performing multiple resuscitation attempts.

Ensuring rapid transport to a capable facility is your top priority when treating a trauma patient.

Traumatic times

If cardiac arrest is associated with uncontrolled internal hemorrhage or pericardial tamponade, immediate surgical intervention in a capable facility is required. In some situations, the number of critical patients may exceed the capability of ACLS providers and the EMS team. If this occurs, a triage process should be instituted, and trauma patients without a pulse should be considered lower in priority for care.

What causes it

Some of the potential causes of cardiac or respiratory arrest in a trauma patient include the following:

- tension pneumothorax; ruptured diaphragm, or pericardial tamponade that causes significant compromise to cardiac output
- exsanguination or internal bleeding with subsequent hypovolemia and inadequate oxygen delivery
- central neurologic injury that causes cardiovascular collapse
- severe hypothermia that complicates injuries occurring in an extremely cold environment
- hypoxia from airway obstruction, severely lacerated or crushed trachea or bronchi, large open pneumothorax, or neurologic injury
- severe direct injury to vital organs, such as the heart, and to such structures as the aorta or femoral artery
- underlying medical problems that led to the traumatic event, such as cardiac arrest precipitating a motor vehicle accident
- cardiac contusion caused by blunt trauma to the chest with ECG changes and rhythm disturbances

What to look for

The signs and symptoms of cardiac arrest may occur suddenly or insidiously, depending on the mechanism of injury and the patient's age and medical history. If the trauma involves multiple injuries, be sure to look past them to assess for circulation, airway, and breathing.

Signs of cardiac arrest in include the following:

- loss of consciousness
- inadequate or absent breathing
- absence of a pulse

How it's treated

If the patient in entrapped in a vehicle, extricate them as soon as possible. As a health care provider, if you suspect cervical injury, remember to immobilize the patient's neck before extrication and transport. Immobilization is usually accomplished by using lateral neck supports and strapping the patient securely to a backboard to assist in transport. You should also apply a hard cervical collar, which has been appropriately sized for the patient. These actions minimize neck and spinal cord injury while caring for, moving, and transporting the patient.

Next, assess for responsiveness, breathing, and a palpable pulse. Keep in mind that several special considerations exist when treating a trauma patient. (See *Assessment of the trauma patient*.) Most emergency interventions for the trauma patient will be performed by a practitioner with special training.

Circulation

Provide chest compressions, as needed, to provide cardiac output. If external hemorrhage is present, apply firm and direct pressure using dry dressing material or a chemically treated hemostasis dressing. A tourniquet may additionally be required for additional hemostasis control. A patient with uncontrollable hemorrhage should be transported immediately to a hospital for surgical intervention.

Trauma to the rib cage increases the risk that chest compressions may cause tension pneumothorax. Be aware of any difficulty providing ventilations, and if a tension pneumothorax is suspected, provide appropriate treatment.

Airway

Remember that you must immobilize the spine for a patient with suspected head or neck trauma or with multisystem trauma. This can make providing required interventions challenging. If possible, have another rescuer support the patient's neck during airway procedures. Follow these steps to ensure a patent airway:

- Open the airway using the modified jaw-thrust maneuver (preferred over the head-tilt, chin-lift maneuver).
- Clear the airway of any obstruction, such as secretions, blood, and vomitus.
- If intubation is needed to obtain or maintain an adequate airway, perform orotracheal intubation.
- Confirm tube placement with continuous waveform capnography.
- Confirm tube placement after the initial intubation and with any movement or transfer of the patient.
- Utilize manual immobilization of the spine when inserting adjunct airways instead of relying on an immobilization device (hard collar). The device may compromise the airway before an adjunct is successfully inserted.
- Cricothyrotomy may be necessary if the patient has experienced massive facial injury, angioedema, or facial damage due to burns.

I'm best given in high concentrations. If I'm not, I get kind of cranky.

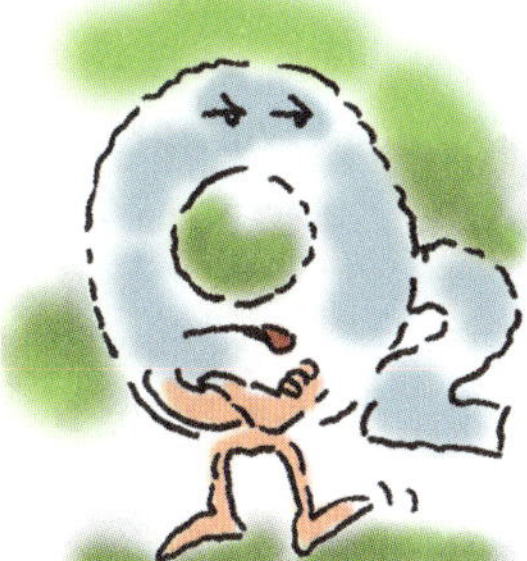

Breathing

Immobilize and maintain the patient's cervical spine when providing ventilations. Provide a high concentration of oxygen, even if the patient's oxygenation status appears adequate. When using a bag-mask device, remember to deliver breaths over 1 second to reduce the chance of gastric distention and regurgitation, which can easily lead to aspiration.

Pitfall potential

Follow these steps if you suspect the presence of conditions that are interfering with the patient's ability to breathe on his own:

- Assess for open pneumothorax and seal the pleural cavity if present.

- If ventilation attempts do not cause the patient's chest to expand despite repeated attempts to open the airway and ventilate, suspect tension pneumothorax or hemothorax.
- If the patient has suffered chest injury, check for asymmetry of breath sounds or resistance to ventilation, which may indicate tension pneumothorax.
- In the presence of tension pneumothorax, immediately perform a needle decompression utilizing a 10-14 gauge catheter at the 2nd intercostal space mid-clavicular or 5-6th intercostal space mid-axillary.
- Once needle decompression is performed chest tube placement on the affected side is required.
- If significant flail chest is present, intubate the patient and provide positive pressure ventilation because they will be unable to maintain adequate oxygenation.
- If penetrating trauma occurred to the patient's left chest and is associated with signs of decreased cardiac output or tamponade (jugular vein distention, hypotension, and muffled heart tones), suspect penetrating cardiac injury. Rapid transportation to a trauma center will provide opportunity for an emergency open thoracotomy, which allows direct cardiac massage as well as management of thoracic hemorrhage and cardiac tamponade. Aortic cross-clamping can also be performed during this procedure.
- Extreme tachycardia, arrhythmias, ST wave changes on the ECG, and impaired function may all be experienced after suffering blunt chest trauma. Diagnosis may be made with a 12-lead ECG, bedside ultrasound, or CT scanner. Diagnosis can be confirmed with an ECG or radionuclide angiography.

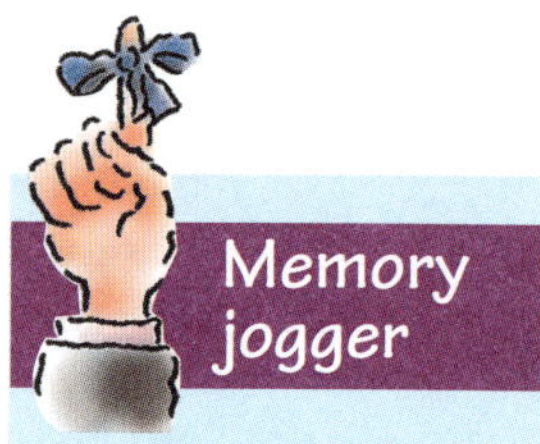

Memory jogger

To help remember what information to obtain during your assessment of the trauma patient, use the acronym **SAMPLE**:

Signs and symptoms

Allergies

Medications

Past medical history

Last meal

Events leading to injury

Turn up the volume

Successful resuscitation may depend on restoring adequate circulating blood volume; however, don't let establishing IV or IO access, fluid resuscitation, or administering medications delay transport of the patient to a trauma facility. Initiate these measures at the scene only if extrication or transport of the patient is prolonged. In all other cases, these actions can be initiated en route to a trauma facility. Keep in mind that aggressive volume replacement may be necessary to obtain adequate perfusion pressures.

Control bleeding as quickly as possible. If external pressure doesn't stop internal bleeding or if you suspect penetrating cardiac injury, surgical exploration is required and cannot be provided at the trauma site. Hemorrhage may require blood replacement.

Explore the possibilities

Surgical exploration is also indicated in trauma patients in the following situations:

- hemodynamic instability despite volume resuscitation

Assessment of the trauma patient

This chart shows what to look for and what to do during the assessment of the trauma patient.

Parameter	Assessment	Interventions
Circulation	• Pulse and blood pressure • Bleeding or hemorrhage • Capillary refill, color of the skin and mucous membranes • Cardiac rhythm	• Perform cardiopulmonary resuscitation, administer medications, and perform defibrillation or synchronized cardioversion. • Control bleeding with direct pressure or tourniquet placement. • Establish intravenous, EZ IO access, or central line access and provide fluid therapy. Fluids may include isotonic crystaloid, plasma, packed red blood cells, and whole blood products. • Treat life-threatening conditions such as cardiac tamponade.
Airway	• Airway patency • Position of the trachea (midline or deviation)	• Position the patient and ensure that their neck is midline and stabilized, then perform the modified jaw-thrust maneuver. • Utilize manual immobilization of the spine rather than a rigid cervical collar during airway management for improved visualization. • Suction the airway as needed. • Remove foreign bodies that are obstructing the airway. • Use airway adjuncts such as nasal and oral airways, extra-glottic airways, endotracheal intubation, or cricothyrotomy.
Breathing	• Respirations (rate, depth, effort) • Breath sounds • Chest wall movement and chest injury	• Administer 100% oxygen using a bag valve mask device. • Treat life-threatening conditions such as simple pneumothorax, tension pneumothorax, or hemothorax.
Disability	• Neurologic assessment, including level of consciousness, pupil reaction, and motor and sensory function	• Provide cervical spine immobilization until X-rays evaluate the cervical spine for injury.
Exposure to environment	• Environmental conditions and exposure (extreme cold or heat)	• Institute appropriate therapy (warming therapy for hypothermia or cooling therapy for hyperthermia).

- excessive thoracic drainage (greater than 300 mL/hour for 3 hours or total drainage of 1.5 to 2 L)
- significant hemothorax on X-ray
- cardiac trauma
- gunshot wound to the abdomen
- penetrating injury
- positive diagnostic peritoneal lavage
- significant solid organ or bowel injury

Defibrillation

If indicated, provide defibrillation for VF and pulseless ventricular tachycardia (VT) following ACLS guidelines.

Differential diagnosis

It's essential that you identify and treat the underlying causes of arrhythmias. Cardiac monitoring may reveal pulseless electrical activity (PEA), bradycardia, VF, or VT. Although epinephrine is typically administered to treat these arrhythmias, it may be ineffective if severe hypovolemia is present and left uncorrected.

Treating PEA requires treating the causes. You may need to reverse hypovolemia, hypothermia, cardiac tamponade, or tension pneumothorax. Bradycardic rhythms are commonly due to hypoxia, severe hypovolemia, or cardiopulmonary failure.

What to consider

- Trauma from a head injury or shock can produce loss of consciousness.
- Spinal cord injuries can result in a conscious patient with neurologic deficits. Monitor the patient's responsiveness closely because deterioration can result from neurologic compromise or cardiopulmonary failure.
- Patients who receive positive pressure ventilations should have a gastric tube placed to decompress the stomach and prevent aspiration.
- Severe maxillofacial injuries are a contraindication for nasogastric tube placement due to the potential for intracranial migration.
- The patient may experience heat loss if their clothing is removed to determine the extent of injuries or if blood or other fluids evaporate. Rewarm the patient as soon as possible to prevent hypothermia induced coagulopathy and subsequent bleeding.

Submersion or drowning

Patients who have been involved in water accidents may be classified according to the type of accident.

- Water rescue: An event in which a patient is alert, experiences distress in the water, and receives timely help. Generally, this patient isn't transported to the hospital for further evaluation unless injured.
- Submersion: An event in which a patient requires support in the field and is transported to a facility for observation and treatment after being rescued from the water. Submersion in liquids other than water may also occur and require emergency treatment.

- Drowning: An event that results in respiratory arrest when a patient is submerged in a liquid medium, usually water. Death may occur at the scene or within 24 hours of the event. (Up to the time of the drowning-related death, the patient is considered a submersion patient.)

Duration determination

When treating a patient who has been submerged, you should first establish the type of fluid the victim was submerged and also determine the duration of the submersion, the water conditions (such as temperature or pollution level), along with the duration and severity of the resultant hypoxia. Hypoxia can cause multisystem complications, such as hypoxic encephalopathy and acute respiratory distress syndrome as well as increased pulmonary capillary permeability, which results in pulmonary edema. The patient may also develop hypothermia if they have been submerged in cold water or has been submerged for a long period of time.

Even if you can't determine the duration of submersion, promptly initiate resuscitation efforts to restore the patient's oxygenation, ventilation, and perfusion unless you note obvious evidence of death, such as rigor mortis, dependent lividity, or putrefaction, which would then be classified as drowning. Submersion patients who require resuscitation should be transported to the hospital and evaluated.

What causes it

Submersion or drowning may occur in such situations as:

- unattended toddler around water
- residential swimming
- injury after diving
- swimming while under the influence of alcohol or drugs
- child abuse
- boating accident
- underlying disease process, such as diabetes, seizure disorder, MI, anxiety, or panic disorder
- suicide or homicide attempt
- scuba diving accident

What to look for

The degree of injury caused by a water incident varies depending on the amount of time that the patient was submerged, the water conditions, the patient's age, and their medical history. Hypothermia is defined as a drop in body temperature to less than 35° C. (Brown, 2020). For example, an elderly patient with a history of lung disease may suffer from water submersion quicker than a healthy adolescent. Additional considerations include injury occurring before submersion and the temperature of the water. For example, cervical injury that occurs while diving may cause drowning due to spinal injury. The CDC (CDC.gov, 2018) noted that the risk of hypothermia can develop in water with temperatures as high as 70 degrees. Water conducts heat away from the body 25 times faster than air, and physical exertion increases heat loss by as much as 50% faster. All of these factors allow hypothermia to set in more quickly.

How it's treated

First, retrieve the patient from the water (or liquid) as quickly as possible while maintaining the safety of the rescuers. Arrange transportation to a nearby facility for further evaluation and treatment, even if resuscitation efforts have already been successful. Attempt to determine the cause of submersion and length of time under water. Although American Heart Association (AHA) guidelines for CPR begin with chest compressions, they recommend that you use the traditional ABC approach for drowning victims and assess the airway first because the cause for the arrest is usually hypoxia. Initiate CPR for this type of victim with two rescue breaths and then provide high-quality chest compressions.

Airway

AHA guidelines state that routine cervical spine immobilization isn't necessary for a submersion patient except in cases when trauma is likely (diving, water slide, signs of injury or alcohol intoxication). If a potential spinal cord injury is suspected, maintain the patient's head and neck in a neutral position while in the water, and immobilize the cervical and thoracic spine before removing the patient from the water.

Remember, you don't have to clear water from the patient's airway before you begin rescue breathing.

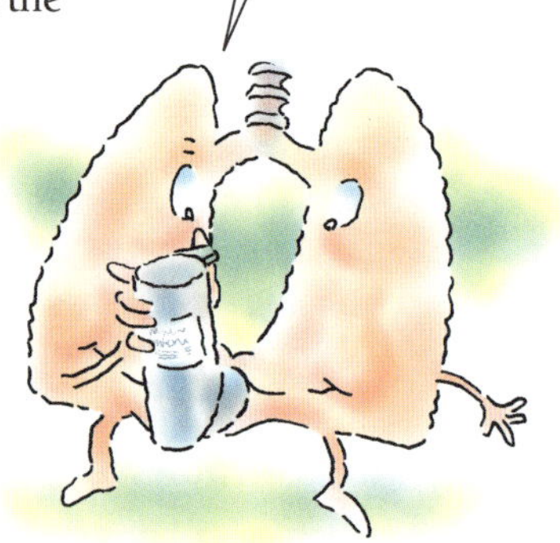

Breathing

Initiate rescue breathing as soon as possible. Remember, you don't need to clear the patient's airway of water before beginning rescue breathing. In most cases, the volume aspirated is small and quickly absorbed by the lung tissue. After an advanced airway is placed, deliver positive pressure ventilation with a bag valve mask device. Continue oxygen administration during transport. Keep in mind that it may take several hours for pulmonary injury to manifest.

Circulation

After rescue breathing has been initiated, assess the patient for a pulse for a maximum of 10 seconds. If you are unable to detect a pulse, provide high-quality compressions. The pulse of a near-drowning patient may be difficult to palpate because of peripheral vasoconstriction. Do not attempt compressions while the patient is still in the water unless special flotation equipment and hard backboard are available to support the patient during the attempt, and until there are available rescuers specifically trained in water-based resuscitation.

Defibrillation

Use defibrillation if a shockable rhythm is identified. Follow electrical safety precautions, remove the patient from the water, and quickly dry their chest before defibrillation. If the patient has a core temperature of 86 °F (30 °C) or less (severe hypothermia), follow standard BLS and ACLS algorithms, including defibrillation, while providing rewarming techniques.

Differential diagnosis

The cause of submersion or drowning should be considered during rescue attempts. If the patient is in VF or has suffered a spinal injury, you should attempt to simultaneously treat that emergency along with providing cardiopulmonary resuscitation and treating hypothermia.

What to consider

- Don't attempt deep-water breathing techniques unless you're specifically trained in their use.
- Be aware that nearly all drowning patients will experience some degree of hypothermia as a result of the submersion and from evaporation during resuscitation.

Electric shock or lightning strike

Electric shock or lightning strike can cause many injuries with varying degrees of severity accompanied by cardiac or respiratory arrest. Initiate treatment immediately after rescuer safety is assured. Although it isn't possible to readily predict a patient's outcome, those without preexisting cardiopulmonary disease, especially the young, have a good potential for survival when immediate support is provided.

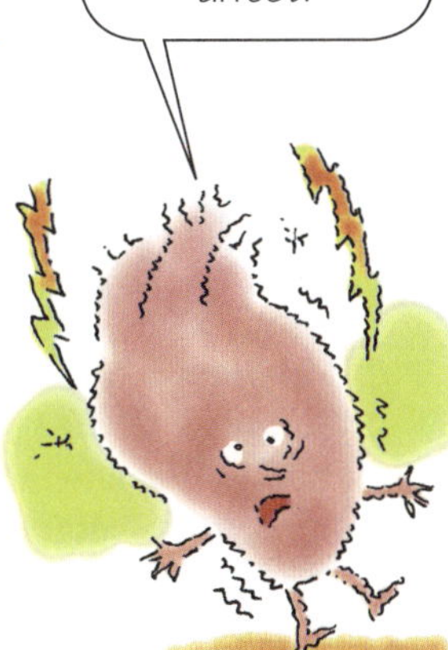

What causes it

Although most electric shocks to children occur in the home, most of the incidents involving adults occur in the workplace. Lightning strikes typically occur when the victim is outdoors during a thunderstorm. Many factors determine the type and severity of injury, including:

- magnitude of energy received
- voltage
- duration of contact (contact with alternating current can cause skeletal muscle contractions that "lock" the patient to the source, leading to prolonged exposure)
- resistance to current flow
- path of current flow

What to look for

Primary respiratory arrest following electric shock or lightning strike can occur due to:

- inhibition of the patient's respiratory center function resulting from electric current passing through the brain
- tetanic contraction of the patient's respiratory muscles during the passing of the electric current
- continued paralysis of the patient's respiratory muscles up to several minutes after the electric current has ended

A lightning strike may also affect the patient's cardiovascular and neurologic systems. Cardiac arrest may present as asystole, VF, or VT. Myocardial injury may occur as a direct effect of the current and from coronary artery spasm. Neurologic injuries may result directly from effects on the patient's brain or secondarily from complications of cardiac or respiratory arrest.

The current may produce such problems as:

- cerebral hemorrhage
- cerebral edema
- small-vessel injury
- neuronal injury
- hypoxic encephalopathy (from cardiac arrest)
- myelin damage to the peripheral nervous system

Shot to the heart

A lightning strike causes an instantaneous, massive direct current countershock. Depolarization occurs to the entire myocardium resulting in VF cardiac arrest. In many cases, cardiac cell automaticity restores organized cardiac activity. Excessive catecholamine release or autonomic nervous system stimulation can result in:

- hypertension
- tachycardia
- nonspecific ECG changes (including a prolonged QT interval and T-wave inversion)
- myocardial necrosis

How it's treated

First, make sure that the electrical current has been turned off or removed before touching a patient who has been shocked. (A victim of lightning strike isn't electrified.) As a health care provider, if you suspect head or neck trauma, maintain the patient's head in a neutral position and immobilize their spine. Spinal injuries can occur with electric shock due to tetanic contraction of skeletal muscles.

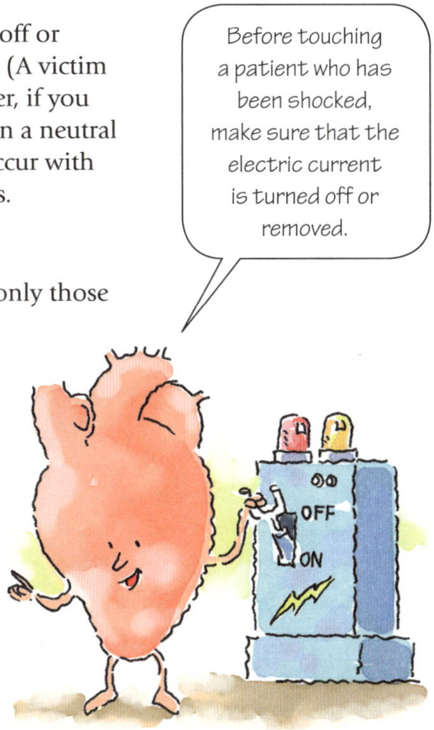

Safety first

If rescuers must remain with the patient near live current, only those specially trained to perform in this circumstance should do so. Remember to maintain the safety of rescuers at all times.

If the patient is in an unsafe environment, such as high on a telephone pole, they must be brought to safety before treatment. After you've ensured the patient's safety, initiate vigorous resuscitative measures.

Circulation

If you don't detect a pulse, initiate high-quality chest compressions as soon as possible. Hypovolemic shock can occur from significant tissue destruction and fluid loss due to increased capillary permeability. Administer adequate IV fluids to support circulating blood volume and to produce diuresis. This will promote excretion of myoglobin and potassium, which are by-products of extensive tissue damage. Edema may occur locally at the site of the patient's injuries. Remove jewelry and other constrictive objects to promote circulation.

Airway

Secure a patent airway if the patient can't maintain one naturally. It's important to intubate the patient early because significant tissue swelling and edema may develop, especially if facial burns are compromising the airway. Insert an endotracheal (ET) tube before signs of airway obstruction become severe. If you suspect head or neck injury, use the jaw-thrust maneuver (preferred over the head-tilt, chin-lift maneuver). Keep in mind that electric burns on the face, mouth, or anterior neck can also result in a compromised airway.

Breathing

Initiate rescue breathing if the patient doesn't spontaneously breathe on their own but has a pulse. Provide ventilatory support and supplemental oxygenation.

Defibrillation

If pulseless VT or VF is present, defibrillate as quickly as possible following ACLS guidelines.

Differential diagnosis

After you treat the patient's injuries, evaluate and address any medical precipitating event.

What to consider

- Electrothermal burns and underlying tissue injury may need surgical treatment. Transport the patient to a burn center if possible for a thorough evaluation of his injuries.
- In addition to potential spinal injuries, the patient may suffer muscular strains or fractures due to the tetanic response of their skeletal muscles.
- The patient may experience thermal damage from smoldering clothing, shoes, and belts. Remove these items as quickly as possible to prevent further injury.

Hypothermia

Patients with severe hypothermia may appear to be clinically dead, with pulses and respiratory efforts difficult to detect. Don't withhold lifesaving procedures unless the patient has obvious lethal injuries or their body is frozen to the point that chest compressions do not produce movement in the chest wall.

What causes it

Hypothermia occurs from exposure to cold temperatures. Unintentional hypothermia may be associated with poverty, mental illness, or the use of drugs and alcohol. Hypothermia may also be a secondary occurrence, such as in the case of submersion, a trauma, or cardiopulmonary arrest patient found in a cold environment.

What to look for

Hypothermia has a physiologic effect on vital organs. Severe hypothermia results in:

- depression of cerebral blood flow
- diminished oxygen requirements
- decreased oxygen demand and consumption
- reduced cardiac output
- decreased arterial pressure.

Keep in mind that mild hypothermia has a protective effect on the brain and vital organs to some extent in cardiac arrest. This is not the case with moderate to severe hypothermia.

Severe hypothermia affects vital organs by causing cerebral blood flow depression and reduced cardiac output.

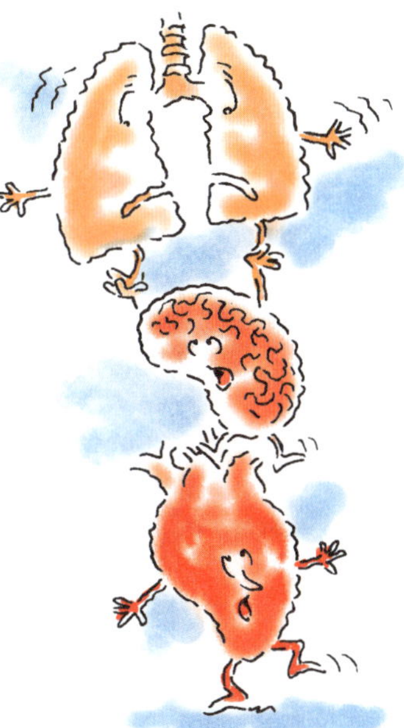

How it's treated

Some patients with hypothermia maintain a perfusing rhythm and only require rewarming. If the patient has maintained a perfusing rhythm:

- Remove wet clothing, insulate their body, and protect them from wind.
- Monitor their core temperature and cardiac rhythm. (You may need to use needle electrodes if adhesive electrodes won't function on very cold skin.)
- Provide additional supportive measures, such as intubation, as needed.

Now we're really warming up!

Institute rewarming for a patient with a core temperature lower than 93 °F (33.9 °C). Rescuers in the field should assess core temperature (tympanic or rectal) if possible, because rewarming techniques vary based on the severity of hypothermia. Rewarming techniques include passive, active external, and active internal.

With passive rewarming, the patient is placed in a warm room and wrapped in blankets. Active external rewarming utilizes heating devices such as forced hot air, warm bath water, warming packs, or warming blankets. Manage a conscious patient with mild or moderate hypothermia with passive and active external rewarming procedures.

Use active internal rewarming for patients with severe hypothermia. Provide these interventions:

- Administer humidified oxygen that has been warmed to 108 °F to 115 °F (42.2 °C to 46.1 °C).
- Administer IV fluids warmed to 110 °F (43.3 °C) at 150 to 200 mL/hour via a central access device.
- Perform peritoneal lavage with potassium-free fluid, 2 L at a time, that has been warmed to 110 °F.
- Use IV warming systems with warmed saline or blood products.
- Use extracorporeal blood warming with partial bypass, if available.

Some patients may experience cardiopulmonary arrest and require resuscitation as well as rewarming. If the patient experiences cardiopulmonary arrest, follow appropriate ACLS guidelines.

Circulation

Assess for a pulse for no longer than 10 seconds. Keep in mind that peripheral vasoconstriction and bradycardia may make the patient's pulse difficult to detect. If there is no detectable pulse, initiate high-quality chest compressions immediately and connect the patient to a cardiac monitor as soon as possible to evaluate the cardiac rhythm.

An extended cold spell

Patients who are hypothermic for 45 minutes or longer have additional interventions that you'll need to provide:

- Administer fluid to counteract the expansion of the vascular space that occurs during vasodilation in rewarming procedures.
- Monitor the patient's heart rate and hemodynamic status to evaluate fluid needs and response to rewarming techniques.
- Monitor the patient's serum potassium level carefully because significant hyperkalemia may develop. Manage a high serum potassium level with IV calcium chloride, sodium bicarbonate, glucose, and insulin or administer a sodium polystyrene sulfonate (Kayexalate) enema. (More aggressive treatments include dialysis or exchange transfusion.)

Airway

Ensure that the patient with hypothermia has a patient airway. There should be visible rise and fall of their chest with each breath or ventilation provided. If this isn't apparent, use the head-tilt, chin-lift maneuver to open the patient's airway. Insert an advanced airway if necessary to provide ventilatory support.

Ahh, this is the life! I get to enjoy the warmth and humidity, and the patient with hypothermia benefits. Talk about a win-win situation!

Breathing

After obtaining and securing a patent airway, assess the patient for breathing. If the patient isn't breathing, provide ventilations with warmed humidified oxygen (108 °F to 115 °F) when possible.

Defibrillation

As soon as a defibrillator is available, assess the patient's cardiac rhythm. Attempt defibrillation if pulseless VT or VF is present, following ACLS guidelines.

Differential diagnosis

Address underlying disorders and coinciding conditions while treating hypothermia. These situations may include drug overdose, alcohol use, and associated trauma.

What to consider

- Administering vasopressors may improve the chance of return of spontaneous circulation, especially if rewarming techniques are also being used. It's reasonable to give vasopressors during cardiac arrest following ACLS guidelines.
- With severe hypothermia, bradycardia may be physiologic, and the heart may not respond to artificial pacing. Pacing isn't indicated unless bradycardia persists after rewarming. Continue to monitor and support the patient.

Toxicologic emergencies

Although exposure to poisons is common, poisoning rarely causes cardiac arrest. However, a toxicologic emergency may result from an overdose of a drug, such as an opioid, and may result in respiratory depression or arrest, with a subsequent cardiac arrest. If you suspect poisoning is the cause of the patient's cardiac arrest, base your treatment on the specific poison or drug involved. In order to provide faster and more appropriate treatment, obtain a careful history from available friends or family members.

Remember that a toxicologic emergency can occur from ingestion of many things. Substances that may cause a toxicologic emergency include the following:

- illicit drugs, such as opioids
- household cleaners
- rodent repellents
- alcohol
- plants
- dangerous gas or fumes

What causes it

A toxicologic emergency can be accidental or intentional. In all cases, it's important to know the drug or substance involved, the approximate amount ingested, and the time that's elapsed since ingestion or exposure. For example, if an ingestion error of opioids occurs, respiratory depression and arrest may occur before cardiac arrest. Also, certain gases, such as carbon monoxide, may cause a toxicologic emergency and resuscitation may be necessary.

What to look for

The symptoms of poisoning vary with the substance that the patient has ingested. (See *Substances that can cause toxicity*.) General symptoms include the following:

Substances that can cause toxicity

Overuse or overdose of a variety of substances can cause life-threatening toxicity. Signs and symptoms of toxicity vary according to the substance ingested.

Substances that cause hypoventilation

- Anesthetics
- Carbon monoxide
- Clonidine
- Cyanide
- Ethanol
- Opioids
- Sedative-hypnotics

Substances that cause bradycardia

- Beta-adrenergic blockers
- Calcium channel blockers
- Clonidine
- Digoxin (Lanoxin)
- Mushrooms
- Opioids
- Organophosphates
- Sedative-hypnotics

Substances that cause tachycardia

- Amphetamines
- Anticholinergic agents
- Antihistamines
- Atropine
- Caffeine
- Cocaine
- Cyanide
- Ethanol
- Nicotine
- Salicylates
- Sympathomimetics
- Theophylline
- Tricyclic antidepressants

- hypoventilation and hypoxia
- bradycardia
- tachycardia
- altered LOC
- hypotension or hypertension
- hypothermia or hyperthermia
- tachypnea

- breath odor
- nystagmus
- miosis
- mydriasis

How it's treated

Keep in mind that standard protocols for toxicologic emergencies may not always result in optimal outcomes. An accurate scene survey may provide valuable information as to the cause of the emergency. ACLS interventions should always be provided if needed.

Circulation

Palpate for a pulse. If unable to palpate a pulse in no more than 10 seconds, initiate high-quality chest compressions. Remember, toxicologic ingestion may cause PEA. Consider specific therapies to reverse the effects of the drug or toxin ingested in order to reverse PEA. (See *Combating drug toxicity*.) Remember that some agents have antidotes. The quicker an antidote is administered, the greater the chance of successful resuscitation.

Resources that may assist with specific antidotal information include the following:

- local poison control center
- poison index
- pharmacist

When treating a patient who has ingested a potentially lethal amount of drug or toxin presenting within 1 hour of ingestion, administer activated charcoal. If a comatose patient requires charcoal, you must intubate them before beginning the charcoal administration to avoid aspiration. (In addition, try to remove and reverse the toxic agent, if applicable.) If the patient presents with an opioid overdose, follow the AHA algorithm developed for this toxicologic emergency. (The opioid-associated emergency for lay responders algorithm can be viewed at https://cpr.heart.org/en/resuscitation-science/cpr-and-ecc-guidelines/algorithms.)

Airway

Assess the patient's airway for patency. If the patient has an altered LOC, there's an increased risk of airway occlusion caused by the tongue. If the patient has vomited, attempt to clear the airway if possible.

Breathing

Assess adequacy of breathing because the poisoned patient's status can deteriorate quickly, depending on the type and amount of drug ingested. This is especially necessary in the case of opioid overdose. If the patient is not breathing adequately, assist with ventilations using a bag valve mask device. If needed, insert an advanced airway.

Defibrillation

Perform defibrillation if the patient with a toxicologic emergency deteriorates to VF or pulseless VT, following ACLS guidelines.

Torsades de pointes

Torsades de pointes can occur with exposure to many drugs. Treatment includes correcting contributing factors, such as hypoxemia and electrolyte abnormalities (especially magnesium imbalance).

Electrical overdrive pacing (100 to 120 beats/minute) or pharmacologic overdrive pacing with isoproterenol (Isuprel) may also be effective when treating torsades de pointes as a result of drug overdose or poisoning.

Differential diagnosis

After ensuring adequate circulation and ventilation, determine further treatment based on the cause of the toxicologic emergency. Consider specific therapies based on the cardiopulmonary effect of the causative agent, such as hemodialysis.

What to consider

- Consult a medical toxicologist or certified regional poison information center for unusual poisoning cases. Receiving specific information quickly will help you treat the patient as effectively and efficiently as possible.
- Activated charcoal administration is recommended for patients who present within 1 hour of ingestion.
- Prolonged resuscitation attempts are warranted in poisoned patients. (If attempts are unsuccessful, organ donation may still be an option.)
- Avoid high-dose epinephrine in cases of sympathomimetic poisoning.
- Evaluation of the patient's liver and kidney function may be warranted as insufficient function of these organs may contribute to inability to clear the toxin.
- The usual criteria for brain death aren't valid during acute toxic encephalopathy and can be used only after drug levels are no longer toxic.

Near-fatal asthma

Severe exacerbation of asthma, with signs and symptoms developing in less than 2½ hours, can lead to sudden death. Commonly, death occurs due to asphyxia from severe bronchospasm and mucus plugging.

The patient's outcome may be affected by:

- whether they have true active asthma or another severe condition
- preexisting conditions, such as cardiac disease, pulmonary disease, acute allergic bronchospasm or anaphylaxis, and pulmonary embolism or vasculitis (Churg-Strauss syndrome)
- medications or illicit drug use (Beta-adrenergic blockers, cocaine, and opioids can cause bronchospasm.)
- discontinuation of long-term corticosteroid therapy, which may result in adrenal insufficiency and other problems.

What causes it

Cardiac arrest can result from hypoxia-induced cardiac arrhythmias and tension pneumothorax. Positive pressure generated in the patient's lungs as a result of air trapping can also induce cardiac arrest.

What to look for

An asthma attack may begin dramatically, with the simultaneous onset of many symptoms, or insidiously, with gradually increasing shortness of breath. An asthma attack typically includes progressively

Combating drug toxicity

Drug classes produce varying signs of toxicity that require different treatment measures. This table shows the signs of toxicity for various drug classes and their treatment options.

Drug class	Signs of toxicity	Treatment options
Beta-adrenergic blockers		
atenolol (Tenormin) carvedilol (Coreg) metoprolol (Lopressor) propranolol (Inderal)	• Bradycardia • Impaired cardiac conduction • Hypotension, shock • Cardiac arrest	• Administer glucagon, high-dose insulin, or calcium IV. • Apply an external pacemaker, insert a temporary pacemaker, or use intra-aortic balloon pump counterpulsation, ventricular assist device, extracorporeal membrane oxygenation. • Administer vasopressors. • Perform CPR.
Calcium channel blockers		
amlodipine (Norvasc) diltiazem (Cardizem) nifedipine (Procardia) verapamil (Calan)	• Bradycardia • Impaired cardiac conduction • Shock • Cardiac arrest	• Administer atropine or dopamine or epinephrine drip. • Infuse calcium IV. • Apply an external pacemaker or insert a temporary pacemaker. • Perform CPR.

(continued)

Combating drug toxicity *(continued)*

Drug class	Signs of toxicity	Treatment options
Cardiac glycosides digoxin (Lanoxin) foxglove oleander	• Bradycardia, atrioventricular (AV) block • Ventricular arrhythmias • Hyperkalemia, hypomagnesemia • Shock • Cardiac arrest	• Administer ovine digoxin immune Fab (Digibind). • Infuse magnesium IV for hypomagnesemia. • Apply an external pacemaker or insert a temporary pacemaker. • Administer glucose and insulin for life-threatening hyperkalemia. • Perform CPR.
Cholinergics carbamates organophosphates nerve agents	• Bradycardia • Impaired cardiac conduction • Shock • Supraventricular and ventricular arrhythmias • Cardiac arrest	• Administer atropine or dopamine or epinephrine drip. • Administer pralidoxime (Protopam). • Perform CPR.
Opioids heroin hydromorphone (Dilaudid) fentanyl (Sublimaze) methadone (Dolophine) oxycodone (OxyContin)	• Bradycardia • Hypotension • Slow, shallow respirations, hypoxia • Cardiac arrest	• Administer naloxone. • Insert an advanced airway and provide oxygen and ventilations. • Administer vasopressors. • Perform CPR.
Sympathomimetics amphetamines cocaine methamphetamine	• Chest pain • Tachycardia • Hypertensive crisis • Impaired cardiac conduction • Shock • Supraventricular and ventricular arrhythmias • Cardiac arrest	• Administer an alpha-adrenergic blocker. • Administer benzodiazepines. • Administer sodium bicarbonate. • Perform CPR.
Tricyclic antidepressants amitriptyline desipramine (Norpramin) nortriptyline	• Bradycardia • Impaired cardiac conduction, AV block • Shock • Tachycardia • Ventricular arrhythmias, torsades de pointes • Cardiac arrest	• Consider sodium bicarbonate. • Administer a mixed alpha-beta agonist or an alpha agonist. • Administer vasopressors. • Administer lidocaine. (Procainamide is contraindicated.) • Perform CPR.

worsening shortness of breath, cough, wheezing, and chest tightness or some combination of these signs or symptoms. Cyanosis, confusion, and lethargy indicate the onset of respiratory failure.

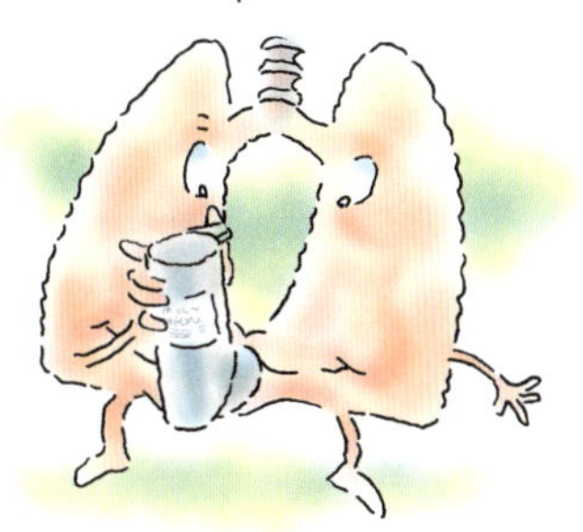

How it's treated

Aggressively treat the severe asthmatic crisis before it deteriorates to full cardiac or respiratory arrest. Administer oxygen to all patients and arrange to transport the patient to a health care facility as soon as possible. Support ventilations with a bag valve mask device as needed or insert an advanced airway if indicated.

Medicate and evaluate

Medications for the treatment of acute asthma include the following:

- beta-agonists such as nebulized albuterol (Proventil)—Give 2.5 to 5 mg every 15 to 20 minutes intermittently or give continuous nebulization of 10 to 15 mg/hour.
- epinephrine (if the patient doesn't respond to albuterol or if the situation is life threatening)—Give 0.01 mg/kg of a 1:1,000 solution divided into three doses subcutaneously at 20-minute intervals.
- corticosteroids—Give initial dose of methylprednisolone (Medrol) 125 mg IV after administering oxygen and initiating beta-agonist therapies.
- nebulized anticholinergics such as ipratropium (Atrovent)—Because these drugs have an onset of 20 minutes, give 0.5 mg in combination with albuterol, which acts immediately.

In addition, magnesium sulfate can improve respiratory function when used in combination with nebulized albuterol and methylprednisolone. For severe refractory asthma in adults, give magnesium sulfate 2 g IV over 20 minutes.

Airway

Because asthma affects airway patency, focus on maintaining a patent airway. The patient with asthma may have difficulty maintaining an adequate airway secondary to bronchospasm and mucus plugging. Oral suctioning may be necessary to open the airway. If you can't maintain a patent airway, insertion of an advanced airway may be necessary.

Breathing

Administer oxygen to achieve a partial pressure of arterial oxygen greater than or equal to 92 mm Hg. Keep in mind that an elevated partial pressure of arterial carbon dioxide doesn't indicate the severity of the asthmatic episode. Always treat the patient according to their clinical symptoms.

It's all positive

Bilevel positive pressure airway pressure can help reduce the work of breathing and help prevent the need for intubation. Studies (Kang, et al., 2020) showed marked improvement in oxygenation, work of breathing, and a decrease in carbon dioxide levels with the initiation of bilevel positive airway pressure. You may also give Heliox (a mixture of 70% helium and 30% oxygen) to delay intubation while other medications are taking effect. Heliox decreases the work of breathing by decreasing the resistance of airflow to the bronchial branches by 28% to 48%.

To intubate or not to intubate

In an asthmatic crisis, intubate the patient, using rapid-sequence intubation, if you note:

- a decline in LOC
- profuse diaphoresis
- poor muscle tone (a clinical sign of hypercarbia)
- severe agitation, confusion, and fighting against the oxygen mask (clinical signs of hypoxemia).

Circulation

Hypoxia resulting from a severe asthma attack may result in cardiac arrhythmias and cardiac arrest. Assess the patient experiencing an asthma attack for adequate perfusion and circulation. Monitor the patient's cardiac rhythm and vital signs. If necessary, initiate CPR, following ACLS guidelines.

Defibrillation

Perform defibrillation if pulseless VT or VF occurs, following ACLS guidelines. These arrhythmias may result from a hypoxic state.

Differential diagnosis

Attempt to identify the trigger for an acute asthma attack. Possible asthma triggers include the following:

- infection
- exercise
- cold weather
- tobacco smoke
- air pollution
- allergens
- chemical odors.

What to consider

- Attempt to identify asthma triggers so that the patient can avoid these triggers, if possible.

- Treating an asthma attack early can help avoid progressive respiratory distress that may compromise the patient's airway and ventilation.
- An asthma action plan should be developed for patients that directs them when to use asthma medications and when to seek medical treatment.

Anaphylaxis

Anaphylaxis is a hypersensitivity reaction triggered by allergens, such as food, medications, insect venom, or latex. Anaphylaxis is life threatening because it causes rapid airway constriction. The time it takes for treatment to be initiated is extremely important to ensure a positive patient outcome. Initial exposure to the allergen may not cause a reaction. Typically, it's the reexposure to an antigen that causes the reaction.

What causes it

The most common causes of anaphylaxis are the following:

- insect venom (especially bees, wasps, yellow jackets, and fire ants)
- drugs (such as antibiotics and aspirin)
- contrast media that contain iodine
- foods (such as peanuts, shellfish, eggs, or dairy products)
- latex, which is contained in a large amount of medical supplies.

What to look for

The sooner a reaction occurs after exposure to an antigen, the more likely it is to be severe. Signs and symptoms of anaphylaxis include the following:

- agitation, feeling faint
- hypotension, tachycardia
- bronchospasm, upper and lower airway edema
- cardiovascular collapse due to vasodilation and increased capillary permeability
- urticaria, rhinitis, pruritus
- abdominal pain, vomiting, and diarrhea
- sense of impending doom.

How it's treated

Depending on the reaction, the patient with anaphylaxis may exhibit various signs and symptoms, which can vary in intensity and severity over time. In the case of an insect sting, scrape away any insect parts at the site of a sting (don't squeeze a venom sac that's intact). Then apply ice to the area to slow absorption. Arrange to transport the patient to a health care facility as soon as possible.

A special kind of pen

You may give epinephrine to treat shock, airway swelling, or difficulty breathing. If the patient is aware of their allergy, he may carry an EpiPen that should be administered as quickly as possible. If there isn't an EpiPen available, administer 0.2 to 0.5 mg (1:1,000) of epinephrine IM and repeat after 5 to 15 minutes if you don't note improvement in the patient's condition. You should also administer epinephrine (1:10,000) 0.05 to 0.1 mg IV over 5 minutes in profound, immediately life-threatening situations. A continuous IV infusion at 5 to 15 mcg/minute may be necessary.

Medication advantage

In addition, you may consider giving the following medications to treat an anaphylactic reaction:

- antihistamines such as diphenhydramine (Benadryl)—Give 10 to 50 mg slowly IV or IM
- inhaled albuterol (Proventil) (if bronchospasm is significant)—If the patient is hypotensive, give epinephrine before inhaled albuterol to prevent a further drop in blood pressure.
- corticosteroids—Give high dose slowly IV or IM. For a severe attack, the effect will not be evident for 4 to 6 hours.
- inhaled ipratropium (Atrovent)—helpful for patients taking beta-adrenergic blockers.

For patients experiencing anaphylaxis, focus initially on obtaining and maintaining a patent airway.

Airway

A typical anaphylactic reaction includes swelling of the tongue and throat, followed by difficulty breathing. Be sure to monitor airway patency if you suspect an allergic reaction. Early and rapid intubation is critical if hoarseness, lingual edema, and posterior or oropharyngeal swelling occur because the patient is at high risk for respiratory compromise. Also, intubate a patient if airway swelling is present, and he doesn't rapidly respond to pharmacologic interventions. Use caution when giving paralytic agents to ease intubation because these drugs deprive the patient of the ability to attempt spontaneous breathing. Manually ventilate the patient with a bag-valve-mask device until spontaneous breathing returns.

Breathing

Deliver 100% oxygen with ventilations, as appropriate. Ventilatory support is essential to maintain oxygen delivery until the effects of anaphylaxis have resolved. Monitor pulse oximetry to make sure that adequate perfusion is occurring.

Deterioration descriptors

Deterioration of the patient is evident with:

- stridor
- severe dysphonia or aphonia

- laryngeal edema
- massive lingual swelling
- face and neck swelling
- signs of hypoxemia (cyanosis, decreased pulse oximetry readings, and abnormal arterial blood gas results).

These symptoms can occur anywhere from 3 minutes to 3 hours after exposure to an allergen.

Consider the alternative

Alternative methods of oxygenation and ventilation include the following:

- fiberoptic tracheal intubation
- digital tracheal intervention (using the rescuer's fingers and a smaller [less than 7-mm diameter] ET tube)
- needle cricothyrotomy followed by transtracheal ventilation
- cricothyrotomy for the patient with massive neck swelling.

Use caution when attempting tracheal intubation or cricothyrotomy because these measures can result in increased laryngeal edema, bleeding, and further narrowing of the glottic opening.

Circulation

If the patient is unresponsive, be sure to check for a pulse. If there is no pulse, initiate CPR and follow the ACLS guidelines for cardiac arrest.

Administer 2 to 4 L of an isotonic crystalloid solution, such as normal saline solution, and high-dose epinephrine to rapidly expand vasculature. Continue to administer isotonic crystalloid IV solutions for hypotension that does not respond promptly to epinephrine. Rapidly infuse IV solutions from 1 to 2 L up to 4 L to maintain circulatory support.

Defibrillation

The patient experiencing anaphylaxis may deteriorate to hypoxia, resulting in myocardial ischemia and arrhythmias. Follow the cardiac arrest algorithm and defibrillate if VF or pulseless VT occurs.

Differential diagnosis

While treating the patient, you should identify and investigate the underlying cause of anaphylaxis. Be sure to check the patient for medical alert information, usually in the form of a bracelet or necklace, that may identify allergy information. If no allergen is identified after investigating patient exposures, the cause may be idiopathic.

What to consider

- Observe the patient for up to 24 hours because signs and symptoms of anaphylaxis may recur in 1 to 8 hours despite effective initial treatment.

- If the practitioner orders an anaphylaxis kit for the patient on discharge, teach the patient and family on how to use it in an emergency situation.
- Recommend that the patient obtain and wear a medical alert bracelet that identifies the allergy.

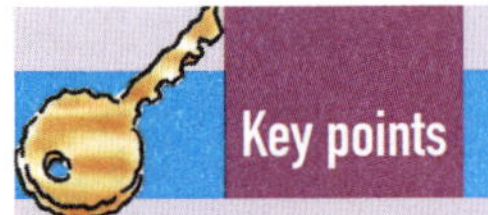

Key points

Critical situations

- Prepare to act quickly in critical situations to prevent respiratory or cardiac arrest.
- Follow standard basic life support and advanced cardiac life support guidelines if indicated.
- Prepare for early intubation in the following critical situations:
  - Anaphylaxis
  - Pregnancy with cardiac arrest
  - Toxicologic emergencies affecting breathing ability
  - Trauma patient in cardiac arrest
  - Hypothermia with minimal or absent respirations

Quick quiz

1. A patient is suspected to be experiencing an opioid overdose. The patient's respiratory rate is approximately 4 breaths per minute, and heart rate is 50 beats per minute. The most effective intervention to reverse this toxicologic situation is:

   A. Initiate high-quality chest compressions.
   B. Administer 0.4 mg of naloxone as soon as it is available.
   C. Perform defibrillation.
   D. Monitor waveform capnography to detect further deterioration.

Answer: B. Naloxone is the antidote or reversal agent effective for opioid overdose. If the patient has a palpable pulse and depressed respirations, administer as soon as available and repeat after 4 minutes if still needed. If there is not pulse or adequate breathing, initiate CPR.

2. A patient in their third trimester of pregnancy experiences a cardiac arrest. This situation requires:

   A. displacement of the uterus to the left when in a supine position.
   B. placing the patient on their right side.
   C. raising the patient's head 30 to 45 degrees.
   D. keeping the patient in a supine position during chest compressions.

Answer: A. A large uterus presses on vital blood vessels and needs displacement to the left when a pregnant patient is in the supine position. They may also be slightly tilted to the left side to assist with this measure.

3. When treating a patient for submersion or drowning after a diving accident:

   A. clear the patient's airway of water before initiating rescue breathing.
   B. initiate chest compressions while the patient is still in the water.
   C. suspect that a spinal cord injury may have occurred.
   D. administer abdominal thrusts.

Answer: C. Consider the submersion or drowning patient to have a head or neck injury, especially after a diving accident, unless proven otherwise. Use the jaw-thrust maneuver to open the patient's airway instead of the head-tilt, chin-lift maneuver, and apply a hard cervical collar as soon as possible.

4. Primary respiratory arrest after electric shock can occur from:
   A. paralysis of respiratory muscles during shock.
   B. pneumothorax from injury.
   C. contraction of respiratory muscles.
   D. cardiac arrhythmias.

Answer: C. Tetanic contraction of respiratory muscles may occur during the passage of the electric current and can result in respiratory arrest.

5. After receiving the second dose of an antibiotic, a patient develops hoarseness and lingual edema. Immediate actions should include:
   A. defibrillation.
   B. administration of epinephrine.
   C. secure a patent airway.
   D. administration of high-dose corticosteroids.

Answer: C. The patient who develops hoarseness and lingual edema after receiving a medication, especially antibiotics, may be experiencing an anaphylactic reaction. Your priority in this situation is to open and protect the airway, as well as provide oxygenation and ventilation. Administering epinephrine as quickly as possible helps reverse the shock and assist with opening the airway.

Scoring

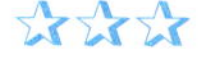 If you answered all five questions correctly, way to go! Your knowledge of ACLS is special.

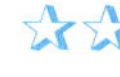 If you answered four questions correctly, great effort! Your understanding of what to do in an emergency is emerging.

 If you answered fewer than four questions correctly, try again! A quick review will make you a "specialist" in no time.

Suggested references

American Heart Association (2020). *Advanced cardiovascular life support provider manual*, E-book edition.

Brown, D. J. A., Brugger, H. (2013). *Accidental hypothermia: Nejm*. New England Journal of Medicine. Retrieved September 21, 2022, from https://www.nejm.org/doi/full/10.1056/nejmra1114208

Centers for Disease Control and Prevention, C. D. C. (2018). Cold stress – cold water immersion. Centers for Disease Control and Prevention. Retrieved September 21, 2022, from https://www.cdc.gov/niosh/topics/coldstress/coldwaterimmersion.html#:~:text=It%20develops%20much%20more%20quickly,temperature%20below%2070%C2%B0F.

Kang, C. M., Wu, E. T., Wang, C. C., Lu, F., Chiang, B. L., Yen, T. A. (2020). Bilevel positive airway pressure ventilation efficiently improves respiratory distress in initial hours treating children with severe asthma exacerbation. *Journal of the Formosan Medical Association, 119(9)*, 1415–1421. https://doi.org/10.1016/j.jfma.2019.11.013

Chapter 10

Megacode review

Just the facts

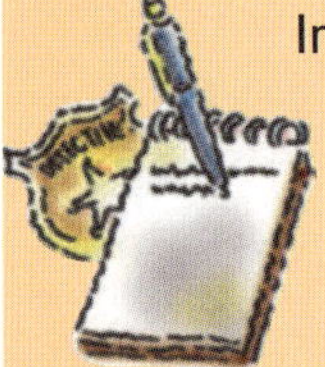

In this chapter, you'll learn:

- the role of the team leader and team members during the Megacode
- the expected ACLS actions, such as airway management, cardiopulmonary resuscitation, and emergency medication administration
- appropriate communication during emergency situations

A look at the megacode

The Megacode station in an advanced cardiovascular life support (ACLS) class or skills session provides an opportunity for team members to rehearse and organize their roles when involved in a real code situation. As a team leader, it's your responsibility to direct and monitor the activities of other team members and delegate actions based on your assessment of the situation. A case study approach is used to present a practice session of what may occur during a code. Each student takes a turn at various roles, based on the number of students in a given session. Types of roles include:

- team leader
- team member responsible for airway management
- team member responsible for cardiopulmonary resuscitation (CPR)
- team member responsible for IV access and drug administration
- team member responsible for use of the defibrillator
- team member responsible for time keeping and documentation

Team leader role

During the Megacode, the team leader serves as the director and coordinator of care activities and assigns responsibilities to the other team members accordingly.

The team leader assesses and oversees the effective delivery of chest compressions, ventilations, and defibrillation. Other components of the team leader role include monitoring the situation for:

- the quality of CPR being performed and appropriate change in compressors
- type of emergent situation and possible causes
- appropriateness and effectiveness of interventions
- changes in cardiac rhythm and patient status.

Additionally, the team leader:

- investigates the existence of advance directives
- incorporates family needs and concerns during and after the resuscitation process
- ensures adequate resources are available
- identifies fatigued team members and ensures relief
- promotes effective communication among team members
- decides when to stop resuscitation
- provides opportunity for a debriefing of the resuscitation event with all team members present

There's no "I" in team

Remember, the team leader needs to be open to suggestions from other team members because many different activities occur simultaneously during a Megacode. Roles that are typically assigned during a code situation include responsibilities of:

- providing high-quality compressions
- airway management and adequate ventilation
- insertion of IV access
- administration of medications
- documentation of events, interventions, and responders
- timekeeper

However, ACLS responders work together as a team. For example, the team member administering drugs may notice that 3 minutes have passed since the last dose of epinephrine was given or the team member who intubated the patient may realize that breath sounds haven't been checked. Team members who respond to code situations frequently, quickly, and smoothly work through algorithms and need infrequent prompting from the team leader to perform appropriately to achieve a positive outcome.

Algorithms

Within the Megacode, algorithms help serve as a guide to patient treatment, pointing the team in a unified direction. However, don't use an algorithm as a replacement for your team's assessment skills. Remember that new research findings may alter the current recommendations, so team members must keep up-to-date and be aware of evidence-based practice.

Megacode testing

At the Megacode testing station, the ACLS instructor will give you a brief patient scenario. This station typically includes equipment that the situation demands. Before testing day, you may be given the opportunity to practice with the equipment.

Instructors typically try to set up scenarios that apply to the student's work situation. For example, if the student is a critical care nurse, the patient situation may take place in an intensive care setting. If the student is employed in a freestanding surgical center, the situation may occur there. However, this isn't always the case. A nurse may be given a scenario that takes place in a patient's home, or an emergency medical services (EMS) provider may be given a scenario that takes place in the hospital. Don't get thrown off; the treatment remains the same.

Raise your hand

When presented with the patient situation, you may find that you need additional information to direct an intervention or make a sound decision. Don't be afraid to ask for that information. If you ordered an arterial blood gas analysis, you can ask if the results have arrived. This information is helpful if you need to make adjustments in oxygenation.

In turn, the instructor may ask you for information that's appropriate to the situation. For example, she may ask you if an alternative medication could be given or remind you that an IV line hasn't been started (or that the team is trying to insert a line). The instructor won't try to trick you, but needs to determine if you're thinking along the correct route or simply guessing. A seasoned instructor can differentiate between an unprepared student and a nervous one and will provide guidance to redirect you back to the algorithm.

Line up!

It may be helpful to review the equipment that is set out as you will need to use some of it for your scenario. Think of the equipment as "props," and if you are unsure of your next intervention, look over the equipment to see if it will trigger your memory. You may also use the equipment to remind yourself about what has occurred during the testing scenario. For example, you might place epinephrine nearer to the patient's IV site as a reminder that one dose has been given.

Manikins

High-fidelity patient simulators are becoming more common in ACLS training. These manikins may have automatic chest rise and fall, palpable pulses, blinking eyes, and many other realistic features that reduce the need for the instructor to provide cues to the student. You will have to respond to the signs and symptoms that the manikin displays. Training programs utilizing high-fidelity manikins may also require you to inject medications and insert an advanced airway. Some manikins are even able to provide feedback to the instructor about your performance, including rate and depth of chest compressions, adequacy of ventilations, and amount of medication injected.

Let's pretend! Sample megacode scenarios

Here are three scenarios to help you prepare for the Megacode section of the ACLS examination. Although a real-life situation may have everyone working simultaneously, for testing purposes, the team leader will need to direct all team members' actions so the instructor can evaluate that person's knowledge of an ACLS situation. Also, the ACLS instructor will typically test the student on more than one algorithm, although these scenarios may only cover one.

Scenario #1

Instructor: A patient arrives in your emergency department (ED) complaining of palpitations and mild dizziness. The patient is visibly anxious and crying. What are your initial actions?

team Leader: I would assess the patient's circulation, airway, and adequacy of breathing. I would direct a team member (if available) to attach the patient to a cardiac monitor and assess the blood pressure, pulse, respirations, and pulse oximetry. I would also assess for orientation.

Instructor: The assessment indicates that the patient is conscious and oriented. the patient has a palpable pulse and her airway is patent, with adequate breathing pattern.

Team Leader: What are the patient's vital signs?

Instructor: The patient has vital signs as follows: blood pressure, 98/50 mm Hg; heart rate, 210 beats/minute; and respiratory rate, 24 breaths/minute with an oxygen saturation of 90%. The patient is placed on the cardiac monitor, which shows the following rhythm:

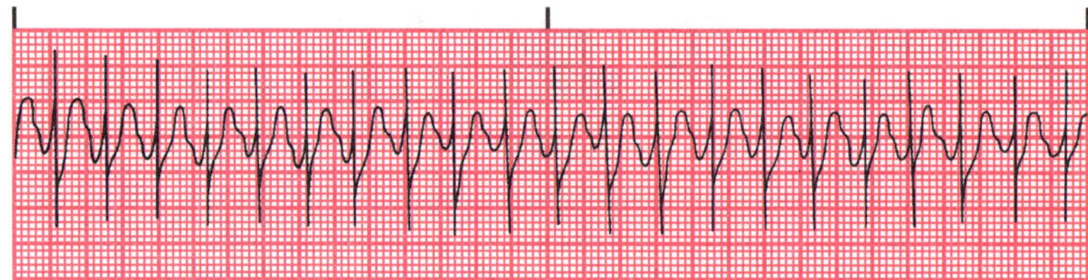

Team leader: The rhythm on the monitor appears to be supraventricular tachycardia (SVT). I would direct a team member to administer oxygen at 4 L/minute via nasal cannula, direct another team member to start an IV, and direct yet another team member to perform a 12-lead electrocardiogram (ECG). I would also ask the patient if they were experiencing any chest pain or shortness of breath.

Instructor: OK. Oxygen is now being administered by nasal cannula at 4 L/minute. An IV line has been started, and a 12-lead electrocardiogram (ECG) is obtained. What is your next intervention?

Team leader: I would ask the patient to perform a vagal maneuver by asking them to bear down or cough.

Instructor: The patient does as you ask, but there is no change in rhythm.

Team leader: I would direct a team member to administer adenosine 6 mg IV push as quickly as possible because of the short half-life of the drug, followed by a 20-mL saline flush.

Instructor: The medication is given, but there is no change in rhythm.

Team Leader: I would then direct giving adenosine 12 mg as quickly as possible followed by a 20-mL saline flush.

Instructor: After the second dose of medication there, is still no change in rhythm. The patient is now complaining of chest pain and is diaphoretic. They are now more difficult to arouse.

Team Leader: I would ask a team member to obtain another set of vital signs.

Instructor: The patient's blood pressure is now 70/20 mm Hg, respiratory rate is 20, and pulse oximetry is 92%.

Team leader: With a systolic blood pressure below 90, she is now considered "unstable." I would direct a team member to place defibrillator pads on the patient's chest. Then I would select the synchronize mode on the defibrillator and direct to charge to 100 joules. I would announce "all clear" and "remove oxygen source from patient" and visually confirm that team members are clear of the patient and the oxygen is turned off before stating "Deliver shock."

Cardioversion is indicated because the patient is now unstable. Remember, synchronization is critical to convert a rapid rhythm with a pulse.

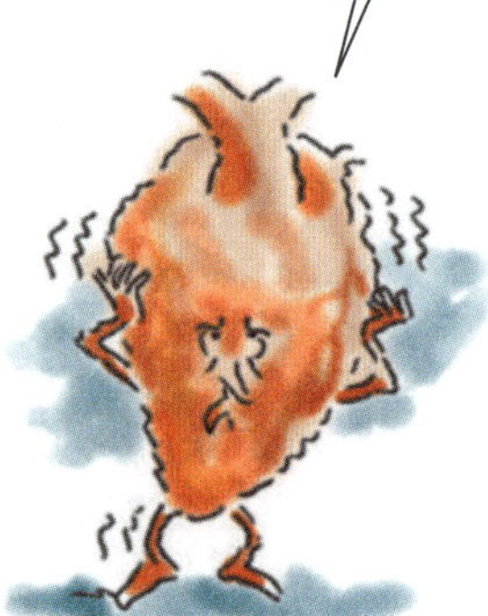

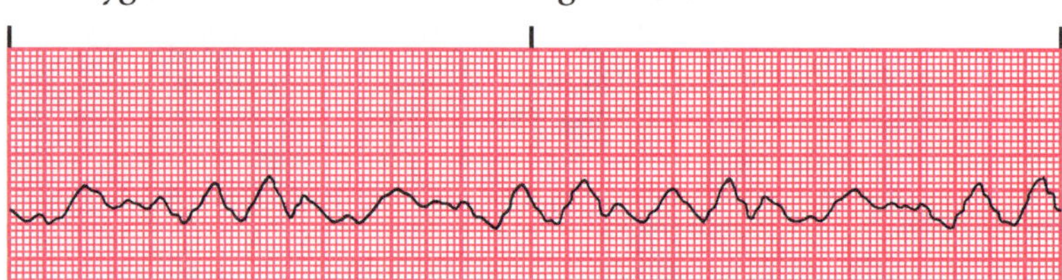

Instructor: The patient converts to this rhythm after cardioversion.

Team leader: The patient now appears to be in ventricular fibrillation. I would assess the patient for a carotid pulse.

Instructor: The patient's carotid pulse is checked and is absent.

Team leader: I would direct one team member to begin chest compressions and another to provide ventilations at a ratio of 30 to 2 and a rate of 100 to 120 compressions per minute. Then, I would then turn off the "synchronize" mode on the defibrillator. Since this is a biphasic defibrillator, I would ask to charge the defibrillator to 200 joules, visually verify and announce "all clear" and "remove oxygen source from patient," and then "deliver shock."

Team leader: After defibrillation I would direct team members to immediately resume CPR and monitor for high-quality compressions, with a depth of 2 to 2.6 cm and full chest recoil between compressions. I would also check for adequate chest rise with the bag valve mask ventilations. I would direct a team member to administer epinephrine 1 mg by IV push, which I can repeat every 3 to 5 minutes. After 2 minutes of CPR, I would recheck the patient's cardiac rhythm.

Instructor: The patient's rhythm is unchanged.

Team leader: I would defibrillate again at 200 joules in the same manner. I would then have the team immediately resume chest compressions, making sure team members switch performing compressions every 2 minutes. I would ask a team member to administer amiodarone 300 mg by rapid IV push followed by a flush of normal saline solution.

Instructor: Amiodarone is administered and epinephrine is administered at 3 minutes.

Team leader: After 2 minutes of CPR, I would check the rhythm on the monitor.

Instructor: The patient has this rhythm on the monitor.

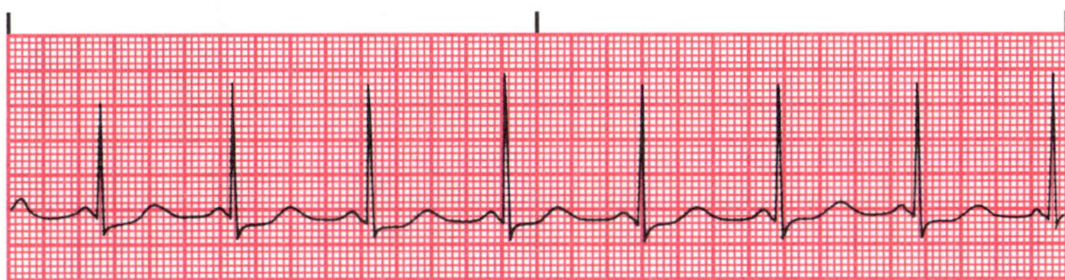

Team leader: The monitor shows what looks like normal sinus rhythm. I would check for a carotid pulse.

Instructor: The patient has a palpable pulse.

Team leader: I would direct a team member to begin a continuous infusion of amiodarone at 1 mg/minute. I would also assess for spontaneous breathing. If the patient is not breathing adequately, I would ask that the patient be intubated. Once the patient is intubated and placement is confirmed by a five-point chest auscultation and waveform capnography, I would order a chest X-ray be done and arterial blood gases after 20 to 30 minutes.

Remember, if the patient's rhythm is successfully converted, an antiarrhythmic may be given by continuous infusion.

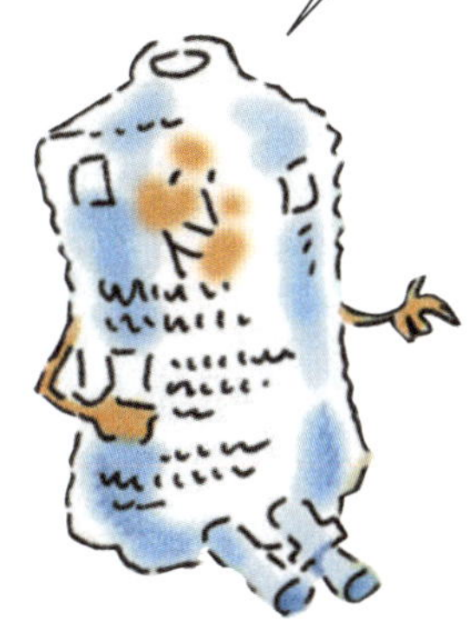

Instructor: What additional actions are appropriate at this time?

Team leader: I would check the patient's vital signs.

Instructor: The patient's blood pressure is 80/50, heart rate is 96, and manual respirations are being delivered at 16 breaths per minute.

Team leader: I would administer a fluid bolus of 1 to 2 L to improve the blood pressure. If that did not help improve the blood pressure, I would administer a vasopressor. Also, at this point I would have a team member draw blood for laboratory analysis and obtain a 12-lead ECG. Is the patient waking up?

Instructor: No, the patient remains unconscious.

Team leader: I would evaluate the patient for therapeutic hypothermia if available and percutaneous coronary intervention if indicated.

Note: This scenario followed the algorithm for adult tachycardia (with pulse), adult cardiac arrest, and post–cardiac arrest care.

Scenario #2

Instructor: A 75-year-old patient is admitted to the intermediate-care unit after a syncopal episode. The patient reports shortness of breath and occasional light-headedness. The patient has vital signs follows: blood pressure, 90/70 mm Hg; heart rate, 38 beats/minute; respiratory rate, 26 breaths/minute; and temperature 98.6°F (37°C). Pulse oximetry is 92%. When the patient is connected to the monitor, it shows this rhythm:

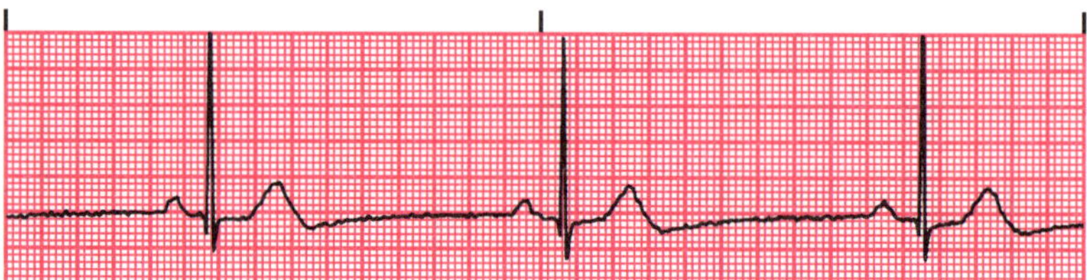

Team leader: The rhythm on the monitor appears to be a sinus bradycardia. I would perform an ABCD assessment.

Instructor: The assessment shows that the patient is alert and oriented and breathing at a rate of 30 breaths per minute. The patient has a palpable pulse.

Team leader: I would direct a team member to administer oxygen via nasal cannula at 4 L/minute. If there's no IV access, I would direct another team member to insert an IV line. If IV access is already present, I would make sure that it's patent. I would also request a 12-lead ECG.

Instructor: Oxygen is on at 4 L/minute and pulse oximetry has increased to 94%. IV access is established and functioning. EKG is complete.

Team leader: Because the patient is complaining of shortness of breath and light-headedness, she would be considered symptomatic.

Order oxygen administration for a patient with cardiac injury or disease to help meet the increased oxygen demands caused by an decreased heart rate.

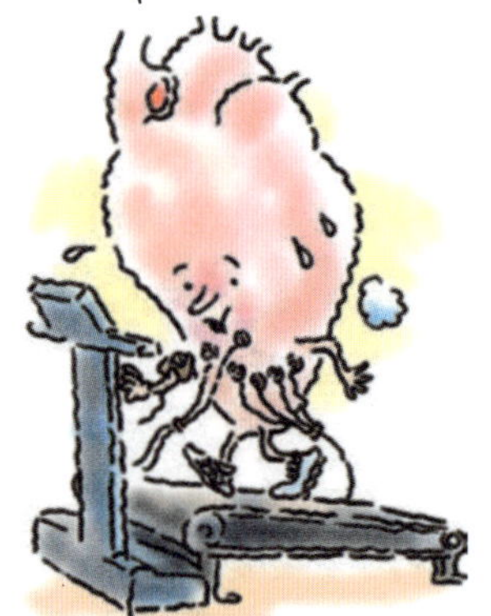

I would direct a team member to administer atropine 0.5 mg IV push, followed by a flush.

Instructor: After administering the medication, the patient's rhythm is unchanged. The heart rate is now 30 beats/minute and the patient now complains of chest pain, along with shortness of breath. Also, the patient is more lethargic than she was previously.

Team leader: I would direct someone to apply the defibrillator pads and ECG cable electrodes for possible transcutaneous pacing. I would also determine if there was a dopamine or epinephrine infusion available, since either pacing or one of these medicated drips is an acceptable treatment option for symptomatic bradycardia.

Instructor: There is a premixed dopamine infusion available. What rate would be appropriate?

Team leader: I would start the infusion at 2 mcg/kg/minute and titrate to a maximum of 20 mcg/kg/minute. If the Epinephrine infusion was available instead, I would start at 2 mcg/minute and titrate to a maximum rate of 20 mcg/minute, based on the patient's response.

Instructor: The infusion is started and is now infusing at 5 mcg/kg/minute. This is what the monitor shows:

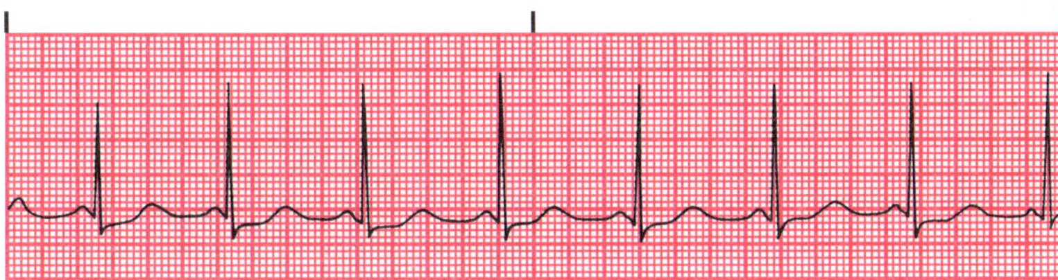

Team leader: The monitor shows normal sinus rhythm. I would make sure that the patient has a palpable pulse and also check the patient's vital signs.

Instructor: The patient's blood pressure is 98/50 mm Hg, and heart rate is 92 beats/minute. The respiratory rate is 20 breaths/minute. Pulse oximetry is 96%. The patient is also more alert.

Team leader: I would consult a cardiologist (expert consultation) and have the team move the patient to the ICU for closer monitoring. Another 12-lead ECG should be obtained.

Note: This scenario followed the algorithm for bradycardia.

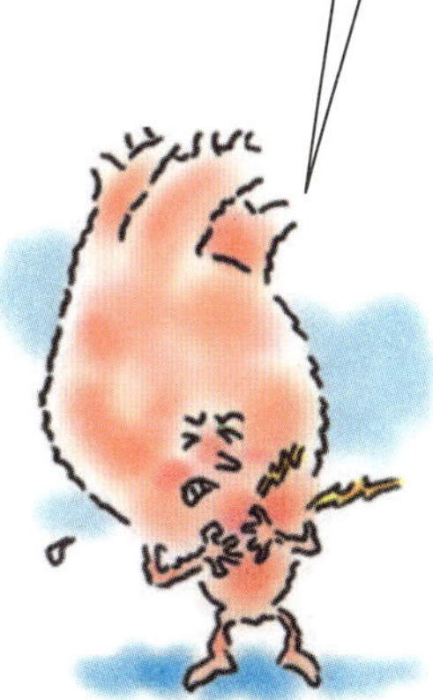

Scenario #3

Instructor: A 66-year-old patient is involved in a motor vehicle crash in which their vehicle hit a telephone pole. The patient complains of pain in the chest and is pale and diaphoretic. A bystander at the scene calls 911. Paramedics arrive, and find the patient conscious with a patent airway. A cervical collar is applied. Oxygen is delivered at 4 L/minute by nasal cannula.

IV access is obtained and a 12-lead ECG is performed. The patient is transported to the ED. He arrives in your ED and is attached to a monitor. The patient has normal saline solution infusing IV, and oxygen is being administered at 4 L/minute. The paramedics report that the patient's chest pain started after the accident occurred and that the patient hit the steering wheel with enough force to bend it. The patient's vital signs are blood pressure, 126/82 mm Hg; heart rate, 84 beats/minute; and respiratory rate, 22 breaths/minute. The patient rates the chest pain as 5 on a scale of 0 to 10, with 0 being no pain and 10 being the worst pain imaginable. A 12-lead ECG is repeated.

The monitor strip shows the following rhythm:

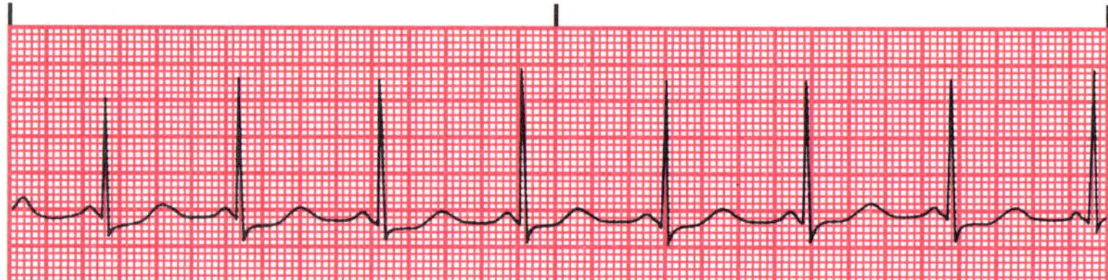

INSTRUCTOR: The patient's 12-lead ECG shows no ST-segment elevation. Please describe your next actions as team leader.

TEAM LEADER: I would quickly assess the patient for injury related to the accident as well as obtain a quick medical history.

INSTRUCTOR: The patient's medical history is unremarkable, and the patient only takes occasional medication for headache or muscle aches. Suddenly, the patient complains of difficulty breathing and then loses consciousness.

TEAM LEADER: I would direct a team member to assess for a pulse and breathing. I would also check the cardiac rhythm displayed on the monitor.

INSTRUCTOR: The patient isn't breathing and has no palpable pulse. The monitor continues to show normal sinus rhythm.

TEAM LEADER: The monitor shows a rhythm with no associated pulse, which indicates that the patient is in pulseless electrical activity (PEA). I would direct team members to immediately begin CPR, pushing hard and fast at a rate of 100 to 120 compressions per minute and a ratio of 30 compressions to 2 ventilations. This would continue for five cycles (2 minutes), at which time I would direct a change of compressors and reassess the patient's status. I would continually monitor for high-quality compressions, full chest recoil between compressions, and adequate chest rise with manual ventilations. I would order epinephrine 1 mg. IV be given. Then, I would assess for a reversible cause of PEA using the "Hs" and "Ts."

Instructor: What possible causes could you relate to this patient's situation? I need you to describe at least three.

Team leader: "Hypoxia" is a possible cause, as the patient suffered chest trauma. I would direct intubation of the patient with either an endotracheal tube or supraglottic airway in order to ensure optimal oxygenation and ventilation. I would check proper placement using a five-point auscultation, capnometer reading, and waveform capnography.

Instructor: Intubation is complete, and tube placement is confirmed. The patient is receiving 100% oxygen with assisted ventilation. The tube is secured. Pulse oximetry is 94%.

Team leader: I would call for a switch of compressors and check for a pulse and any change in cardiac rhythm.

Instructor: The patient has no palpable pulse. The monitor now shows this rhythm:

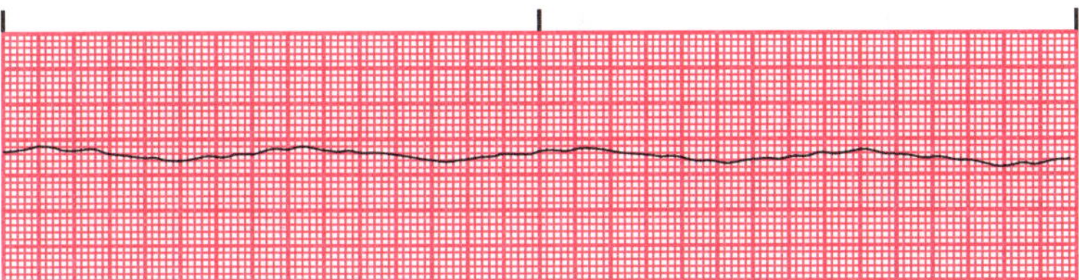

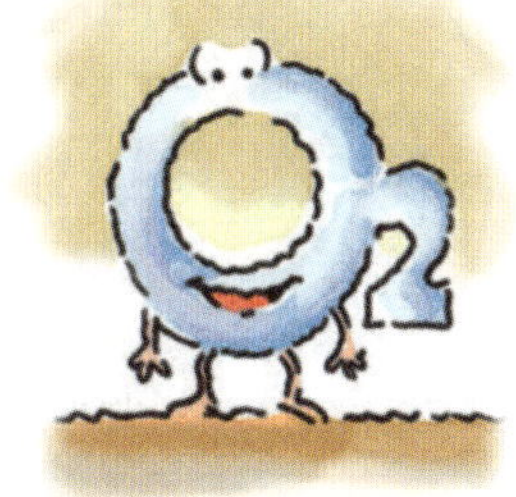

Team leader: The rhythm looks like asystole. I would confirm it in a different lead. I would direct team members to continue CPR. Then I direct a team member to administer epinephrine 1 mg at the 3-minute mark. I would continue my assessment of possible causes. Since this patient was involved in a motor vehicle crash, there may be internal bleeding occurring and the patient may be hypovolemic. I would direct team members to administer a 500-mL IV bolus of normal saline solution. Additionally, I would have someone assess for bilateral breath sounds and equal chest rise to rule out a tension pneumothorax.

Instructor: The IV bolus is infusing. Chest auscultation reveals that the patient has absent breath sounds and decreased chest expansion on the right side with ventilations.

Team leader: I would then order a needle compression to relieve the tension pneumothorax.

Instructor: Needle decompression is complete with an audible release of air.

Team leader: I would check for a pulse while checking the rhythm on the monitor.

INSTRUCTOR: The patient has a palpable pulse. You check the monitor, and this rhythm appears on the screen:

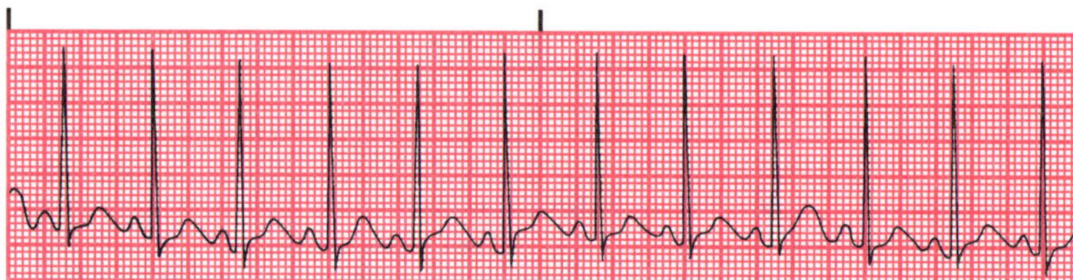

TEAM LEADER: I would ask for a pulse check.

INSTRUCTOR: The patient has a palpable pulse.

TEAM LEADER: Is the patient regaining consciousness?

INSTRUCTOR: The patient remains unconscious.

TEAM LEADER: I would ask a team member for the patient's vital signs (blood pressure, pulse, respirations, and pulse oximetry).

INSTRUCTOR: The patient's blood pressure is 70/20 mm Hg; heart rate, 115 beats/minute; and respiratory rate, 12 breaths/minute with a bag valve mask device. Pulse oximetry is 96%.

TEAM LEADER: I would instruct the team to now administer a fluid bolus of 1 to 2 L, and then I would recheck the blood pressure. If it did not improve, I would direct that a vasopressor be administered. I would also direct insertion of a chest tube, followed by a chest X-ray to confirm endotracheal tube placement and status of the pneumothorax.

INSTRUCTOR: Is there any other action that would be appropriate?

TEAM LEADER: I would check a 12-lead ECG.

INSTRUCTOR: The EKG shows ST elevation in two contiguous leads.

TEAM LEADER: I would direct the team to obtain laboratory specimens to check cardiac enzymes and troponin levels, as well as hemoglobin and hematocrit levels, electrolytes, and a coagulation panel. I would also contact the cardiac cath lab for percutaneous intervention. Is the patient still unconscious?

INSTRUCTOR: The patient remains unconscious.

TEAM LEADER: I would evaluate for therapeutic hypothermia therapy and if the patient meets inclusion criteria, direct that it begin as soon as possible as it is able to be administered in the cardiac cath lab.

INSTRUCTOR: Ok—you are finished! Great job!

Note: This scenario followed the algorithm for asystole/PEA and post–cardiac arrest care.

Quick quiz

1. A patient has a history of rapid atrial fibrillation nonresponsive to medication. The patient is in the cardiac cath lab for an elective cardioversion and suddenly goes into ventricular fibrillation. An important step before performing defibrillation (with a biphasic defibrillator) is:
   A. providing continuous oxygen, even when defibrillating.
   B. setting the defibrillator to 50 joules.
   C. setting the defibrillator on synchronize mode.
   D. making sure the defibrillator is not set on synchronize mode.

Answer: D. To defibrillate, you first need to make sure that the machine is not set to "synchronize," as the synchronize mode requires the patient to have an "R" wave in order to deliver the shock. Since the patient is in V-fib, the defibrillator would not function if it is in the synchronize mode.

2. You are assigned the role of team leader at the ACLS skills testing session. As team leader you are responsible for:
   A. directing the other team members to deliver care following appropriate ACLS algorithms.
   B. administering medications to the patient as needed.
   C. recording team member activities and patient response during resuscitation.
   D. checking all equipment as it's used.

Answer: A. It's the team leader's responsibility to direct and monitor the activities of other team members and delegate actions based on the overall assessment of the patient's response.

3. The code team is providing CPR for a 75-year-old patient who was found in asystole. An endotracheal (ET) tube is inserted. What is the most reliable method for confirming and monitoring ET tube placement?
   A. Continuous cardiac output monitoring
   B. Continuous waveform capnography
   C. Pulse oximetry
   D. Measuring resistance with a bag valve mask device

Answer: B. Continuous waveform capnography is the most reliable method of confirming and monitoring correct placement of ET tubes.

4. A patient was brought to the emergency room by paramedics after they collapsed at the grocery store. The cardiac monitor displayed sinus tachycardia at a rate of 135. Suddenly, the monitor alarms and displays a flat line, and the patient is found to be

unresponsive. Which of the following is the most important action to perform when there's a change in cardiac rhythm on the monitor?

A. Check the oxygen delivery system is in place and the setting is correct.
B. Check for adequate breathing and a palpable carotid pulse.
C. Check the patient's cardiac enzymes and electrolytes.
D. Check the patient's chest X-ray and obtain an arterial blood gas.

Answer: B. When there's a change in cardiac rhythm, check the patient for responsiveness, adequate breathing, and a palpable pulse.

5. An 80-year-old patient was successfully resuscitated following cardiac arrest in the emergency room. What action is an important part of immediate post–cardiac arrest care?

A. Collecting all the patient's belongings to deliver to the family
B. Initiating hemodialysis
C. Evaluating for therapeutic hypothermia therapy
D. Discontinuing IV bolus if infusing

Answer: C. If the patient remains unresponsive after return of spontaneous circulation, therapeutic hypothermia should be considered, if available.

Scoring

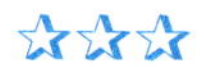 If you answered all five questions correctly, impressive! You have a "mega" command of the Megacode.

 If you answered four questions correctly, not bad! You'll make a fine team leader.

 If you answered fewer than four questions correctly, don't sweat it! After a quick review, you'll be a Megacode megastar in no time.

Suggested references

American Heart Association. (2022). *Highlights of the 2020 American Heart Association guidelines update for CPR and ECC*. Retrieved from https://cpr.heart.org/en/resuscitation-science/cpr-and-ecc-guidelines.

American Heart Association. (2022). COVID-19 *Resuscitation Algorithms*. Retrieved from https://cpr.heart.org/en/resuscitation-science/cpr-and-ecc-guidelines/covid-19-resuscitation-algorithms

Knight, B. P. (2022). Basic principles and techniques of cardioversion and defibrillation. In R.L. Page (Ed.). *UpToDate*. Retrieved from www.uptodate.com

Kviklte, G. (2021). Cardioversion vs. Defibrillation: What's the Difference? *Advanced Medical Certification*. Retrieved from https://advancedmedicalcertification.com/cardioversion-vs-defibrillation-whats-the-difference/

Appendices

Practice makes perfect

1. After an advanced airway is inserted, you should:
   A. deliver ventilations in sync with chest compressions.
   B. deliver ventilations at a rate of 20 to 30/minute.
   C. immediately secure the tube to the patient to prevent dislodgement.
   D. deliver ventilations asynchronously with chest compressions at a rate of 10 ventilations/minute (1 breath every 6 seconds).

2. A 75-year-old patient presents to the emergency room with signs and symptoms of sepsis. You go in to assess the patient and find them unresponsive and pulseless. After calling for help, you begin chest compressions. How many compressions per minute should you provide?
   A. 100 to 120
   B. 80 to 100
   C. At least 100
   D. As many as you can do

3. A 60-year-old patient calls EMS because they are experiencing chest pain. EMS providers arrive, and their immediate actions include:
   A. administration of an aspirin.
   B. completing the Cincinnati Prehospital Stroke Assessment.
   C. administration of hydromorphone.
   D. synchronized cardioversion.

4. You're assisting with a pericardiocentesis. It's most important to notify the practitioner if:
   A. the patient complains of dyspnea.
   B. blood enters the syringe.
   C. jugular vein distention develops.
   D. cardiac arrhythmias are noted on the monitor.

5. Emergency treatment of a tension pneumothorax includes:
   A. needle thoracostomy.
   B. pericardiocentesis.
   C. emergency thoracotomy.
   D. intubation

6. Death occurs from a tension pneumothorax due to:
   A. excessive compression of the heart.
   B. massive hemorrhage into the pleural space.
   C. increased venous return.
   D. collapse of the lungs.

7. The most common initial rhythm in sudden cardiac arrest is:
   A. VT.
   B. atrial fibrillation with rapid ventricular response.
   C. bradycardia.
   D. VF.

8. An indication for cardiac pacing would be:
   A. hemodynamically unstable bradycardia.
   B. asystole.
   C. sinus arrhythmia.
   D. PACs.

9. You find an unresponsive patient in the parking lot. Which action should you take first?
   A. Defibrillate the patient.
   B. Activate the EMS.
   C. Open the patient's airway.
   D. Initiate cardiac compressions.

10. A 27-year-old patient is brought to the emergency room with a suspected overdose. The respiratory rate is approximately 6 per minute and appears agonal; however, you can palpate a pulse. You call for help and immediately do the following:
   A. Initiate chest compressions.
   B. Open the airway and provide rescue breaths.
   C. Insert an IV
   D. Obtain a more thorough history from the family.

11. Which ECG component gives you information about impulse conduction from the atria to the ventricles?
   A. P wave
   B. PR interval
   C. ST segment
   D. QRS complex

12. You arrive on the scene of a Code Blue call and find that the patient is in asystole. Which medication should be given as soon as possible?
   A. Atropine
   B. Adenosine
   C. Epinephrine
   D. Amiodarone

13. A patient presents with symptomatic sinus bradycardia. Which drug is appropriate to treat this patient?
   A. Atropine
   B. Heparin
   C. Cardizem
   D. TPA

14. A patient is found to be in VF and is defibrillated with 200 J. What is the next immediate action of the code team?

A. Administer amiodarone.
B. Initiate cardiac pacing.
C. Resume CPR.
D. Administer a second shock.

15. Administer amiodarone 300 mg by IV push for:

A. refractory pulseless VT.
B. symptomatic supraventricular tachycardia.
C. symptomatic bradycardia.
D. asystole.

16. Your patient calls you to the room with the complaint of chest pain. You assess that their blood pressure is 110/72 mm Hg, heart rate is 92 beats/minute, respiratory rate is 18 per minute, and pulse oximetry is 97%. Your next intervention should be:

A. administer atropine IV.
B. obtain an ECG.
C. call for a stat cardiology consult.
D. call a rapid response.

17. Asking the patient to perform a vagal maneuver is to:

A. prevent the continual development of PACs.
B. increase the ventricular rate in AV block.
C. convert paroxysmal atrial tachycardia to sinus rhythm.
D. treat VT.

18. You are performing CPR on a patient in cardiac arrest. After 2 minutes of compressions, the team leader calls for a switch of compressors and pulse check. How long should these actions take?

A. No longer than 20 seconds
B. No longer than 10 seconds
C. As long as is needed
D. Only 1 second

19. The team leader in an ACLS situation is responsible for:

A. contacting the patient's family.
B. obtaining arterial blood gas values.
C. monitoring the quality of CPR being performed.
D. signing the death certificate.

20. After you deliver a synchronized cardioversion shock to a patient with rapid SVT, the rhythm changes to VF. What's the treatment of choice for a patient with VF?

A. Defibrillation
B. Transesophageal pacing
C. Synchronized cardioversion at the same rate
D. Synchronized cardioversion at a higher rate

21. Which treatment is appropriate for a patient in third-degree AV block with a ventricular rate of 30 beats/minute?

A. Lidocaine
B. Dobutamine
C. Transcutaneous pacing
D. Diltiazem

22. You are shopping at the mall and another shopper collapses in the store. You initiate CPR while the store owner calls EMS. Another shopper knows CPR and comes to assist. The ratio of compressions to ventilations with two rescuer CPR is:

A. 15:1.
B. 15:2.
C. 30:1.
D. 30:2.

23. Which agent should be given to a patient exhibiting signs of anaphylaxis?

A. A corticosteroid
B. Epinephrine
C. An antihistamine
D. A histamine-2 blocker

24. An 80-year-old patient with a history of diabetes is admitted with new onset Afib. You are called to the room but the patient has trouble speaking. They are diaphoretic. What further assessment should be performed?

A. Administer nitroglycerin sublingually.
B. Obtain an ECG.
C. Obtain an expert consultation.
D. Perform a glucose check.

25. When delivering lunch trays, you find a patient who is unresponsive and pulseless. You call for help and initiate chest compressions. When the patient is placed on the monitor, the rhythm shows sinus tachycardia; however, the patient does not have a palpable pulse. What should the team leader tell the code team regarding care of this patient?

A. Stop CPR because the patient shows a cardiac rhythm.
B. Continue CPR until a pulse is obtained.
C. Obtain a stat ECG.
D. Initiate cardiac pacing.

26. A patient complaining of chest pain and is found to be in SVT and has a blood pressure of 80/50 mm Hg. The next appropriate intervention is:

A. synchronized cardioversion.
B. administration of 2 mg of morphine.
C. initiation of dopamine drip.
D. administration of 12 mg of adenosine.

27. Naloxone is recommended for:
   A. all patients who have ingested lethal amounts of drugs, regardless of time.
   B. overdose of an opioid.
   C. a patient who present within 1 hour of ingestion of a toxic substance.
   D. a patient in asystole.

28. A patient suffering a cardiac arrest has a return of spontaneous circulation. The patient's blood pressure is presently 88/56 mm Hg, and their HR is 65. Initial postresuscitation care includes:
   A. administration of 1 mg atropine IV push.
   B. administration of D5W at 100 mL/hour.
   C. administration of 1 mg epinephrine IV push.
   D. administration of 1 to 2 L of NSS.

29. Which first-line agent should be administered to treat torsades de pointes?
   A. Magnesium
   B. Calcium chloride
   C. Glucagon
   D. Epinephrine

30. A 68-year-old patient suddenly goes into SVT at a rate of 250 beats/minute. The vital signs are BP 125/80 mm Hg, RR 20 per minute, and pulse oximetry 95% on 2 L oxygen. Vagal maneuvers are not successful in converting the rhythm. The next expected action is:
   A. administration of 6 mg adenosine by rapid IV push.
   B. administration of 6 mg adenosine by slow IV push.
   C. administration of 6 mg atropine by rapid IV push.
   D. administration of 6 mg atropine by slow IV push.

31. You arrive at a scene of a cardiac arrest with an AED. What is your first action concerning the AED?
   A. Attach the pads.
   B. Check the battery.
   C. Turn it on.
   D. Charge it for a shock.

32. A 74-year-old patient presents to the emergency department with a cardiac rhythm determined to be stable, monomorphic, wide complex tachycardia. Which of the following medications should the team leader consider administering at this time?
   A. Adenosine
   B. Atropine
   C. Vasopressin
   D. Epinephrine

33. A 72-year-old patient is experiencing the sudden onset of mental status change, right arm paralysis, slurred speech, and vision changes. You should immediately evaluate the patient for:

A. anaphylaxis.
B. unstable angina.
C. stroke.
D. MI.

34. Which tool is useful for an EMS responder to rapidly identify a patient with stroke?

A. Glasgow coma scale
B. Hunt and Hess prehospital scale
C. Cincinnati Prehospital Stroke Scale
D. NIH stroke scale

35. A 78-year-old female with suspected COVID-19 is leaving the doctor office and collapses outside. After calling for help and an AED, you find the patient has a pulse and agonal respirations. You open the airway with a jaw thrust maneuver. What would your next action be?

A. Begin CPR using a 30:2 ratio of compressions to breaths.
B. Give rescue breaths using a HEPA filter with bag-mask ventilation.
C. Continue to monitor pulse until AED arrives.
D. Insert an oral airway.

36. Which of the following may be an appropriate treatment for an unresponsive cardiac arrest patient with return of spontaneous circulation?

A. Maintaining a temperature of at least 99°F (37°C) at all times
B. Providing therapeutic hypothermia
C. Discussing placement in a long-term care facility
D. Administering an atropine drip

37. When providing chest compressions, the best way to optimize the amount of cardiac output is to:

A. lift your hands off the chest between compressions.
B. administer ventilations with as much strength as possible.
C. provide faster compressions.
D. allow for complete chest recoil between compressions.

38. An 80-year-old patient develops signs of stroke and the family of the patient calls EMS. On transport to the closest stroke center, the EMS team learns that the CT scanner is being repaired. The best action for the EMS team to take is:

A. continue to the stroke center—they will have a back-up plan.
B. ask the patient's family where they would prefer the patient to go.

C. divert to the next closest stroke center with a functioning CT scanner.
D. take the patient home until the CT scanner is fixed.

39. A post-op CABG patient goes into PEA. During resuscitation, the team leader asks for input as to the possible cause of this patient's PEA. A reasonable cause may be:
A. hypothermia.
B. hyperkalemia.
C. tamponade.
D. toxins.

40. The ACLS team is resuscitating a patient in cardiac arrest. The team leader calls for 1 mg of epinephrine to be given IV push. The team member assigned to medications repeats the request. This is an example of:
A. closed-loop communication.
B. echoing.
C. questioning.
D. summarization.

41. EMS providers are transporting a patient who is unresponsive and in possible hypovolemic shock. They are unable to obtain an IV access. Their next best option intervention to deliver fluids is:
A. insert a central line.
B. insert an NG tube.
C. insert an ET tube.
D. insert an intraosseous needle.

42. Cardiac pacing may be initiated for:
A. pulseless electrical activity.
B. asystole.
C. hemodynamically unstable bradycardia.
D. ventricular tachycardia.

43. Treatment of PEA usually includes:
A. defibrillating the patient.
B. administering amiodarone.
C. treating the underlying cause.
D. applying an external pacemaker.

44. A 70-year-old patient is in atrial fibrillation with a rapid ventricular rate of 175. The patient's blood pressure is 70/50 mm Hg, and they are losing consciousness. It is determined that synchronized cardioversion must be performed. The recommended joules (biphasic device) to deliver to this patient is:
A. 120 to 200 J.
B. 300 to 360 J.
C. 50 to 75 J.
D. 100 J.

45. You arrive with an AED to find a 63-year-old man unresponsive. You turn on and attach the AED while your partner checks for a pulse and respirations. The AED does not promptly recognize the rhythm. What is your next action?

A. Check the AED connections and reanalyze.
B. Begin chest compressions.
C. Attach new electrodes and restart AED.
D. Shock the patient.

46. A patient suddenly goes into VF. How many joules would be appropriate to deliver to the patient when using a biphasic defibrillator?

A. 100 J.
B. 200 J.
C. 300 J.
D. 360 J.

47. You are participating in resuscitating a patient. The team leader tells you to defibrillate the patient. Before delivery of the shock, it is your responsibility to:

A. ensure that oxygen is not flowing over the patient's chest.
B. administer a dose of epinephrine IV.
C. make sure that no one is touching the patient while the machine charges.
D. record the joules that will be delivered.

48. While performing synchronized cardioversion on a patient with symptomatic tachycardia, you note that the patient's cardiac rhythm changes to VF. The defibrillator fails to deliver a shock of 200 J. Which of the following is the most likely cause?

A. The defibrillator's battery failed.
B. The defibrillator is in SYNC mode.
C. The defibrillator monitor didn't recognize the VF rhythm.
D. The defibrillator has malfunctioned.

49. Which of the following is the AHA-recommended method for confirming and monitoring ET tube placement?

A. Serial arterial blood gas sampling
B. Daily chest X-ray
C. Assessment of breath sounds every 15 minutes
D. Continuous quantitative waveform capnography

50. An 81-year-old patient is in sinus bradycardia with a heart rate of 40 beats/minute. The patient is complaining of slight chest pain and is lightheaded. Atropine has been ineffective in increasing the heart rate. What is the next appropriate intervention?

A. Initiate a diltiazem drip.
B. Initiate an amiodarone drip.
C. Initiate a dopamine drip.
D. Initiate a Levophed drip.

Answers

1. D. You should give ventilations asynchronously with chest compressions at 8 to 10 ventilations/minute. Secure the tube after positive confirmation and monitor placement with continuous waveform capnography.

2. A. Current 2020 AHA guidelines recommend providing 100 to 120 chest compressions per minute for a patient in cardiac arrest.

3. A. Initial actions when treating a patient with chest pain include administration of aspirin, oxygen, nitroglycerin, and morphine, if necessary. The Cincinnati Prehospital Stroke Assessment is done when stroke is suspected. Hydromorphone administration and synchronized cardioversion are actions that would need a more complex assessment of the patient presenting with chest pain.

4. D. During pericardiocentesis, arrhythmias may occur if the needle touches the myocardium. Echocardiography or cardiac ultrasound may be used to definitely identify the location of the needle.

5. A. Immediate needle thoracostomy is indicated for a patient with tension pneumothorax to allow air to escape and organs to return to their original position.

6. A. With a tension pneumothorax, the heart is compressed, resulting in decreased ventricular filling and decreased cardiac output. This condition can be fatal if not treated promptly.

7. D. The most common rhythm seen in sudden cardiac arrest is VF. The only effective treatment is defibrillation.

8. A. Bradycardia that causes hemodynamic changes, such as hypotension and shock, may require cardiac pacing.

9. B. You should immediately activate the EMS after discovering an unresponsive person. Next, initiate chest compressions at a rate of 100 to 120/minute at a depth of 2.0 to 2.4 inches.

10. B. Immediate interventions for a patient who is not adequately breathing but has a pulse is to open the airway and provide rescue breaths. Once help arrives, an IV access can be established and history obtained from the family regarding any medication taken so as to provide the correct antidote. Chest compressions should be initiated if the patient becomes pulseless.

11. B. The PR interval measures the interval between atrial depolarization and ventricular depolarization. A normal PR interval is 0.12 to 0.20 seconds.

12. C. Epinephrine is the only recommended medication for asystole. Atropine is used to treat bradycardia. Adenosine is administered for SVT, and amiodarone is an antiarrhythmic.

13. A. Atropine is the standard treatment for symptomatic sinus bradycardia.

14. C. CPR should be resumed immediately after defibrillation. After 2 minutes of high-quality chest compressions, check for a pulse.

15. A. You may administer amiodarone 300 mg by IV push for pulseless VT or VF that isn't responsive to multiple shocks. For recurrent VT or VF, consider administrating an additional dose of 150 mg IV and starting an infusion at 1 mg/minute.

16. B. The patient complaining of chest pain should have an ECG to evaluate for cardiac changes. Based on the ECG reading, a cardiologist ("expert consultation") may be called.

17. C. A vagal maneuver stimulates the vagus nerve to inhibiting the firing of the SA node and slowing AV conduction. This allows the SA node to reestablish itself as the primary pacemaker.

18. B. Interruption of CPR should be no longer than 10 seconds for optimal patient outcomes.

19. C. The responsibilities of the team leader include monitoring the quality of CPR being performed as well as assessing the outcome of the actions.

20. A. A patient with VF is in cardiac arrest and requires defibrillation.

21. C. Transcutaneous pacing is a temporary way to increase the patient's heart rate and improve cardiac output.

22. D. The ratio of compressions with both one and two rescuer CPR is 30 compressions to 2 ventilations.

23. B. Epinephrine is the drug of choice for the patient in anaphylactic shock. You should also give oxygen at a high flow rate.

24. D. Hypoglycemia can mimic signs of stroke. A bedside capillary glucose level should be obtained when a patient demonstrates signs of possible stroke. If the patient's glucose level is low, provide sugar rapidly to prevent further deterioration. If the patient's glucose level is normal, perform a rapid stroke assessment.

25. B. The patient who displays a cardiac rhythm but does not have a pulse is in PEA. Compressions should be continued until a pulse is obtained.

26. A. A patient in SVT with a systolic B/P less than 90 is considered unstable. The appropriate intervention is synchronized cardioversion.

27. B. Naloxone is indicated for patients who have ingested a potentially lethal amount of an opioid.

28. D. The postcardiac arrest care algorithm recommends administration of 1 to 2 L of NSS or lactated Ringers for systolic blood pressure less than 90 mm Hg, followed by administration of a vasopressor if this action is not successful in improving the patient's BP.

29. A. Magnesium (1 to 2 g IV) is usually effective in converting torsades de pointes, even if the patient's magnesium level is normal.

30. A. If vagal maneuvers do not successfully convert a patient in SVT with stable vital signs, then 6 mg adenosine by rapid IV push, followed by a flush, should be given. Because of the rapid half-life of adenosine, it should not be given slowly.

31. C. The first step in using an AED is to turn it on. Then follow the instructions given by the device.

32. A. Adenosine is now recommended as an initial treatment of stable, regular, monomorphic wide-complex tachycardia.

33. C. The patient is experiencing the early signs of stroke. Immediate evaluation and treatment will improve his outcome.

34. C. The Cincinnati Prehospital Stroke Scale checks for facial droop, arm weakness, and speech abnormality and can rapidly identify patients with stroke.

35. B. Per the American Heart Association 2021 guidelines, a HEPA filter with a bag-mask is to be used. Other PPE, such as gowns, gloves, and face shields are to be worn for suspected aerosol-generating procedures, such as intubation.

36. B. Post–cardiac arrest care includes therapeutic hypothermia, along with percutaneous coronary interventions, electroencephalogram, and cardiopulmonary and neurologic support.

37. D. Allowing for complete chest recoil between compressions allow the heart to fill, increasing cardiac output with the next compression.

38. C. Having a CT scan performed rapidly allows for faster, more accurate interventions that result in better patient outcomes.

39. C. Because the patient had recent heart surgery, a complication of bleeding around the heart may be causing cardiac tamponade. Treatment for this cause is immediate pericardiocentesis.

40. A. Closed-loop communication allows for confirmation of messages. Emergency situations may be chaotic and stressful, so utilization of closed-loop communication prevents impairment of treatment.

41. D. An intraosseous access is an appropriate option for delivery of fluids and medications in the hemodynamically compromised patient.

42. C. Bradycardia that causes hemodynamic changes, such as chest pain, hypotension, and altered mental status, may require cardiac pacing.

43. C. You must treat the underlying causes of PEA—known as the "H's" and "T's." They include hypovolemia, hypothermia, hydrogen ion (acidosis), hyperkalemia, hypokalemia, tamponade, toxins, pulmonary and cardiac thrombus, and tension pneumothorax.

44. A. The recommended joules for a biphasic device for irregular narrow complex tachycardia is 120 to 200.

45. B. It is important to minimize interruptions of high-quality CPR. Effective compressions increase the patient's chance of survival.

46. B. When defibrillating a patient in VF using biphasic defibrillator, you should use 200 J. Deliver one shock and then immediately resume CPR for five cycles or 2 minutes.

47. A. Before delivery of a shock, be sure that the oxygen source is not blowing over the patient's chest as the shock could cause a spark and subsequent fire.

48. B. When performing synchronized cardioversion, if the patient's rhythm changes to VF, you need to switch off the synchronize mode. Cardioversion delivers an electric charge to the myocardium at the peak of the R wave because synchronizing the electrical charge with the R wave ensures that the current won't be delivered on the vulnerable T wave and disrupt repolarization. VF is irregular and doesn't have an R wave with which to synchronize; therefore, the defibrillator won't deliver a shock.

49. D. Continuous quantitative waveform capnography is recommended by the AHA for confirming and monitoring correct ET tube placement based on end-tidal volume carbon dioxide values.

50. C. If the first-line treatment of atropine (for bradycardia) is ineffective, it is appropriate to initiate a dopamine or epinephrine drip.

BLS guidelines: obstructed airway management (adult)

Choking—conscious adult

Symptoms

- Grabbing throat with hand
- Inability to speak
- Weak, ineffective coughing
- High-pitched sounds while inhaling

Interventions

1. Ask the person, "Are you choking? Can you speak?" and "Can I help you?" Assess for airway obstruction. Don't intervene if the person is coughing forcefully and can speak; a strong cough can dislodge the object. Quickly activate emergency medical services if the person is having difficulty breathing.
2. Stand behind the person and wrap your arms around the person's waist. (If the person is pregnant or obese, wrap your hands around the chest.)
3. Make a fist with one hand and place the thumb side of your fist just above the person's navel and well below the sternum.
4. Grasp your fist with your other hand.
5. Perform quick, upward and inward thrusts with your fist. (If the person is pregnant or obese, use chest thrusts.)
6. Continue thrusts until the object is dislodged or the person loses consciousness.
7. If the person loses consciousness, activate the emergency response system and provide cardiopulmonary resuscitation. (Each time you open the airway to deliver rescue breaths, look in the person's mouth and remove any object you see. Never perform a blind finger sweep.)

Guide to common antiarrhythmic drugs

Antiarrhythmic drugs are categorized into four main classes based on their electrophysiologic actions and how they affect the action potential. The mechanism of action of antiarrhythmic drugs can vary, and some drugs exhibit properties common to more than one class. Several drugs don't fall into any of the classes and are, therefore, listed as miscellaneous antiarrhythmics.

Drugs	Indications	Special considerations
Class IA antiarrhythmics Disopyramide phosphate, procainamide hydrochloride, quinidine	• Ventricular tachycardia (VT) • Atrial fibrillation with rapid rate in Wolff-Parkinson-White syndrome • Paroxysmal atrial tachycardia • Monomorphic wide-complex tachycardia	• Check the patient's apical pulse rate before starting therapy. If you note extremes in pulse rate, withhold the dose and notify the prescriber. • Monitor for electrocardiogram (ECG) changes (widening QRS complexes, prolonged QT interval).
Class IB antiarrhythmics Lidocaine, mexiletine, tocainide	• VT • Ventricular fibrillation (VF)	• IB antiarrhythmics may potentiate the effects of other antiarrhythmics. • Use an infusion pump to administer IV infusions.
Class IC antiarrhythmics Flecainide, moricizine, propafenone	• VT • VF • Supraventricular arrhythmias • Atrial fibrillation • Atrial flutter	• Correct electrolyte imbalances before administration. • Monitor the patient's ECG before and after dosage adjustments. • Monitor for ECG changes (widening QRS complexes, prolonged QT interval) and new atrioventricular block (AV) blocks.
Class II antiarrhythmics Acebutolol, atenolol, esmolol, propranolol	• Atrial flutter • Atrial fibrillation • Paroxysmal atrial tachycardia	• Monitor the patient's apical heart rate and blood pressure. • Abruptly stopping these drugs can exacerbate angina and precipitate myocardial infarction. • Monitor for ECG changes (prolonged PR interval). • Use cautiously in patients with asthma.
Class III antiarrhythmics Amiodarone, dofetilide, ibutilide, sotalol	• VF, pulseless VT • Atrial arrhythmias	• Monitor the patient's blood pressure and heart rate and rhythm for changes. • Amiodarone increases the risk of digoxin toxicity in patients taking digoxin. • Monitor for signs of pulmonary toxicity (dyspnea, nonproductive cough, and pleuritic chest pain) in patients taking amiodarone. • Monitor for ECG changes (prolonged QT interval) in patients taking dofetilide, ibutilide, and sotalol.
Class IV antiarrhythmics Diltiazem, verapamil	• Supraventricular arrhythmias • Atrial fibrillation and atrial flutter	• Carefully monitor the patient's blood pressure and heart rate and rhythm when initiating therapy or increasing the dosage. • Calcium supplements may reduce effectiveness.

(continued)

Drugs	Indications	Special considerations
Miscellaneous antiarrhythmics		
Adenosine	• Paroxysmal supraventricular tachycardia • Regular, monomorphic wide-complex tachycardia	• Adenosine must be administered over 1–2 seconds, followed by a 20-mL flush of normal saline solution. • Record rhythm strip during drug administration.
Atropine	• Symptomatic sinus bradycardia, AV block	• Monitor the patient's heart rate and rhythm. • Use cautiously in patient's with myocardial ischemia; not recommended for third-degree AV block or type II AV block. • In adult patients, avoid doses <0.5 mg because of the risk of paradoxical slowing of the heart rate.
Epinephrine	• VF, pulseless VT, asystole, PEA • Symptomatic bradycardia (after atropine administration)	• Carefully monitor the patient's blood pressure and heart rate and rhythm. • Don't mix IV dose with alkaline solutions. • Give the drug into a large vein to prevent irritation or extravasation at site.

NIH stroke scale

You can use a neurologic flow sheet, such as the National Institutes of Health (NIH) Stroke Scale, to record frequent neurologic assessments. For each item, choose the score that reflects what the patient can actually do at the time of the assessment. Add the scores for each item and record the total. The higher the score, the more severe the neurologic deficits.

Category	Description	Score	Date/time *3/3/12 1100*	2 hours posttreatment
1a. Level of consciousness (LOC)	Alert Drowsy Obtunded Unresponsive	0 1 2 3	*1*	
1b. LOC questions (Ask patient what month it is and their age.)	Answers both correctly Answers one correctly Incorrect	0 1 2	*0*	
1c. LOC commands (Have patient open/close the eyes, make a fist, and then let go.)	Obeys both correctly Obeys one correctly Incorrect	0 1 2	*1*	
2. Best gaze (Eyes open; have patient follow your finger or face.)	Normal Partial gaze palsy Forced deviation	0 1 2	*0*	
3. Visual (Introduce visual stimulus/threat to patient's visual field quadrants.)	No vision loss Partial hemianopsia Complete hemianopsia Bilateral hemianopsia	0 1 2 3	*1*	
4. Facial palsy (Have patient show his or her teeth, raise the eyebrows, and squeeze the eyes shut.)	Normal Minor Partial Complete	0 1 2 3	*2*	
5a. Motor arm—left (Elevate extremity to 90 degrees and score drift/movement.)	Normal, no drift Drift Some effort against gravity No effort against gravity No movement Not tested (amputation, joint fusion) (explain)	0 1 2 3 4 UN	*4*	
5b. Motor arm—right (Elevate extremity to 90 degrees and score drift/movement.)	Normal, no drift Drift Some effort against gravity No effort against gravity No movement Not tested (amputation, joint fusion) (explain)	0 1 2 3 4 UN	*0*	

(continued)

Category	Description	Score	Date/time *3/3/12* *1100*	2 hours posttreatment
6a. Motor leg—left (Elevate extremity to 30 degrees and score drift/movement.)	Normal, no drift	0	*4*	
	Drift	1		
	Some effort against gravity	2		
	No effort against gravity	3		
	No movement	4		
	Not tested (amputation, joint fusion) (explain)	UN		
6b. Motor leg—right (Elevate extremity to 30 degrees and score drift/movement.)	Normal, no drift	0	*0*	
	Drift	1		
	Some effort against gravity	2		
	No effort against gravity	3		
	No movement	4		
	Not tested (amputation, joint fusion) (explain)	UN		
7. Limb ataxia (Perform finger-nose, heel down shin testing.)	Absent	0	*1*	
	Present in one limb	1		
	Present in two limbs	2		
	Not tested (amputation, joint fusion) (explain)	UN		
8. Sensory (Pinprick patient's face, arm, trunk, and leg—compare side to side.)	Normal	0	*0*	
	Partial loss	1		
	Severe loss	2		
9. Best language (Have patient name items, describe a picture, and read sentences.)	No aphasia	0	*1*	
	Mild to moderate aphasia	1		
	Severe aphasia	2		
	Mute	3		
10. Dysarthria (Have patient repeat listed words—evaluate speech clarity.)	Normal articulation	0	*1*	
	Mild to moderate dysarthria	1		
	Near to intelligible or worse	2		
	Intubated or other physical barrier (explain)	UN	*0*	
11. Extinction and inattention (Use information from previous testing to identify neglect or double simultaneous stimuli testing.)	No abnormality	0		
	Partial	1		
	Profound	2		
		Total	*16*	

Individual administering scale: Helen Horeson, RN

Source: National Institute of Neurologic Disorders and Stroke. NIH Stroke Scale. Available at www.ninds.nih.gov.

Managing electrolyte disturbances associated with cardiac arrest

Life-threatening electrolyte disturbances are often associated with cardiac arrest. In addition to standard advanced cardiovascular life support (ACLS) interventions, additional ACLS interventions may be necessary to improve the patient's cardiovascular stability during the cardiac arrest and hemodynamic recovery afterward.

Electrolyte disturbance	Causes	Signs and symptoms	ECG changes	Possible additional ACLS interventions
Severe hyperkalemia (serum potassium level >6.5 mmol/L)	• Kidney failure or injury • Excess potassium administration • Drug therapy	• Flaccid paralysis • Paresthesia • Depressed reflexes • Respiratory distress or failure	• Peaked T waves • Long PR interval • Wide QRS complex • Merging of S and T waves • Flat or absent T waves • Idioventricular rhythm • Asystole	• Calcium chloride (10%) 5–10 mL (500–1,000 mg) IV over 2–5 minutes, or calcium gluconate (10%) 15–30 mL IV over 2 minutes • Sodium bicarbonate 50 mEq IV over 5 minutes • 25 g (50 mL of D50) glucose followed by 10 units regular insulin and given IV over 15–30 minutes • Albuterol 10–20 mg nebulized over 15 minutes • Furosemide 40–80 mg IV • Kayexalate 15–50 g plus sorbitol PO or PR. • Hemodialysis
Severe hypokalemia (serum potassium level <2.5 mmol/L)	• GI losses (severe vomiting, diarrhea, laxatives, GI tube drainage) • Renal losses (high-dose thiazide diuretics [furosemide] without potassium replacement) • Adrenal adenoma • Drug toxicities (chloroquine, risperidone, albuterol, terbutaline, digoxin, amphotericin B) • Epinephrine release during stress response (coronary ischemia)	• Muscle weakness • Hypoventilation • Respiratory arrest • Muscle cramps • Rhabdomyolysis • Myoglobinuria	• Decreased ST segment • Decreased amplitude of T waves with flattening • Increased amplitude of U wave • Atrial and junctional tachycardia Sinus bradycardia • Atrioventricular block • Ventricular tachycardia (VT) • Ventricular fibrillation • Pulseless electrical activity • Asystole	• Treating hypomagnesemia if present • Estimating potassium deficit based upon underlying cause • Replacing potassium by slow IV infusion

(continued)

Electrolyte disturbance	Causes	Signs and symptoms	ECG changes	Possible additional ACLS interventions
Hypermagnesemia (serum magnesium level >2.2 mEq/L)	• Kidney failure or injury • Excess magnesium replacement therapy • Magnesium laxative abuse	• Nausea and vomiting • Muscle weakness • Decreased deep tendon reflexes • Ataxia • Paralysis • Decreased level of consciousness (LOC) • Hypoventilation • Respiratory arrest • Hypotension • Cardiac arrest	• Bradycardia • Prolonged PR interval • Wide QRS duration • Prolonged QT interval • Complete heart block	• Calcium chloride (10%) 5–10 mL IV over 2–5 minutes, or calcium gluconate (10%) 15–30 mL IV over 2–5 minutes
Hypomagnesemia (serum magnesium level <1.3 mEq/L)	• Thyroid hormone dysfunction • Diarrhea • Drug toxicities (cisplatin, diuretics, pentamidine, alcohol, amphotericin B, cyclosporine, proton pump inhibitors) • Malnutrition • Kidney dysfunction (acute tubular necrosis, renal transplantation) • Bartter and Gitelman syndromes	• Anorexia • Generalized weakness • Positive Chvostek and Trousseau signs • Seizures • Decreased LOC	• Prolonged PR interval • Wide QRS complex • Peaked or flat T waves • Polymorphic VT (including torsades de pointes)	• Magnesium sulfate 1–2 g diluted in 10 mL D_5W IV or IO.

Glossary

aberrant conduction: the abnormal pathway of an impulse traveling through the heart's conduction system

accelerated idioventricular rhythm: wide ventricular complex originating from the ventricle at a rate of 40 to 120 beats/minute

adrenergic: medication used to restore heart rate and rhythm and blood pressure during resuscitation of the patient

afterload: resistance that the left ventricle must work against to pump blood through the aorta

amplitude: the height of a waveform

analgesic: medication used primarily to help alleviate pain and promote relaxation

anaphylaxis: severe allergic reaction to a foreign substance; life threatening

angiotensin-converting enzyme (ACE) inhibitor: medication that prevents the body from converting angiotensin I to angiotensin II, which causes narrowing of the blood vessels; used to reduce mortality and improve left ventricular function in postacute myocardial infarction (MI) patients, prevent adverse left ventricular remodeling, delay progression of heart failure, and decrease sudden death and recurrent MI

antiarrhythmic: medication used to treat, suppress, or prevent three major mechanisms of arrhythmias: increased automaticity, decreased conductivity, and reentry

antiplatelet drug: medication used to block the final common pathway of platelet aggregation and thrombus formation

arrhythmia: a disturbance of normal cardiac rhythm due to abnormal origin, discharge, or conduction of electrical impulses

artifact: waveform interference in an electrocardiogram tracing that results from sources other than the electrical signals from the heart, such as patient movement or poorly placed or malfunctioning equipment

asthma: chronic disorder in which airways are hyperresponsive to a particular trigger

asystole: the total absence of ventricular activity

atrial fibrillation: chaotic, asynchronous, electrical activity in atrial tissue that stems from impulses firing in reentry pathways at a rate of 400 to 600 times/minute, causing the atria to quiver instead of contract

atrial flutter: a cardiac rhythm characterized by an atrial rate of 250 to 400 beats/minute that originates in a single atrial focus, resulting from reentry and, possibly, increased automaticity

atrial kick: the force incurred by the atrial contraction immediately prior to ventricular contraction that increases the amount of blood flowing into the ventricle; contributes about 30% of total cardiac output

atrioventricular node: the node situated low in the septal wall of the right atrium that slows the impulse conduction between the atria and ventricles, providing time for the contracting atria to fill the ventricles with blood before the lower chambers contract

automaticity: the ability of a cardiac cell to initiate an impulse on its own

bigeminy: a premature beat occurring every other beat that alternates with normal complexes

biphasic: a complex containing both an upward and a downward deflection; usually seen when the electrical current is perpendicular to the observed lead

bundle-branch block: the slowing or blocking of an impulse as it travels through one of the bundle branches of the heart

capture: successful pacing of the heart, represented on an electrocardiogram by a pacemaker spike followed by a P wave or QRS complex

cardiac output: the amount of blood ejected from the left ventricle in 1 minute (the normal value is 4 to 8 L/minute)

cardioversion: the restoration of normal rhythm by synchronized electric shock or drug therapy

carotid sinus massage: manually rubbing the carotid sinus (of the carotid artery) to slow the heart rate

compensatory pause: the period following a premature contraction during which the heart regulates itself, allowing the sinoatrial node to resume normal conduction

conduction: the transmission of electrical impulses through the myocardium

conductivity: the ability of one cardiac cell to transmit an electrical impulse to another cell

contractility: the ability of a cardiac cell to contract after receiving an impulse

couplet: a pair of premature beats that occur together

defibrillation: delivery of a dose of electrical current to the heart through the use of a defibrillator during ventricular tachycardia or fibrillation with the goal of the heart returning to normal electrical conduction

deflection: the direction of a waveform, based on the direction of a current

depolarization: the response of a myocardial cell to an electrical impulse that causes movement of ions across the cell membrane, which triggers myocardial contraction

diastole: the phase of the cardiac cycle during which both atria (atrial diastole) or both ventricles (ventricular diastole) are at rest and filling with blood

ectopic beat: a contraction that occurs as a result of an impulse generated from a site other than the sinoatrial node

electrocardiogram complex: waveform representing the electrical events of one cardiac cycle, consisting of five main waveforms (labeled P, Q, R, S, and T), a sixth waveform (labeled U) that occurs under certain conditions, the PR and QT intervals, and the ST segment

endotracheal intubation: oral or nasal insertion of a flexible tube through the larynx into the trachea to control the airway and mechanically ventilate the patient

enhanced automaticity: a condition in which pacemaker cells increase the firing rate above their inherent rate

excitability: the ability of a cardiac cell to respond to an electrical stimulus

first-degree atrioventricular (AV) block: a cardiac rhythm that occurs when impulses from the atria are consistently delayed during conduction through the AV node; identified by a prolonged PR interval of greater than 0.20 seconds

hypoxemia: oxygen deficit in arterial blood (lower than 80 mm Hg)

hypoxia: reduction of oxygen in body tissues to below normal levels

idioventricular rhythm: wide ventricular complex originating from the ventricle at a rate of 20 to 40 beats/minute

intrinsic: naturally occurring electrical stimulus from within the heart's conduction system

inverted: a negative or downward deflection on an electrocardiogram

junctional tachycardia: three or more premature junctional contractions occurring in a row, caused by an irritable focus from the atrioventricular junction that enhances automaticity and overrides the sinoatrial node to function as the heart's pacemaker, which depolarizes the atria by means of retrograde conduction (usually the rate measures between 100 and 200 beats/minute)

lead: perspective of the electrical activity in a particular area of the heart through the placement of electrodes on the chest wall

monomorphic ventricular tachycardia: a form of ventricular tachycardia in which the QRS complexes have a uniform appearance from beat to beat

multifocal atrial tachycardia: a cardiac rhythm that results from an extremely rapid firing of multifocal ectopic sites

multiform or multifocal: a type of premature contraction that has differing QRS configurations as a result of originating from different irritable sites in the atria or ventricles

nonrebreather mask: type of oxygen delivery system involving a one-way inspiratory valve, which opens on inhalation and directs oxygen from a reservoir bag into the mask, allowing the patient to breathe high concentrations of oxygen from the bag

nonsustained ventricular tachycardia: ventricular tachycardia that lasts less than 30 seconds

normal sinus rhythm: the standard against which all other rhythms are compared; an impulse that starts in the sinus node and progresses to the ventricles through a normal conduction pathway—from the sinus node to the atria and atrioventricular node, through the bundle of His, to the bundle branches, and on to the Purkinje fibers; heart rate is between 60 and 100 beats/minute

oropharyngeal airway: curved rubber or plastic device inserted into the mouth to the posterior pharynx to establish or maintain a patent airway

pacemaker: a group of cells that generate impulses to the heart muscle or a battery-powered device that delivers an electrical stimulus to the heart to cause myocardial depolarization

paroxysmal: an episode of an arrhythmia that starts and stops suddenly

pneumothorax: collapse of part or all of the lung due to air in the pleural space

polymorphic ventricular tachycardia: a type of ventricular tachycardia in which the QRS complexes change from beat to beat

preload: a stretching force exerted on the ventricular muscle by the blood it contains at the end of diastole

proarrhythmia: a rhythm disturbance caused or made worse by drugs or other therapy

pulmonary edema: a life-threatening condition in which an abnormal amount of fluid accumulates in the lungs

pulmonary embolism: sudden obstruction of a pulmonary artery by a foreign substance or a blood clot

pulse oximetry: noninvasive device used to measure arterial oxygen saturation

pulseless electrical activity: a cardiac rhythm in which isolated electrical activity occurs sporadically without evidence of effective myocardial contraction; commonly caused by a clinical condition that can be reversed when identified quickly and treated appropriately

quadrigeminy: a premature beat occurring every fourth beat that alternates with three normal complexes

reentry mechanism: the failure of a cardiac impulse to follow the normal conduction pathway; instead, it follows a circular path

refractory: a type of arrhythmia that doesn't respond to usual treatment measures

refractory period: a brief period during which excitability in a myocardial cell is depressed

repolarization: the recovery of myocardial cells after depolarization during which the cell membrane returns to its resting potential

rhythm strip: the length of electrocardiogram (ECG) paper that shows multiple ECG complexes representing a picture of the heart's electrical activity in a specific lead

second-degree atrioventricular (AV) block (type I, Wenckebach or Mobitz I): a cardiac rhythm that occurs when diseased tissues in the AV node delay conduction of impulses to the ventricles; each impulse from the sinotrial node is delayed slightly longer than the previous impulse with a pattern of progressive prolongation of the PR interval, eventually leading to a dropped beat when the impulse isn't conducted to the ventricles; the pattern then repeats after the dropped beat

second-degree atrioventricular block (type II): a cardiac rhythm produced by a conduction disturbance in the His-Purkinje fibers, causing an intermittent conduction delay or block (the PR and R-R intervals remain constant before the dropped beat)

sinoatrial (SA) node: the node located on the endocardial surface of the right atrium near the superior vena cava, which serves as the heart's normal pacemaker by firing an impulse throughout the right and left atria, resulting in atrial contraction (under normal conditions, the SA node generates an impulse 60 to 100 times/minute)

sinus bradycardia: a cardiac rhythm in which the sinus rate is below 60 beats/minute, and all impulses come from the sinoatrial node

sinus tachycardia: an acceleration of the firing of the sinoatrial node beyond its normal discharge rate, resulting in a heart rate of 100 to 150 beats/minute (rates greater than 150 beats/minute may indicate an ectopic focus)

status asthmaticus: life-threatening situation resulting from an acute asthma attack that goes untreated or in which the person doesn't respond to drug therapy after 24 hours

Stokes-Adams attack: a sudden episode of light-headedness or loss of consciousness caused by an abrupt slowing or stopping of the heartbeat

systole: the phase of the cardiac cycle during which both atria (atrial systole) or both ventricles (ventricular systole) are contracting

tension pneumothorax: air trapped within the pleural space that can be fatal without prompt treatment

third-degree atrioventricular block: a cardiac rhythm in which all supraventricular impulses are prevented from reaching the ventricles; the atria and ventricles beat independently of each other

torsades de pointes: a polymorphic ventricular tachycardia characterized by a prolonged QT interval and QRS polarity that seem to spiral around the isoelectric line

trigeminy: a premature beat occurring every third beat that alternates with two normal complexes

triplet: three premature beats occurring together

uniform or unifocal: a type of premature ventricular contraction that has the same or similar QRS configuration and originates from the same irritable site in the ventricle

vagal stimulation: the pharmacologic or manual stimulation of the vagus nerve to slow the heart rate

Valsalva's maneuver: a technique of forceful expiration against the closed glottis that's used to slow the heart rate

ventilation: gas distribution into and out of the pulmonary airways

ventricular fibrillation: a chaotic pattern of electrical activity in the ventricles in which electrical impulses arise from many different foci, producing no effective muscular contraction and no cardiac output

ventricular tachycardia: rapid heart rate originating from the ventricle; may occur with or without a pulse

Venturi mask: type of oxygen delivery system that allows for the mixture of a specific volume of air and oxygen to deliver a highly accurate oxygen concentration

Wolff-Parkinson-White syndrome: abnormality of cardiac rhythm that occurs when an anomalous atrial bypass tract (bundle of Kent) develops outside the atrioventricular junction, connecting the atria and ventricles and causing impulses to be conducted to either the atria or ventricles

Index

Note: i refers to an illustration; t refers to a table.

Note: i refers to an illustration; t refers to a table.

Note: i refers to an illustration; t refers to a table.

Note: i refers to an illustration; t refers to a table.

Note: i refers to an illustration; t refers to a table.

Note: i refers to an illustration; t refers to a table.

Note: i refers to an illustration; t refers to a table.